The Acoustic Analysis of Speech

i

The Acoustic Analysis of Speech

Ray D. Kent, Ph.D.
and
Charles Read, Ph.D.
University of Wisconsin—Madison

SINGULAR

THOMSON LEARNING

Australia Canada Mexico Singapore Spain United Kingdom United States

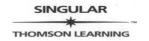

SINGULAR

TM

THOMSON LEARNING

The Acoustic Analysis of Speech, 2nd edition
by
Ray D. Kent, Ph.D.
and
Charles Read, Ph.D.

Health Care Publishing Director:
William Brottmiller

Executive Editor:
Cathy L. Esperti

Acquisitions Editor:
Candice Janco

Editorial Assistant:
Maria D'Angelico

Executive Marketing Manager:
Dawn F. Gerrain

Channel Manager:
Jennifer McAvey

Production Editor:
Mary Colleen Liburdi

Cover Design:
Mary Colleen Liburdi

COPYRIGHT © 2002 by Delmar, a division of Thomson Learning, Inc. Thomson Learning™ is a trademark used herein under license

Printed in Canada
3 4 5 XXX 06 05 04 03

For more information contact Delmar, 3 Columbia Circle, PO Box 15015, Albany, NY 12212-5015.

Or find us on the World Wide Web at http://www.delmar.com

For permission to use material from this text or product, contact us by
Tel   (800) 730-2214
Fax   (800) 730-2215
www.thomsonrights.com

Library of Congress Cataloging-in-Publication Data on file

ISBN 0-7693-0112-6

NOTICE TO THE READER

Publisher does not warrant or guarantee any of the products described herein or perform any independent analysis in connection with any of the product information contained herein. Publisher does not assume, and expressly disclaims, any obligation to obtain and include information other than that provided to it by the manufacturer.

The reader is expressly warned to consider and adopt all safety precautions that might be indicated by the activities herein and to avoid all potential hazards. By following the instructions contained herein, the reader willingly assumes all risks in connection with such instructions.

The Publisher makes no representation or warranties of any kind, including but not limited to, the warranties of fitness for particular purpose or merchantability, nor are any such representations implied with respect to the material set forth herein, and the publisher takes no responsibility with respect to such material. The publisher shall not be liable for any special, consequential, or exemplary damages resulting, in whole or part, from the readers' use of, or reliance upon, this material.

Contents

Author Biographies

Ray D. Kent is Professor of Communicative Disorders at the University of Wisconsin [em]Madison. His current primary research interest is neurogenic speech disorders in children and adults, especially the disorders associated with amyotrophic lateral sclerosis, Parkinson's disease, cerebellar disease, stroke, and cerebral palsy. Other research interests include speech development in infants and young children, measuring speech intelligibility and quality, acoustic analyses of speech, and theories of speech production. In addition to more than 150 journal articles, book chapters, and reviews, he has authored or edited the following books: *Clinical phonetics* (with L.D. Shriberg), *Decision making in speech-language pathology* (with D.D. Yoder), *Papers in speech communication (Vols. 1-3)* (with J.L. Miller and B.S. Atal), *Intelligibility in speech disorders: Theory, measurement, and management, the acoustic analysis of speech* (with C. Read), Reference manual for communicative sciences and disorders: Speech-language pathology, the speech sciences, the new phonologies (with M.J. Ball), Dictionary of speech-language pathology (with S. Singh), and Handbook of voice quality measurement (with M.J. Ball). His journal editing experience includes: editor of the Journal of Speech and Hearing Research, associate editor of Clinical Linguistics and Phonetics, and associate editor for motor speech disorders for Folia Phoniatrica et Logopaedica. Kent received the Honors of the American Speech-Language-Hearing Association in 1994 and was awarded the Docteur Honoris Causa (Honorary Doctorate) from the Faculte de Medecine, Universite de Montreal, in 1995. He is a fellow of the American Speech-Language-Hearing Association, the Acoustical Society of America, and the International Phonetics Association.

Charles Read is Professor of Linguistics and Associate Dean of the Graduate School at the University of Wisconsin[en]Madison. He directs the Phonetics Laboratory in Linguistics and conducts research on the phonetic foundations of reading and writing. Perhaps best known for his research on children's beginning spelling, Professor Read has also studied how children and adults use prosody in recognizing the syntactic structure of sentences, as well as the linguistic and cognitive skills of adults of low literacy.

Preface to the Second Edition

This book is intended for readers who need an introduction to the acoustics of speech. Little in the way of mathematics or physics is required, although an occasional formula is used. In this respect, the book is written especially for those readers who do not have an extensive quantitative background. Elementary acoustic concepts are assumed. For example, readers should be familiar with the concepts of waveforms and spectra, resonance, and decibels.

The philosophy behind this book is that speech acoustics should be understood from three complementary perspectives: theory, analysis methods, and data sources. The acoustic theory of speech production not only accounts for how speech sounds are made, but it also is the foundation for understanding some of the most important methods of speech analysis and the interpretation of acoustic data. Modern methods of speech analysis rely on the digital computer, and discussion is included of how the acoustic signal of speech is analyzed by digital signal processing. A variety of methods are described, and abundant references guide the interested reader to other sources of information. Theory and analysis lead to the generation of data on speech acoustics. It is difficult to collect and interpret acoustic data without a basic understanding of acoustic theory and the strengths and limitations of analysis methods. Although this book is by no means an encyclopedic archive of acoustic data, it does include data summaries for a number of acoustic variables pertinent to speech production and speech perception. The primary focus is on American English but selected information for other languages is mentioned as well. A special effort has been made to include data for speakers of both sexes and various ages. Because speech is used by nearly everyone, the methods for its analysis must be universal.

This second edition represents a substantial updating of the first. The text is expanded in virtually all major areas, and new information is included on acoustic theory, methods of acoustic analysis, acoustic properties of vowels and consonants, acoustic correlates of speaker variables and suprasegmentals, and speech synthesis. The text also has been reorganized to achieve a more effective grouping of topics. The updating is reflected especially by the addition of many new references and by the addition of several new tables of acoustic data.

Above all, this book is witness to a remarkable technologic achievement—the ability to analyze speech as an acoustic signal, to interpret that signal in terms of its biologic and psychologic origins, and to design machines that share spoken communication with humans.

The Authors (RK and CR)
Madison, Wisconsin, January 2001

An Introduction to the Study of Speech Acoustics

CHAPTER

What is Speech?

Raymond H. Stetson, a pioneer in the study of speech, wrote that *speech is movement made audible* (Stetson, 1928). The movements of the speech organs—structures such as the tongue, lips, jaw, velum and vocal folds—result in sound patterns that are perceived by the listener. However, speech is more than audible sounds; otherwise, we would not bother to distinguish the sounds of speech from those of other bodily processes, such as hand clapping or breathing. Speech gains its unique importance as the primary means by which language is expressed in all human cultures except for people who are deaf. Speech is a modality of language. Speech communication is common to nearly all humans in every culture, in every part of the earth—except the deaf. The end product of speech is an acoustic signal. This signal represents the communicative message of the speaker. Under ordinary circumstances, the signal perishes rapidly as the sound vibrations are damped by the physical world, but modern recording techniques enable us to preserve speech signals and this capability opens new horizons for the study of speech.

The famous linguist, Charles Hockett, defined what he considered to be the design features of communication. These are summarized in Table 1–1 and, taken together, they characterize the uniqueness of human language. As far as is known, no other species has a communication system with all these attributes. Considering these features individually, we gain an appreciation of speech as a human faculty and a means of communication. Several of the design features pertain directly and uniquely to speech as a modality of language, for example, items 1, 2, 3, 6, and 9 in Table 1–1. By combining these features, we might define speech as an auditory–vocal channel that has a rapidly fading broadcast transmission; is specialized to convey meaning with arbitrary sound symbols; and is composed of discrete units or elements that can be formed into an infinite number of messages. This definition refers to both the limits and the power of speech. The fact that speech fades rapidly presents challenges to its analysis. Fortunately, modern equipment makes it possible to store and analyze the fleeting signal of speech. With this capability, it is possible to conduct studies of the way in which speech sounds relate to language.

In the scientific laboratory, speech has three major arenas of study: the physiologic arena (or *physiologic phonetics*), the acoustic arena (or *acoustic phonetics*), and the perceptual arena (typically called *speech perception*). A unified understanding of speech requires the study of each of these areas in relation to the others. The discussion in this book will be concerned primarily with the acoustic arena but references necessarily will be made to the other two arenas. Of particular importance is the need to understand how the acoustic analysis of speech can aid the study of the physiologic phenomena, on the one hand, and perceptual phenomena, on the other. Because the acoustic signal intermediates between a speaker's production of speech and a listener's perception of the speech, acoustic analysis helps in the understanding of both speech production and speech perception. In many important ways, the acoustic signal helps to give a unified understanding of speech.

The Physiologic Arena of Speech

The physiologic arena is identified physically with the speech apparatus, consisting of

TABLE 1–1

Hockett's Design Features of Communication (these characterize all human languages but do not apply in their entirety to the communication systems of other species)

Feature	Definition
1. Auditory-vocal channel	Sound is transmitted from the mouth to the ear.
2. Broadcast transmission and directional reception	An auditory signal can be detected by any perceiver within hearing range, and the perceiver's ears are used to localize the signal.
3. Rapid fading	In contrast to some visual and olfactory signals, auditory signals are transitory.
4. Interchangeability	Competent users of a language can produce any signal that they can comprehend.
5. Total feedback	All signals produced by an individual can be reflected upon.
6. Specialization	The only function of the acoustic waveforms of speech is to convey meaning.
7. Semanticity	A signal conveys meaning through its association with objects and events in the environment.
8. Arbitrariness	The speech signal itself bears no relationship with the object or event that it is associated with.
9. Discreteness	Speech is composed of a small set of acoustically distinct units or elements.
10. Displacement	Speech signals can be used to refer to objects or events that are removed from the present in both space and time.
11. Productivity	Speech allows for the expression of an infinite variety of meaningful utterances as a result of combining discrete elements into new sentences.
12. Traditional	Language structure and usage is transmission passed from one generation to the next via pedagogy and learning.
13. Duality of patterning	The particular sound elements of language have no intrinsic meaning but combine from structures (e.g., words, phrases) that do have meaning.

three major anatomic subsystems: respiratory (including the lungs, chest wall, diaphragm), phonatory (larynx or voice box), and articulatory (tongue, lips, jaw, and velum). Figure 1–1 is a simplified diagram of these subsystems. This tripartite division is justified on both anatomic and physiologic grounds, but it should be emphasized that the three subsystems work closely together in speech and are often highly interactive. Speech articulation is a complex movement

phenomenon, the understanding of which has been hindered by many obstacles, not the least of which is the difficulty of observing the structures of interest, hidden as they are in the cavities of the mouth, neck and thorax. The following three paragraphs give a highly simplified summary of these subsystems. The reader who is not acquainted with speech production may find it helpful to read this material before proceeding with the balance of the book.

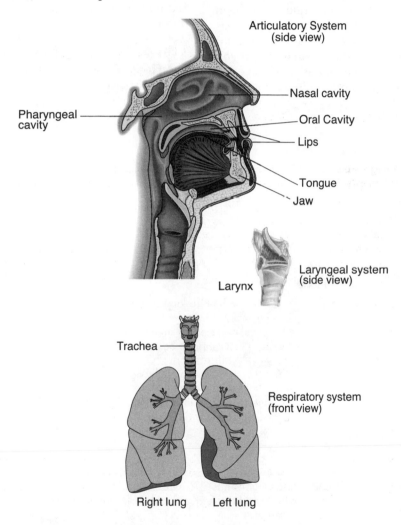

Articulatory System
(side view)

Nasal cavity

Pharyngeal cavity

Oral Cavity

Lips

Tongue

Jaw

Larynx

Laryngeal system
(side view)

Trachea

Respiratory system
(front view)

Right lung   Left lung

FIGURE 1–1. The system of speech production, divided into three primary subsystems: respiratory, laryngeal, and articulatory. The different systems are drawn to different scales and with different orientations (e.g., the articulatory system is enlarged relative to the other two and is shown in a lateral rather than frontal view). From *The speech sciences. A volume in the speech sciences* (1st ed.), by Kent, copyright 1998. Reprinted with permission of Delmar, a division of Thomson Learning.

The Respiratory Subsystem

The respiratory subsystem consists of the trachea, lungs, rib cage, and various muscles (Figure 1–1 and 1–2). Besides providing for ventilation to support life, this system produces most of the aerodynamic energy of speech. The basic *aerodynamic parameters* are *air volume, flow, pressure,* and *resistance.* Volume is a measure of the amount of air and is measured with units such as liters (l) or milliliters (ml). Flow is the rate of change in volume and is expressed in units such as liters/minute or milliliters/millisecond (ml/ms), which expresses a change in volume per unit of time. Pressure is force per unit area and is commonly expressed in

pascals, a unit which replaced earlier units such as dynes per square centimeter. In speech studies, pressure often is recorded with a different unit, such as centimeters of water (cm H_2O) or millimeters of mercury (mm Hg). The reason is that manometers are a convenient way of measuring pressure as the displacement of a column of liquid. Resistance is a variable that relates flow and pressure, according to an important law called *Ohm's law*. This law may be expressed in the following alternative forms:

Pressure = Flow x Resistance
Flow = Pressure / Resistance
Resistance = Pressure / Flow

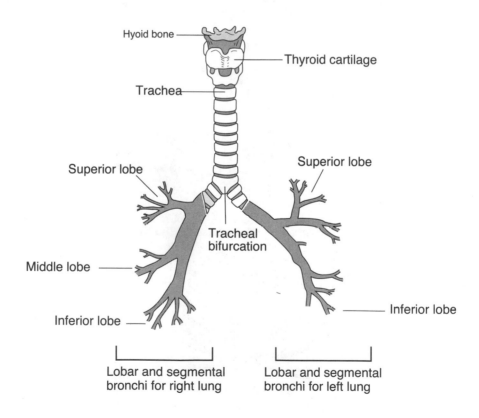

FIGURE 1–2.   The respiratory and laryngeal subsystems of speech production. These two subsystems combined are called the lower respiratory tract. The larynx is situated directly above the trachea and below the pharynx. The trachea bifurcates into bronchi that lead to the lungs. From *The speech sciences. A volume in the speech sciences* (1st ed.), by Kent, copyright 1998. Reprinted with permission of Delmar, a division of Thomson Learning.

Note, for example, that flow is directly proportional to pressure but inversely proportional to resistance. If resistance is held constant, an increase in air pressure will result in an increase in air flow. If air pressure is held constant, an increase in resistance will cause a decrease in air flow.

Speech is produced with a relatively constant lung pressure of about 6–10 centimeters of water or about one kPa (kPa = kilopascal, or 1000 pascals.) To get an idea of how much pressure this is, dip a straw to a depth of 6 centimeters in a water-filled glass (Figure 1–3). Then, blow into the straw until bubbles just begin to form at the end of the water-immersed straw. This con-

dition corresponds to a pressure of 6 centimeters of water. There is only a small loss of air pressure from the tiny air sacs of the lungs up to the larynx at the top of the trachea, so that the subglottal air pressure (the pressure just below the vocal folds) is approximately equal to the air pressure in the lungs. Of course, if there were not closure at the larynx or in the upper airway of the articulatory system, air pressure developed by the respiratory system would be immediately released through the open tract into the atmosphere. Speech is produced by valving or regulating the air pressures and flows generated by the respiratory subsystem. In simple terms, the

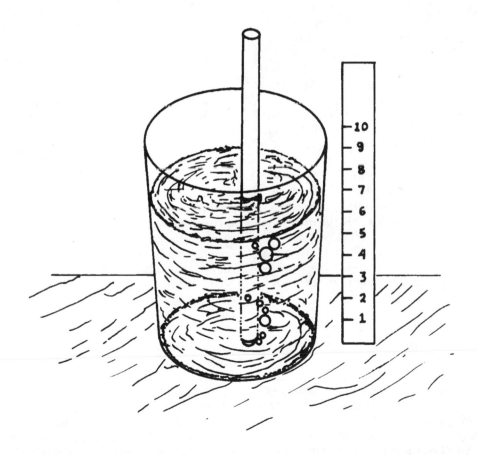

FIGURE 1–3. Simple demonstration of the air pressure requirement of speech production. Place a straw into a cup of water to a depth of 6 cm. Then blow through the straw until bubbles begin to rise up through the water. This condition corresponds to a water pressure of 6 cm, which is adequate for the purposes of conversational speech.

respiratory subsystem is an air pump, providing aerodynamic energy for the laryngeal and articulatory subsystems. The basic pattern of respiratory support for speech is that the speaker inspires air by muscular adjustments that increase the volume of the respiratory system. Air is then released from the lungs by combinations of passive recoil and muscular activity, depending on the actual volume of air in the lungs and the aerodynamic requirements.

The essential point is that respiratory function for speech is understood in terms of aerodynamic events—air volumes, pressures, and flows. The mechanical events of speech thus begin as a speaker uses the respiratory system to generate aerodynamic energy. In most languages, speech is produced on expired air, which means that speech production must be interrupted whenever the speaker takes in a breath. The typical pattern in speech is a quick inspiration followed by a much slower expiration on which speech is produced. During rest breathing, the inspiratory and expiratory phases of a breathing cycle are nearly equal in duration, but for speech the expiratory phase is prolonged relative to the inspiratory phase. These differences in inspiratory and expiratory patterning may be represented as shown below, where insp = inspiration, exp = expiration, rest breathing is shown to the left of the double vertical line and speech breathing is shown to the right of the double line. The dashed lines represent the prolonged expiratory phase of speech breathing.

insp | exp | insp | exp | insp | exp | |
   insp | exp——————— | insp | exp—
   ———————|

The necessity to interrupt speech for the purpose of inspiration means that speech is produced in *breath groups*, which are groups of words or syllables produced on a single breath. In general, the units produced within a breath group have an overall coherence, such as fitting within an intonational pattern (a pattern of pitch rises and falls).

The Laryngeal Subsystem

As shown in Figure 1–2, the larynx is situated on the top of the trachea and opens into the pharynx above. The larynx consists of a number of cartilages and muscles. Of particular importance are the vocal folds, small muscular cushions that adduct (come together) to close the laryngeal airway or abduct (separate) to open this airway. A drawing of a coronal section of the larynx is shown in Figure 1–4. The true vocal folds are the vibrating structures of interest here. These have a complex layered structure shown in the enlargement of Figure 1–4. The opening between the vocal folds is called the **glottis** (Figure 1–5), and the term *glottal* has come to be used as a general term for laryngeal function, especially the function of the vocal folds. For example, the laryngeal tone is often called the glottal source. If the vocal folds are tightly closed, air is prevented from escaping from the inflated lungs. The vocal folds are typically tightly closed during intensive physical tasks such as lifting, defecating and childbirth, so as to make the respiratory subsystem rigid as a foundation for pushing.

The fact that people often grunt during the lifting of a heavy object is evidence that the vocal folds are closed. The occurrence of the grunt also tells us that voiced sound is produced with abducted vocal folds. The sound results from the vibration of the folds, which alternately snap together and apart, colliding with one another in a basically periodic fashion. The rate of vibration of the vocal folds basically determines the perception of a speaker's *vocal pitch*. A speaker with a high-pitched voice has a relatively high frequency of vocal fold vibration, and a speaker with a low-pitched voice has a relatively low frequency of vocal fold vibration.

The larynx is important to speech not only because it is the source of voicing energy but also because it valves the air moving into or out of the lungs. The valving functions are described in terms of *adduction* and *abduction*. When the vocal folds are adducted tightly, no air movement

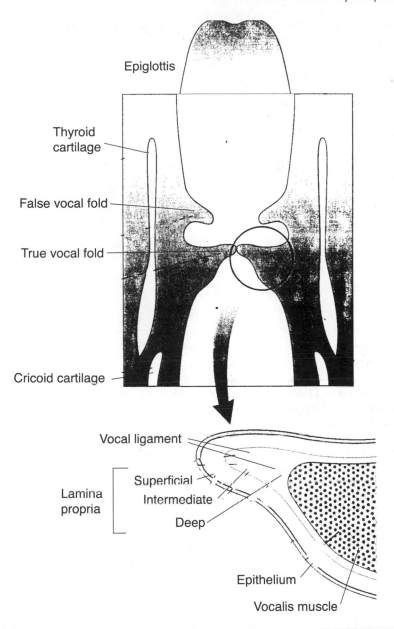

FIGURE 1–4. Coronal section of the larynx, showing the false and true vocal folds. The enlargement shows the layered structure of the latter, which are the source of vibratory energy for voice. From *The speech sciences. A volume in the speech sciences* (1st ed.), by Kent, copyright 1998. Reprinted with permission of Delmar, a division of Thomson Learning.

will occur. Tight adduction is important for certain strenuous physical tasks, as described earlier, but it also is used to interrupt the air stream for some speech sounds.

Adduction with less resistance to air flow enables vocal fold vibration. A large degree of abduction allows air to move readily from the lungs into the upper airway. Voice-

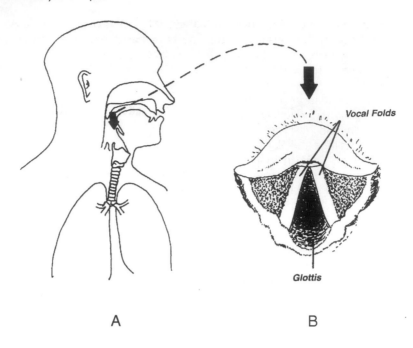

A   B

FIGURE 1–5. Superior view of the larynx to show the vocal folds and glottis. The folds are observed from the perspective shown in A, and the enlarged view of the folds is in B. From *The speech sciences. A volume in the speech sciences* (1st ed.), by Kent, copyright 1998. Reprinted with permission of Delmar, a division of Thomson Learning.

less sounds, such as the [s] in *see*, require that air pressure be impounded within the mouth as a source for noise energy. Abduction of the vocal folds satisfies this requirement by permitting the pressure in the mouth to approximate that in the lungs. Finally, a partial abduction of the vocal folds is used to generate voiceless noise energy, such as that of whispering.

As important as the larynx is, it contributes relatively little to the phonetic differentiation of speech sounds. Certainly, laryngeal action differentiates voiced from voiceless sounds, such as the initial sounds in the contrasting pair *bill-pill*. But laryngeal function is highly similar within major grouping of sounds. For example, vocal fold vibration differs little across vowels, which gain their distinctiveness by the shaping of the articulatory system above the larynx. For this reason, the phonetic description of speech is based largely on supraglottal articulatory features.

The Articulatory System

This system extends from the larynx up through the lips or nose, that is, the two openings through which air and acoustic energy can pass (Figure 1–6). Transmission of energy through the lips involves the oral cavity as a conduit, and transmission of energy through the nose involves the nasal cavity as a conduit. The *articulators* are movable structures and include the tongue, lips, jaw, and velum (or soft palate), as illustrated in Figure 1–6. Movements of these structures shape the vocal tract. The shape of the tract determines its resonance properties. When a speaker makes the vowel sound in the word *he*, the physical process may be understood as a shaping of the vocal tract to produce a particular pattern of resonance frequencies. In this process, energy from the vibrating vocal folds activates the resonance system of the vocal tract. Changing the vocal tract shape changes its resonance frequencies. The articulatory system also may be used to obstruct air flow (as in the case of the consonants in the word *pop*) and to generate noise (as in the case of the consonants in the word *seethe*).

Speech articulation typically is described in terms of articulatory contacts and positions. For example, a phonetician might describe the consonant [s] in *see* as a lingua-alveolar fricative. Lingua-alveolar denotes the place of articulatory constriction. *Lingua* means tongue and *alveolar* indicates a ridge on the bony ceiling of the mouth. **Fricative** indicates a sound that is produced with significant noise energy. The phonetician usually describes vowels with respect to the position of the tongue and the status of the lips. The vowel in *see* is termed a high-front and unrounded vowel because the tongue is relatively high and front in the mouth and the lips are unrounded. These articulatory descriptions are a convenient way to characterize the differences among speech sounds. Readers who are not familiar with phonetic descriptions should read Appen-

dix A before moving on to the other chapters of this book. Appendix A also lists the phonetic symbols that will be used in discussing speech sounds.

The Acoustic Arena of Speech

The acoustic arena is the major focus of this book but it is difficult to understand the acoustics of speech independently of speech physiology and perception. The acoustic signal of speech is the physical event that is transmitted in telecommunications or is recorded on magnetic tape, laser disc, or other mediums. That is, when we transmit or store speech, we almost always do so on the basis of the acoustic signal. This signal contains the linguistic message of speech. The listener may recover this message by hearing it. This may seem like an obvious statement. Is there any other way by which speech might be understood? To answer

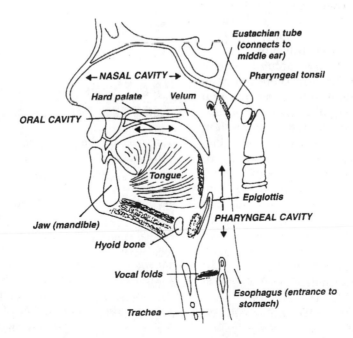

FIGURE 1–6. Drawing of a midsagittal section of the vocal tract. Note the major cavities, articulators, and related structures. From *The speech sciences. A volume in the speech sciences* (1st ed.), by Kent, copyright 1998. Reprinted with permission of Delmar, a division of Thomson Learning.

this question, imagine a person who is born deaf and blind. This person can neither hear speech nor see its articulation. Yet, persons with these joint disabilities can learn to produce and perceive speech. One technique used by the deaf and blind is called *Tadoma*. Users of this method place a hand over the speaker's face in such a way as to sense the actions of speech production—vocal fold vibrations, puffs of air escaping from the nose or mouth, movements of the jaw or lips, and so on. Practiced users of Tadoma can carry on conversations. That is, speech communication can be accomplished without perception of an acoustic signal. For these rare individuals, speech is movement only, not movements made audible.

However, for the great majority, speech is audible and necessarily so. Few of us can understand a televised speaker when the sound is turned off. We might guess a few words by observing the visual information (*lip reading* or *speech reading*), but understanding is at best difficult and uncertain. On the other hand, if the video is faded to black while the audio signal is maintained, we continue to understand the spoken message, usually with little difficulty.

The primary objective of this book is to describe how speech sounds are carried in the acoustic signal. This objective will involve (a) an account of how the physiologic events of speech production result in various types of sounds, (b) the description of speech sounds in terms of acoustic variables, (c) the description of techniques for the study of speech acoustics, and (d) a consideration of how acoustic cues are used in the perception of speech. A full understanding of speech acoustics requires that acoustic patterns be related to the physiologic patterns of speech production and to the perceptual decisions that are based on the acoustic signal.

Readers who do not have at least an introductory background in acoustics should read Appendix B before proceeding with this book.

The Perceptual Arena

The study of speech perception is in large part an attempt to identify the acoustic cues that are used by a listener in reaching phonetic decisions. For example, what are the acoustic cues that enable a listener to decide that the consonant [b] was produced in the word *bye*? The understanding of speech perception has been advanced greatly by improvements in the acoustic analysis of speech and the synthesis of speech by machines. The ability to analyze the acoustic signal of speech and the ability to produce synthetic replicas of speech have been complementary in the modern understanding of how humans perceive speech. Although many questions remain to be answered about speech perception, the basic acoustic cues are sufficiently understood that speech synthesizers are becoming highly intelligible and sometimes even quite natural. Great progress also has been made in machine speech recognition. As we learn how humans perceive speech, we are better able to design machines that have the capability of deriving linguistic decisions from the acoustic signal.

The Three Forms of the Acoustic Speech Signal

Progress in the study of speech and the development of speech technologies, such as speech synthesis and machine speech recognition, is rooted in the capabilities to record the speech signal and then play back the stored signal for analysis. Modern acoustic analysis is highly dependent on the digital computer, so much so that digital signal processing is at the heart of contemporary acoustic analysis of speech. Therefore, it is essential to understand how the acoustic signal is entered into a computer. This matter will be taken up in some detail in Chapter 3, but some background information is needed.

The Acoustic Wave

It is convenient to regard the signal of speech as having three interchangeable forms. The first of these is the airborne *acoustic wave*, or the signal that can be heard by the ear or sensed by a microphone. An acoustic wave is a longitudinal wave, meaning that the particles move in the same direction as the propagation of the wave. Our ears and most microphones respond to sound as pressure variations in the atmosphere. These variations take the form of condensations and rarefactions. Figure 1–7 shows a pattern of condensations and rarefactions for a simple sinusoid. The ear converts the air pressure variations into neural impulses that are sent to the brain for interpretation. Microphones convert the air pressure variations into electrical signals. Microphones are one kind of *transducer*. A transducer is an element that converts one form of energy into another. A microphone transduces acoustic energy into electrical energy.

Technically, the airborne acoustic signal of speech is called the *propagated* or *radiated* acoustic signal. This signal propagates or radiates into space after it emerges from a speaker's vocal tract. Because this signal quickly vanishes, it is not a convenient form of speech for analysis. The acoustic analysis of speech requires stored forms of speech, or replicas of the original sound pattern, that can be examined at length.

The Stored Analog Signal

The second form of speech is the stored **analog signal**, a common example of which is an audiotape recording. An analog signal varies continuously in its basic properties. The analog signal of speech varies continuously in its pressure and time properties. This continuous variation is evident in the usual waveform representation of speech (Figure 1–8), which displays amplitude variations over time. Both the time and pressure dimensions may be divided into infinitely many points because of their continuous variation. Magnetic tape stores the speech signal as a magnetic field, which, like the original airborne acoustic signal,

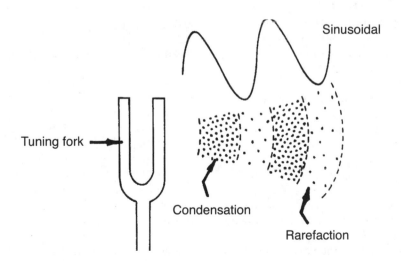

FIGURE 1–7. Wave of condensations and rarefactions produced by a vibrating tuning fork, which produces a sinusoid or pure tone. From *The speech sciences. A volume in the speech sciences* (1st ed.), by Kent, copyright 1998. Reprinted with permission of Delmar, a division of Thomson Learning.

varies continuously in its properties The advantage of the stored analog signal in a magnetic tape recording is that it may be played back for listening or analysis. Playback is accomplished by converting the magnetic energy back to electrical energy, which, in turn, is converted to acoustic energy by a loudspeaker or headphone. Each of these energy forms preserves the analog or continuous nature of the signal.

The Stored Digital Signal

The third form is another stored form, the **digital** (or *digitized*) **signal**. This form can be stored in a digital computer or on digital magnetic tapes or disks. Digital means numerical. Digital computers store information as numbers. To store a speech signal in a digital computer, it is necessary to convert the analog (continuous) signal to a series of numbers. This is accomplished by a process called *digitization*. An **analog-to-digital (A/D) converter** is a process or device that changes an analog signal to a digital one. In the reverse process, a *digital-to-analog (D/A) converter* changes the digital signal to an analog form. For example, D/A conversion would be required to play back the digitally stored signal through earphones or a loudspeaker. The abbreviations ADC and DAC are sometimes used for the two types of conversion. The digital representation of speech is very important because it permits the analysis of speech with the computational power of modern digital computers. Even personal computers are capable of some sophisticated speech analyses.

The three forms of speech—airborne acoustic signal, stored analog signal, and stored digital signal—are interchangeable in the sense that one form may be converted to another form and back again. For example, the airborne acoustic signal may be recorded with a microphone, then stored in analog form on audiotape, then converted to digital form for storage in a computer, and finally converted back to analog form to drive a loudspeaker and be heard again as an airborne acoustic signal. Both analog and digital storage are virtually permanent, so that a speech signal may be held indefinitely.

With modern digital processing techniques, it is not necessary to use analog storage devices like audiotape recorders at all. The digital computer can store the signal and analyze it, and, through D/A conversion, play it back as needed. But in whatever form the speech signal is stored, it is important to recognize some basic properties of speech to be certain that the stored signal really retains the important characteristics of the airborne acoustic signal.

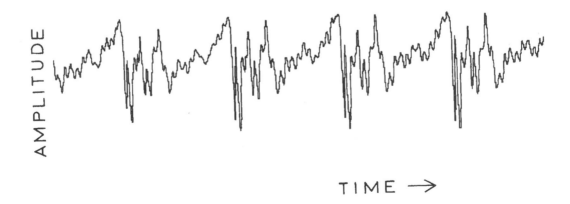

FIGURE 1–8. The waveform of speech. The vertical axis represents the amplitude of vibration and the horizontal axis represents time. The waveform shown is for a vowel sound.

Valuable information may be lost in the operations of transduction and storage. Unfortunately, many people have discovered that signals that were thought to be safely recorded are badly distorted upon playback. For both the storage and analysis of speech, it is important to know some basic characteristics of the signal in question. This issue is taken up next.

Considerations of the Acoustic Properties of Speech

The energy of speech extends over a bandwidth of more than 10 kHz. Figure 1–9 shows the long-term spectrum of speech, that is, the energy distribution across frequencies for a long sample of speech, say, several seconds or even minutes. Although most of the long-term energy is in the lower frequencies, energy is spread quite widely over the frequency range. In fact, the energy in speech can extend beyond 10 kHz, but for most purposes it is sufficient to consider a much smaller frequency range. The bandwidth for telephone transmission is only about 500–3500 Hz, and a readily intelligible speech signal can be transmitted with a total

bandwidth of less than 5 kHz. But whenever any speech is recorded or analyzed, it is important to know how frequency limitations in recording or analysis may affect the results. The frequency response of the recording or analyzing equipment should be known before quantitative analyses are performed. It should never be simply assumed that a tape recording is faithful in its reproduction of a sound. Recorders advertised as "high fidelity" aren't necessarily so. For the purposes of this tutorial, it will be assumed that a frequency range of at least 5 kHz is needed for even modest objectives in speech analysis. But a range of 10 kHz is much more appropriate for the study of various sounds produced by different speakers, including men, women and children.

The *dynamic range of speech*—its range of energy—is about 60 dB, meaning that the weakest sounds are about 60 dB less intense than the strongest sounds. Vowels, especially the low vowels, are the most intense sounds, and the fricatives that begin the words *fin* and *thin* are typically the weakest. When a V-U (*volume units*) meter on a tape recorder is used to monitor the peak intensity of a speech sample, it is responding mainly to the energy in vowels. If recording and analyzing instruments are not properly adjusted, the dynamic range of recording or

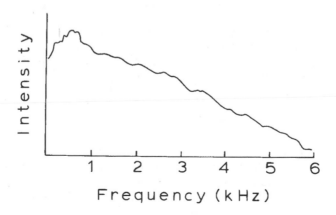

FIGURE 1–9. Sketch of the long-term average spectrum of speech. The energy is spread over a range of frequencies, but the region of greatest energy is in the low frequencies.

analysis may not be matched to the dynamic range of the sounds of interest. As a rule of thumb, the dynamic range for a given speaker may be estimated from the sounds in the word *thaw*, which consists of a weak fricative and an intense vowel. If both the fricative and the vowel are satisfactorily represented in a recording or analysis, then the procedures are at least roughly suitable. It will be assumed in this tutorial that a dynamic range of about 60 dB is appropriate for the storage and analysis of speech. Within this range, it usually is desirable that recordings be sensitive to variations of 1 dB. The human ear responds to variations of about this magnitude and it is for this reason that a 1–dB sensitivity is required.

Time also is an important dimension to consider in speech recording and analysis. The minimal time resolution for general analysis purposes is about 10 ms. This is the shortest duration of important speech events, such as the transient burst associated with the release of stop consonants (e.g., the initial sounds in the words *pat*, *tap*, and *cat*). Analyses that cannot achieve this resolution may miss significant information about the temporal structure of speech.

Finally, it should be remembered that both the frequency and energy of speech sounds can change very rapidly. Instants of rapid change may be especially important in the information carried by the speech signal, and, therefore, storage and analysis operations should be able to follow these rapid changes with little or no distortion.

With these thoughts in mind, we can see that the study of speech acoustics involves the analysis of a signal whose energy (a) is distributed over a range of about 10 kHz for most purposes, (b) possesses a dynamic range of about 60 dB, and (c) has significant variations in time that occur in 10 ms or less. Bear in mind also that the speech signal is lost quickly as its acoustic energy dissipates into the atmosphere. We may repeat what was said but we can never retrieve the original production.

Speech Acoustics as the Intermediary Between the Expression and Comprehension of Spoken Language

The acoustic signal of speech is at once the product of the operations of language expression and the input to the processes of language comprehension. As such, the acoustic representation of speech is a basic referent for understanding how humans use language. To some degree the processes of language production and understanding can be related to acoustic patterns, and the study of these relationships is a major reason for the application of acoustics to fields such as linguistics, psycholinguistics, speech-language pathology, and communication engineering. Figure 1–10 is a simplified diagram of the operations of language expression and comprehension. In several places in this book, we examine the possibility that various language structures are reflected in the acoustic signal. The encoding of various kinds of information—linguistic, emotional, and personal—into the acoustic speech signal invites analysis of this signal as a primary means to understand human communication.

Theory, Instruments, and Measures

This book takes up issues related to the acoustic theory of speech production, the laboratory instruments suited to acoustic analysis, and measurements of the acoustic signal of speech. These three—theory, instruments and measures—are interrelated. The use of tools and measures is influenced by the acoustic theory of speech. Test of the theory depends on the availability of laboratory instruments and measures. The application of measures requires that the signal be stored and appropriately displayed by laboratory instruments. The

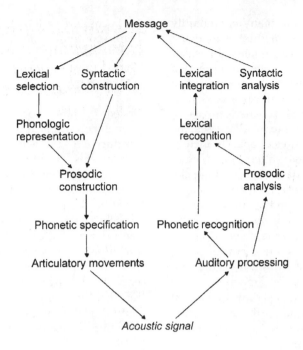

FIGURE 1-10. Diagram of the major operations in language expression and comprehension. The acoustic signal of speech is the intermediary between these two facets of spoken language.

proper use of acoustic analysis requires an understanding of how speech is produced (the acoustic theory of speech production), a knowledge of laboratory instruments available for acoustic analysis of signals like speech, and a familiarity with various measures that can be made of the acoustic signal of speech.

Chapter 2 presents basic concepts of the acoustic theory of speech production. Knowing what speech is—how it is generated as an acoustic signal—helps in the design and use of analysis instruments and in the selection of measures to characterize the signal. The acoustic theory of speech production summarized in Chapter 2 is a first step in understanding the acoustic analysis of speech. Chapter 3 considers the instruments and methods used for the analysis of the acoustic signal of speech. Contemporary speech analysis relies heavily on the digital computer. Therefore, to understand speech analysis, one needs to

know about the digital processing of signals. Chapter 3 describes the procedures by which the acoustic signal, as obtained with a microphone, is converted to a form that can be stored in a digital computer. Chapter 3 also describes the modern acoustic analyses used in the study of speech. These analyses are typically available on systems that run on digital computers or that are provided by stand-alone systems based on microprocessors. In both cases, digital signal processing is involved. Chapters 4 and 5 pertain to the acoustic characteristics of vowels and consonants, respectively. These two chapters define the acoustic measures that are typically used in acoustic phonetics and also present data on some of the more commonly used of these measures. Although the emphasis is on American English, an attempt is made to show how these measures apply to other languages as well. However, it should be noted that acoustic data are not abundant for the world's languages, and many have hardly been studied by this method. Chapter 6 considers the acoustic correlates of speaker characteristics such as age and gender. Because the acoustic patterns of speech vary considerably across speakers, it is important to understand the sources of these variations. Chapter 7 discusses the suprasegmental features of speech, including intonation, stress patterns, and emotional attributes. Speech is more than the phonetic (segmental) constituents discussed in Chapters 4 and 5, and Chapter 7 presents information on the suprasegmental properties by which speech gains its full richness and communicative power. Chapter 8 discusses speech synthesis, or the generation of speech by machine. The Appendices and Glossary may be helpful for occasional referral, so the reader may want to take a quick look at these materials to become familiar with their contents before continuing on to the next chapter.

Summary

Speech is the vocal/aural channel of human communication. Speech sounds are produced by the actions of three primary subsystems (respiratory, laryngeal, and articulatory). The acoustic signal of speech is of particular interest because it intervenes between the production and perception of speech. That is, the acoustic signal is at once the output of the production system and the input to the processes of perception. Because the acoustic signal of speech encodes linguistic, emotional, and personal information in the act of human communication, it is an important goal to develop effective means for its analysis.

Acoustic Theory of Speech Production

2

CHAPTER

The Linear Source–Filter Theory of Speech Production

The primary goal of this chapter is to summarize a theory commonly known as the *linear source–filter theory of speech production*. Gunnar Fant's classic book, *Acoustic Theory of Speech Production* (1970; first published in 1960) is a basic reference as is the article by Stevens and House (1961). This theory is useful in understanding articulatory-acoustic relationships, and it also provides a foundation for many procedures for the acoustic analysis of speech, and for popular methods of speech synthesis. Only broad outlines of the theory are presented here. The reader who seeks a more complete presentation should read Fant's book or the more recent book by Stevens (1998). The books by Fant and Stevens are essential sources for the theoretical bases of speech production, but they can be challenging for readers who do not have a background in mathematics and physics. (Also recommended is Stevens, 1989 and Pickett, 1999.)

In this chapter, the acoustic theory of speech is discussed in terms of the following major sound classes: vowels, fricatives, nasals, stops, affricates, liquids, diphthongs and semivowels. The first three of these—vowels, fricatives, and nasals—are discussed at length because they involve principles that can be generalized to the other sound classes. For example, the semivowel [w] as in *way*, can be understood as a modification of the theory for vowel production, and affricates such as the initial and final sounds in the word *judge* can be understood as a combination of a stop (silence) and a fricative. Therefore, vowels, fricatives, and nasals form the essential foundation of the acoustic theory for speech in this chapter.

Some simple diagrams help to identify the major features of interest. Ordinarily, vowels are sounds produced with laryngeal vibration (so that voicing is the energy source) and a relatively open vocal tract that is shaped to produce particular patterns of resonances (so that the entire vocal tract functions as a filter, or frequency-selective transmission system). A general diagram for vowels is given in Figure 2–1A, which is a fairly simple pipe, with one end at the larynx and the other opening to atmosphere. Modifications of this diagram are used to model liquids and semivowels, which are similar to vowels in their acoustic properties. Fricatives are produced with a narrow constriction somewhere in the vocal tract, as depicted in Figure 2–1B. Air passing through this constriction generates turbulence noise that is the energy source for sound production. The noise source is filtered (modified) by the vocal tract, especially by the section of the vocal tract anterior to the constriction. The model of Figure 2–1B is modified for stop and affricative consonants, both of which involve a brief closure of the vocal tract and the generation of noise similar to that of fricatives. As shown in Figure 2–1C, nasal sounds are produced with the velopharynx open so that sound is radiated through the nasal cavity. If the mouth is closed, the resultant sound is a nasal consonant, like *m* and *n* in the word *man*. If the mouth is open, the resultant sound is a nasalized vowel. Nasals, like vowels, typically have voicing as an energy source. However, nasals differ from oral vowels in that the filtering of the source energy is determined by both the oral and nasal passages.

Acoustic Theory for Vowels

Tube Resonance as a Model of Vowel Production

To introduce the acoustic theory of speech production, we begin with an apparatus that may not look very much like the human vocal tract. As shown in Figure 2–2, this apparatus consists simply of a vibrator (a rubber membrane with a slit cut into it will do) and a length of straight pipe. The vibrator is stretched to fit over one end of the pipe and the other end of the pipe is left open. The vibrator is a source of acoustic energy that travels through the pipe. The pipe is a resonator, in fact, an example of a very important class of resonators. The pipe is a tube closed at one end (where the vibrating source is located) and open at the other. Such a pipe has an infinite number of resonances, located at frequencies given by the *odd-quarter wavelength* relationship:

$$F_n = (2n-1) \ c \ / \ 4l,$$

where *n* is an integer,

c is the speed of sound (about 35,000 cm/sec), and

l is the length of the pipe.

The formula shown above gives the resonance frequencies of the pipe. If the formula is restated in words, it says that a

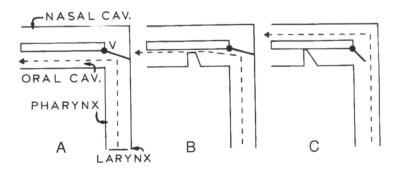

FIGURE 2–1. Vocal tract models for three classes of speech sounds: (A) vowels, (B) fricatives, and (C) nasals. Note the partial constriction in (B) and the total obstruction in (C).

Vibrating membrane

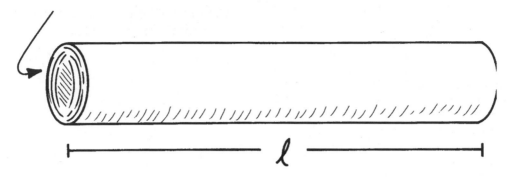

FIGURE 2–2. Simple model of vowel production: a straight tube of uniform cross section closed at one end (by a vibrating membrane to simulate the vocal folds) and open at the other (corresponding to the mouth opening).

pipe resonates with maximal amplitude a sound whose wavelength is 4 times the length of the tube. In fact, such resonances occur in multiples and that is why the expression (2n-1) is used to generate the set of odd numbers. Resonances occur at c/4l, 3c/4l, 5c/4l, 7c/4l, and so on. Let's assume that the pipe has a length l of 17.5 cm. Then the first resonance will have a frequency given by:

$$F1 = c/4l$$

$$= 35,000 \text{ cm/sec} / (4 \times 17.5 \text{ cm})$$

$$= 500 \text{ 1/sec, or 500 Hz.}$$

The second resonance will have a frequency calculated as:

$$F2 = 3c/4l$$

$$= 3 \times 35,000 \text{ cm/sec} / (4 \times 17.5 \text{ cm})$$

$$= 1500 \text{ 1/sec, or 1500 Hz.}$$

Higher resonances can be determined by continuing the calculations for different solutions of (2n-1). Doing so results in the following resonance frequencies: 500, 1500, 2500, 3500, 4500 Hz (far enough for our purposes). Note that the resonance frequencies fall at intervals of 1000 Hz.

To make this example relevant to the production of human speech, we need to note two things: (1) the average vocal tract of a man has a length of about 17.5 cm running from glottis to lips, and (2) the vocal tract has approximately the same resonance frequencies as a straight tube of the same length and cross-sectional area. That is, the simple pipe apparatus shown in Figure 2–2 is a satisfactory model of one particular vowel of human speech. The vowel in question is produced with the tongue and other articulators positioned so as to create a uniform cross-sectional area along the length of the vocal tract. This vowel is depicted in Figure 2–3. As you might have guessed, the vibrating membrane in the pipe apparatus is analogous to the vibrating vocal folds. The pipe is analogous to the vocal tract, at least for the one particular vowel shown in Figure 2–3. In a sense, the rubber membrane and pipe apparatus is a one-vowel sound generator. It has an energy source (the vibrating membrane) and a resonator (the pipe).

Changing the length of the resonating pipe changes the resonance frequencies as indicated in the odd-quarter wavelength formula. If the pipe length is doubled from 17.5 cm to 35 cm, the resonance frequencies would assume much lower values, namely,

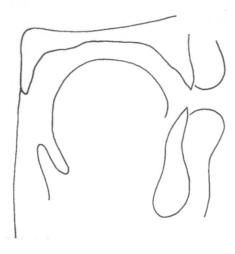

FIGURE 2–3. Vocal tract configuration of a vowel that roughly corresponds to the idealized tube in Figure 2–2. The cross–sectional area is essentially the same from glottis to lips.

250, 750, 1250, and 1750 Hz for the first (or lowest) resonances. If the pipe length is halved to make a new pipe only 8.75 cm long, then the lowest four resonance frequencies would be 1000, 3000, 5000 and 7000 Hz. These results explain why the longest pipes in a pipe organ sound the lowest tones whereas the shortest pipes sound the highest tones. Similarly, we have an explanation for the changes in resonance frequencies of the vocal tract as a child grows into an adult. An infant has approximately half the vocal tract length of an adult and has much higher resonance frequencies. In fact, the resonance frequencies for an infant's vowel corresponding in vocal tract shape to Figure 2–3 are about 1000, 3000, 5000 and 7000 Hz, or the values calculated above for a pipe that is 8.75 cm in length. Obviously, then, the length of a speaker's vocal tract will determine the relative location of the resonance frequencies. The longer the vocal tract, the lower the resonance frequencies and the smaller their separation in frequency. Conversely, the shorter the vocal tract, the higher the resonance frequencies and the larger their separation in frequency.

We have seen that the length of the vocal tract determines the average spacing of the resonance frequencies. This means that resonance frequencies vary with speaker characteristics that determine the length of the vocal tract. The two main factors are age and sex. In most of this chapter, the examples pertain to the speech of adult males, and it should be remembered that adjustments are needed to account for the speech patterns of women and children. Samples of acoustic data from speakers of both sexes and various ages are included in several chapters of this book.

Extending the Tube Resonance Model

The results so far pertain to just a single vowel, the so-called mid-central vowel in which the cross-sectional area is the same along the length of the vocal tract. What are the resonance frequencies for other vowels? The answer can be determined experimentally by discovering the resonance frequencies for various shapes of pipes that have the same length. As noted above, the resonance frequencies are not affected appreciably by whether the pipe is straight or curved (the differences that occur were described by Sondhi, 1986). However, it is easier to draw a straight pipe, so straight pipes of different shapes will serve as models for this discussion. Some examples of different pipe shapes are shown in Figure 2–4. Each one of the shapes corresponds roughly to the vocal tract shape of a vowel in English. Figure 2–4A corresponds to vowel [i] (as in *he*), Figure 2–4B to vowel [u] (as in *who*), and Figure 2–4C to vowel [a] (as in *ha*). Also shown in Figure 2–4 are spectra for each of these simple vowel models. The spectral peaks are the resonance frequencies of the pipes. Notice that, on average, the resonance frequencies are separated by about 1000 Hz, but that the individual resonance frequencies vary about the frequency locations for the mid-central vowel. For example, compared to the first resonance for the mid-central vowel, the first resonance for [i] has a lower frequency, but the first resonance frequency for [a] has a higher frequency.

This is a good point to review what has been discovered so far:

1. A uniform pipe that is closed at one end and open at the other has resonance frequencies determined by the length

of the pipe (assuming constant atmospheric conditions). The resonance frequencies are relatively lower for long pipes and relatively higher for short pipes.

2. For non-uniform pipes (that is, pipes for which the cross-sectional area is not constant over pipe length), the individual resonance frequencies vary around the values determined for a uniform pipe.

3. The uniform pipe closed at one end and open at the other is an acoustic model for one vowel, namely the mid-central vowel.

4. In order that the pipe model can represent other vowels, the cross-sectional area must be varied as a function of pipe length in a way that approximates the vocal tract shape for a particular vowel.

At this point, you might be wondering if simple pipes like those depicted in Figure 2–4 actually do sound like vowels produced by humans. In fact, they do sound

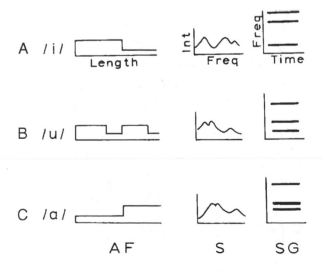

FIGURE 2–4. Shown for each of three vowels is an idealized area function (AF), spectrum (S) and spectrogram (SG). The closed end of the area function represents the glottis, and the open end, the lips. Formants are represented in the spectra by peaks and in the spectrogram by horizontal bands.

something like human vowels, provided that an appropriate source of vibratory energy is applied to them. (Remember that resonators do not generate sound energy but only respond to energy that is delivered to them.) Moreover, all the other vowels in English can be modeled, at least roughly, by appropriate shape modifications of a straight pipe.

What is the relationship between the resonator (such as a pipe) and the source of energy (such as a vibrating rubber membrane)? To a large degree, the energy source and the resonator are independent, except for special conditions. This is an important principle, and it explains why a speaker can produce a low-pitched vowel [i] or a high-pitched vowel [i] without losing the phonetic distinctiveness of the vowel. Vocal pitch is determined almost entirely by the vibrating frequencies of the vocal folds. The lower the rate of vibration, the lower the

pitch. Therefore, a bass voice has a lower vibratory frequency than a soprano voice. However, the frequency of vibration of the vocal folds does not affect the properties of the resonator. The resonance frequencies of a pipe resonator are determined almost entirely by just two factors: the length of the pipe and its cross-sectional area as a function of length. Changing the frequency of the energy source *does not* change the resonance frequencies of the pipe receiving the energy.

The Source–Filter Theory of Vowel Production

The principles introduced to this point may be summarized in a conceptualization called the **source–filter theory** (Figure 2–5). This theory, as applied to vowel production, states that the output energy (or what was called the radiated speech signal in an

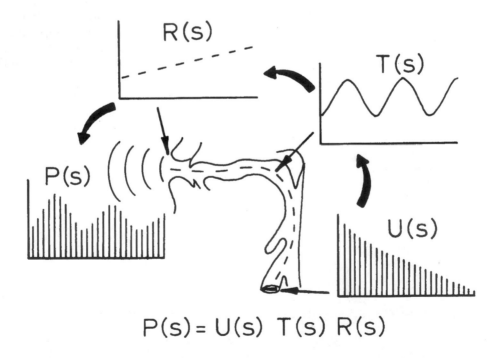

$$P(s) = U(s) \ T(s) \ R(s)$$

FIGURE 2–5. Diagrammatic representation of the source–filter concept for vowels. The laryngeal source spectrum, U(s), is filtered by the vocal tract transfer function, T(s), and the radiation characteristic, R(s), to yield the output spectrum, P(s). Mathematically, P(s) is a coproduct of U(s), T(s) and R(s) where s = frequency.

earlier section) is a product of the source energy and the resonator or filter. We might more accurately refer to this theory as *linear source–filter theory*, because it is based on a linear mathematical model. The assumption of linearity opens the door to powerful yet relatively simple mathematical operations. In the simplest sense, linearity obtains when the input–output function of a system is described by a straight line. Still one more adjective might be included to describe the theory as *linear time–invariant source–filter theory*. *Time invariance* means that if the input to the system is advanced (or delayed) in time, the output is similarly advanced (or delayed). The assumptions of linearity and time invariance are commonly made in many applications of physics and engineering, especially because they make the system under consideration mathematically tractable.

It is convenient to think of the source energy in the form of a spectrum. The vibrating vocal folds produce a sound spectrum like that in Figure 2–6. The energy falls at discrete frequencies determined by the rate of vibration. The result is called a *line spectrum*, or a spectrum in which the energy distribution takes the form of lines. The spectrum of voicing energy can be ide-

alized as a line spectrum in which the individual lines fall at integer multiples of the fundamental (lowest) vibratory frequency. For example, the average man's voice has a fundamental frequency of about 120 Hz, and the energy of this source spectrum will fall at the frequencies of 120, 240, 360, 480 Hz and so on. However, a man can produce much lower or higher frequencies of vibration than this average value. If a man's fundamental frequency increases to 300 Hz, then the energy in the source spectrum will fall at the frequencies of 300, 600, 900, 1200 Hz and so on. The same principles apply to women's and children's voices. The average fundamental frequency for a woman is about 230 Hz, so the energy of the idealized spectrum would fall at the frequencies of 230, 460, 690 Hz, and so on. These changes in vibratory frequency are changes in the source only and do not necessarily have any effect on the resonator or filter. Similarly, the amplitude of vocal fold vibration can be changed. A speaker can produce a soft voice or a loud voice. Such changes affect the resonator only in that they determine the level of energy which the resonator will receive. The relative independence of source and filter makes it possible for us to produce intelligible

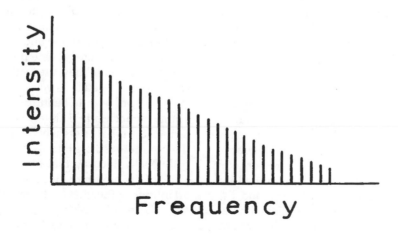

FIGURE 2–6. Idealized laryngeal spectrum in which the energy is located at discrete frequencies which are integer multiples of the fundamental frequency. The amplitudes of the successive harmonics decrease with frequency.

speech with a variety of energy sources, including low- and high-pitched voices, whisper, gravelly voices, and other phonatory variations.

To extend the source–filter model to the production of all vowels (and eventually to other speech sounds as well), it is helpful to make some changes in terminology. First, different kinds of sources are involved in speech production, but for the moment we are concerned with only one kind of source, the vibrating vocal folds. We now refer to this source as the **laryngeal spectrum** (frequency domain) or the *laryngeal waveform* (time domain). The laryngeal spectrum can be idealized as a line spectrum, as discussed above. It is characteristic of the laryngeal spectrum that the energy in its harmonic components (each line is a harmonic of the fundamental frequency) declines as frequency increases. This decline in the energy of the higher harmonics is shown in Figure 2–6 and means that most of the energy in voiced speech is in the lower frequencies. The rate of decline in energy is 12 dB per octave, or a drop in energy of 12 dB for every doubling of frequency. We may say, then, that the laryngeal spectrum can be ideally regarded as a line spectrum in which the energy of the harmonics falls with frequency at a rate of 12 dB/octave. (This value should not be taken as an absolute constant for all speakers, because it can differ between males and females and between speakers with different voice qualities).

The next terminologic change applies to the filter. Instead of referring to resonance, we now refer to **formant**. A formant is a natural mode of vibration (resonance) of the vocal tract. Theoretically, there is an infinite number of formants, but for practical purposes only the lowest three or four are of interest. Formants are identified by formant number (e.g., F1, F2, F3, and F4, numbered in succession beginning with the lowest-frequency formant). Each formant can be described by two characteristics: center frequency (commonly called the **formant frequency**) and bandwidth (**formant bandwidth**, which is a measure of the

breadth of energy in the frequency domain, or a measure of the rate of damping in the time domain).

The term formant is used somewhat differently by different authors. Some refer to a formant as a peak in the acoustic spectrum. In this usage, a formant is an acoustic feature that may or may not be evidence of a vocal tract resonance. Others use the term formant to designate a resonance, whether or not actual empirical evidence is found for it. In this book, formant will be used synonymously with vocal tract resonance. A formant often is associated with a peak in the acoustic spectrum, but not necessarily so. One of the goals of acoustic analysis is to estimate the formant structure of a sound segment.

Taken together, the formants constitute the *transfer function* of the vocal tract. A transfer function is the input–output relation and is one way of describing the operation of a process like filtering. Because each formant is associated with a peak in the transfer function (Figure 2–4), each formant is potentially associated with a peak in the output spectrum (or radiated spectrum). There would, of course, be no peak in the radiated spectrum at a given formant region if the laryngeal source did not supply energy in the frequency region corresponding to the formant location. Formants do not supply energy, but only modify energy supplied by a source. Formants are determined by the shape and length of the vocal tract, but they become physically evident only when they are activated by a source of sound such as voicing or whisper.

The final term to be introduced is **radiation characteristic**. This term refers to a filtering effect that arises when sounds escape the mouth to radiate into space. An acoustic engineer would say that the acoustic coupling of the mouth to the atmosphere is like an infinite baffle, that is, the radiated sound spreads in all directions as it leaves the mouth. This kind of radiation characteristic acts like a high-pass filter (reducing energy more in the low frequencies than in the high frequencies). A reasonable approximation to this effect is to assume that the output sound increases in frequency at a rate of 6 dB/octave. Because this is a constant characteristic, it is sometimes combined with the 12 dB/octave drop in the laryngeal spectrum to yield a resultant –6 db/octave. (The −12dB/octave characteristic of the laryngeal spectrum and the +6db/octave characteristic of radiation often are taken as constants in the acoustic theory of speech production).

The source–filter theory of vowel production is summarized in Figure 2–5 and in the following equation:

$$P(f) = U(f)\ T(f)\ R(f).$$

P(f) is the radiated sound pressure spectrum of speech. P stands for pressure and (f) simply indicates a function of frequency. Recall from an earlier discussion that most microphones and the human ear respond to pressure variations. Therefore, it is useful to describe the output signal of speech as a sound pressure waveform (in the time domain) or a sound pressure spectrum (in the frequency domain). The three terms on the right side of the equation refer, respectively, to the laryngeal source spectrum, the transfer function of the vocal tract, and the radiation characteristic. U refers to volume velocity and is used because the vocal folds act like a source of air pulses. Volume velocity is analogous to current in an electrical circuit. T represents transfer function, and R denotes radiation characteristic. Putting this equation into words, we can say that the radiated sound pressure waveform of speech is the product of the laryngeal spectrum, the vocal tract transfer function and the radiation characteristic.

For the present, we consider the terms U(f) and R(f) to be constant as different vowels are produced. That is, different vowels will be described as variations in the transfer function, T(f), and the radiated spectrum, P(f). Because T(f) consists of the vowel formants, the discussion boils down to the formant patterns of different vowels.

A brief historical note is in order. Credit already has been given to the highly influential work by Gunnar Fant, particularly his book *Acoustic Theory of Speech Production* (1970). Another important contribution to the understanding of vowel acoustics was a book first published in 1946. This book, Chiba and Kajiyama's *The Vowel: Its Nature and Structure*, was unfortunately not widely distributed because of complications associated with World War II. Although copies of the book are hard to find, its influence should be noted in the modern understanding of speech acoustics.

Articulatory–Acoustic Relations for Vowels

Shown in Figure 2–7 is an X-ray picture of the vocal tract. It is, in fact, the vocal tract of a prominent phonetician named Peter Ladefoged. This kind of picture is called a lateral X-ray because the image obtained represents a projection of X-rays from one side to the other of the object under study. This X-ray picture of the vocal tract corresponds anatomically to a *midsagittal section*, or a plane that runs through the head from front to back, cutting the head into right and left halves. The entire vocal tract, extending from larynx to lips, is the resonating cavity of vowel production. This cavity can be described in terms of its cross-sectional area as a function of length. Of course, the X-ray picture in Figure 2–7 provides only partial information because the vocal tract is seen in only two dimensions. Precise determination of the area over the length of the vocal tract requires information on the third dimension, the width of the cavity over its length. However, by some simplifying assumptions, such as an assumption that the vocal tract is essentially circular along its length, we can estimate the area of the vocal tract for any given distance along its length. The result of such an estimation is sketched in Figure 2–8A. What we have accomplished is to determine the three-dimensional shape of the vocal tract. This is equivalent to creating a mold by filling the vocal tract with a semi-liquid material that gradually hardens so as to retain the shape of the tract. As noted earlier in this chapter, the fact that the actual vocal tract is curved is not of critical significance to its function as an acoustic resonator. Therefore, we can straighten the curved model of the vocal tract in Figure 2–8A to produce the version in Figure 2–8B.

The labors described in the preceding paragraph are necessary to obtain an accurate acoustic model of the resonating cavity of the human vocal tract. However, for purposes of discussion, it is sufficient to represent the vocal tract shape as a graph of its cross dimension over its length. Such a graph is depicted for four vowels in Figure 2–9. In making these graphs, we have neglected the third dimension. Clearly, the vocal tract configurations for these vowels have some relatively constricted regions and other regions that are widely flared. For example, vowel /i/ (as in *beam*) has a constricted region near the lip opening but a large open region near the larynx and pharynx. In contrast, vowel /ɑ/ (as in *bomb*) has a constricted region in the pharyngeal portion of the model but a large open region near the lip opening. It is possible to calculate the resonance frequencies of such configurations using formulas from acoustic theory. When such calculations are performed, the results generally conform to measured formants of the human vowels on which the models are based. The agreement between the formant frequencies of the vowel models and those of the human vowels being modeled is evidence of the validity of the approach.

The same four vowels are shown again in Figure 2–10, but this time in the form of acoustic spectra. The spectral peaks in each graph represent vowel formants. Notice that the high vowels /i/ and /u/ have in common a relatively low frequency of the first formant (F1), whereas the low vowels

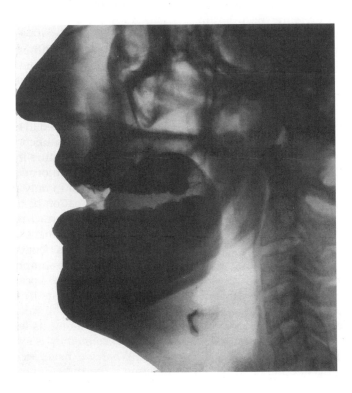

FIGURE 2–7. Lateral (side–view) X–ray of the vocal tract. (Courtesy of Peter Ladefoged, of the Phonetics Laboratory, University of California at Los Angeles.)

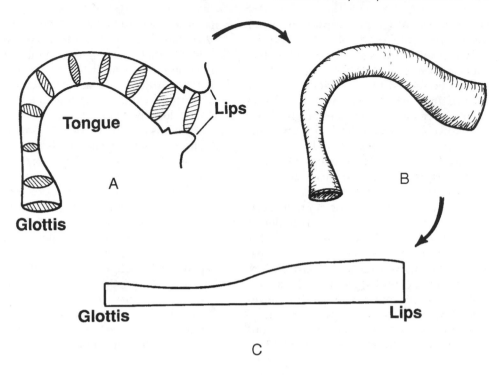

FIGURE 2–8.   Derivation of the vocal tract area function. In *(A)* the cross–sectional diameter is determined for length increments of the vocal tract, proceeding from glottis to lips. The curved tube *(B)* can be straightened to form the straight tube in *(C)*.

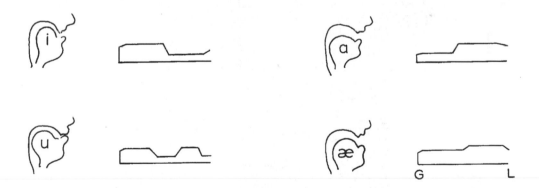

FIGURE 2–9.   Vocal tract configurations and corresponding area functions (idealized) for the four vowels /i/ as in *beam*, /u/ as in *boom*, /æ/ as in *bomb*, and /æ/ as in *bam*. G = glottis and L = lips.

/a/ and /ae/ have in common a relatively high frequency of this formant, that is, the frequency of the first formant varies inversely with **tongue height** of the vowel. Next, notice that the back vowels /u/ and /a/ share a relatively low frequency of the second formant (F2), whereas the front vowels /i/ and /ae/ have a relatively high frequency for this formant, that is, the frequency of the second formant varies with the posterior–anterior dimension of vowel articulation. This result points to an articulatory–acoustic correspondence: the frequencies of the first two formants, F1 and F2, can be related to dimensions of vowel articulation. The frequency of F1 is inversely related to tongue height (e.g., high vowels have a low F1 frequency), and the frequency of F2 is related to tongue advancement (e.g., F2 frequency increases as the tongue position moves forward in the mouth).

All the vowels of American English can be plotted as shown in Figure 2–11 to depict their F1 and F2 values. Note that in this F1–F2 plot (or F1–F2 chart), the axes have two labels. The F1 axis has the articulatory label of tongue height, and the F2 axis has the articulatory label of **tongue advancement** (or posterior–anterior position). These paired articulatory–acoustic labels are consistent with the discussion in the preceding paragraph. In general, the frequency of F1 varies with tongue height and the frequency of F2 varies with tongue advancement. This articulatory–acoustic correspondence makes it possible to draw articulatory inferences from acoustic data on vowel formant frequencies. When the F1 frequency decreases, it is usually safe to conclude that the tongue

has moved to a higher position. When the F2 frequency increases, it is usually safe to conclude that the tongue has moved to a more anterior position. It should be noted that this articulatory–acoustic relationship is only approximate, and other relationships will be described later.

The lips also are involved in vowel production. Labial participation is quite simple for English vowels. Lip rounding occurs for some back and central vowels, such as the vowels in the words *who*, *hoe*, and *her*. Front vowels are not rounded in English. The effect of lip rounding is to lower all formant frequencies. The reason follows directly from the fact that formant frequencies depend on the length of the vocal tract. The longer the length, the lower the formant frequencies. Because lip rounding tends to extend the length of the vocal tract, rounded vowels tend to have lower formant frequencies relative to nonrounded vowels.

Perturbation Theory

Perturbation theory allows the prediction of formant–frequency changes resulting from perturbations (local constrictions) of a tube resonator. This is a very powerful theory in

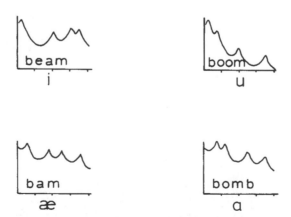

FIGURE 2-10. Spectra for the four vowels shown in Figure 2–9. The four peaks in each spectrum reflect formants. Hence, the frequency location of each peak is an estimate of a formant frequency. The frequency axis represents a range of 0–4 kHz.

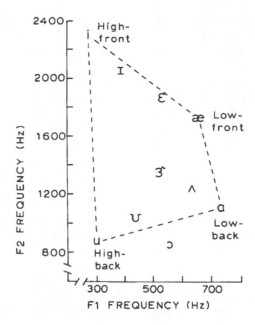

FIGURE 2-11. Classic F1–F2 chart in which a vowel is represented acoustically by its F1 and F2 frequencies. The values shown are for an average adult male. The phonemic symbols are positioned to show the F1 and F2 values for that vowel. An articulatory–acoustic relationship is suggested by the labels in the figure. Low vowels have a high F1 frequency; high vowels have a low F1 frequency; front vowels have a high F2 frequency; and back vowels have a low F2 frequency.

acoustics and is particularly important for the acoustics of speech production in its ability to explain the formant frequencies of vowel sounds. Perturbation theory is discussed here as a way of determining how variations in vocal tract shape affect vowel formants. The discussion begins with formant frequencies and then proceeds to the determination of formant amplitudes.

To see how this theory applies to vowel production, we will use a single-tube representation of the vocal tract, as shown in Figure 2–12. This tube model should be quite familiar by now. Such a tube will have at each of its resonance frequencies a standing wave distribution of volume velocity or the inverse of volume velocity, pressure. Basically, volume velocity variations during resonance in the pipe reflect the way in which individual particles vibrate at various positions in the pipe. At certain positions, particle vibration is minimal (and pressure has its maximum). At other posi-

tions, particle vibration is maximal (and pressure has its minimum). Regions where the particles vibrate with minimum amplitude are regions of volume velocity minima, or *nodes*. Regions where the particles vibrate with maximum amplitude are regions of volume velocity maxima, or *antinodes*. It is characteristic of pipe resonance that volume velocity or its inverse, pressure, will have a stationary distribution along the length of the pipe. Because the pipe has an infinite number of resonances, a volume velocity or pressure distribution can be described for each resonance. We will restrict our discussion to the first three resonances, corresponding to the first three formants of vowels. Incidentally, it is possible to verify these standing wave distributions experimentally. The 1960 Nobel laureate Georg von Bekesy demonstrated pressure variations within the vocal tract by slowly moving a miniature microphone into the vocal tract as the speaker phonated a vowel. The output of the microphone had maxima and minima corresponding to the standing wave pressure variations.

As shown in Figure 2–13, the first resonance has a standing wave distribution with a volume velocity maximum, or antinode, at the open end (the lip ending of the vocal tract) and a volume velocity minimum, or node, at the closed end (the glottal end of the vocal tract). For the second resonance, there are two volume velocity maxima (antinodes) and two volume velocity minima (nodes). For the third resonance, there are three volume velocity maxima and three minima. In other words, each formant, Fn, of the vocal tract has *n* nodes and *n* antinodes.

Suppose that the single-tube resonator in Figure 2–12 is pliable so that it can be squeezed at various points along its length.

Each local constriction of the tube produced by squeezing is a perturbation, and the effect of the perturbation on a formant frequency Fn depends on whether the constriction is proximal to a node or antinode. We will not explain the reasons here (except to say that electrical circuit models are very useful in the explanation), but the general relation is as follows:

1. A local constriction of the tube near a volume velocity maximum *lowers* the formant frequency.

2. A local constriction of the tube near a volume velocity minimum *raises* the formant frequency.

Now Figure 2–12 can be redrawn as shown in Figure 2–14 to resemble the human vocal tract with nodes and antinodes located

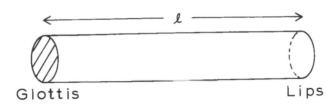

FIGURE 2-12. Straight-tube model of the vocal tract for vowel production.

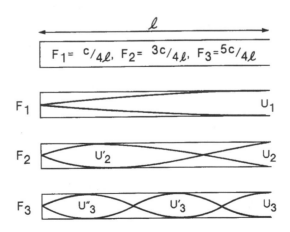

FIGURE 2-13. Straight–tube model of the vocal tract showing spatial distribution of volume velocity for each of the first three formants. U indicates a volume velocity maximum.

by the symbols N and A, respectively. The subscript for each N or A indicates the formant number for which the region is a node or antinode. For example, $N_{1,2}$ is a node, or volume velocity minimum, for the first two formants F1 and F2. The effect of a vocal tract constriction is to change the formant pattern from that for the neutral vowel according to the relations just described. A constriction at antinode A tends to lower both F1 and F2 (in fact, all formant frequencies are lowered by lip constriction). A constriction at node B raises F2. A constriction at antinode C lowers F2. Consider how these relations apply to individual vowels. Vowel [i] (*he*) has a constriction in the palatal region (near antinode B) and therefore has a high F2 frequency. The vowel [ɑ] (*ha*) has a constriction in the pharyngeal region (near antinode C) and therefore has a low F2 frequency. The vowel [u] has a labial constriction (near antinode A) and therefore has lowered frequencies of both F1 and F2. In this way, perturbation theory

allows a prediction of the effects of constriction of the vocal tract on the formant frequencies for the resulting configuration.

As a final way of showing the predictions of perturbation theory, Figure 2–15 illustrates how the location of a constriction along the length of a single-tube resonator affects F1, F2 and F3 frequencies. A positive sign indicates that the constriction at that point raises the formant frequency and a negative sign indicates that the constriction at that point lowers the formant frequency. Notice in particular the following effects:

1. All three formant frequencies are lowered by labial constriction.

2. All three formant frequencies are raised by a constriction near the larynx.

3. The curve for F2 has a negative region corresponding to the tongue constriction for [ɑ] and a positive region corresponding to the tongue constriction for [i].

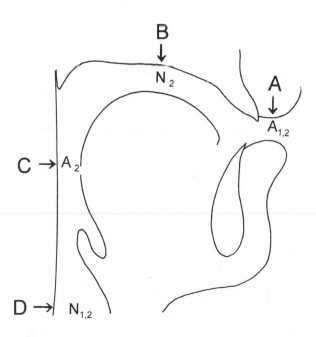

FIGURE 2–14. Drawing of vocal tract showing nodes (N) and antinodes (A) for volume velocity distribution (or the inverse, pressure distribution). Subscripts indicate formant numbers.

4. The curve for F3 has negative regions corresponding to constrictions at the lips, the palate and the pharynx (this result is helpful in understanding the different articulations of the American English [r] (as in *ray*), which can be rounded, is sometimes produced with a palatal constriction and sometimes with a pharyngeal constriction—all 3 of these constrictions are associated with a lowering of F3).

The first conclusion deserves additional comment. It was mentioned previously that lip rounding tends to lower all formant frequencies because rounding usually lengthens the vocal tract. However, some speakers accomplish a lowering of formant frequencies merely by constricting the lips without protrusion. How is this possible? Examination of Figures 2–13, 2–14 and 2–15 gives the answer: the lips are a volume velocity maximum for each formant; therefore, constriction in this region will lower all formant frequencies. In fact, there are three general ways by which a speaker can accomplish a lowering of all formant frequencies: (1) protrude the lips to

lengthen the vocal tract, (2) constrict the lips, and (3) lower the larynx, an action that also lengthens the vocal tract.

Formant Amplitudes

Recall that the vocal tract, like all pipe resonators, has an infinite number of resonance frequencies. However, because most of the laryngeal energy that activates the resonances is at frequencies below about 5kHz, the usual discussion of vowel formants is limited to the lowest four or five formants—F1, F2, F3, F4, and F5. However, the higher formants cannot be neglected without introducing errors into acoustic analysis of the vocal tract. Following Fant, we can consider the formants of vowel production in terms of the graph shown in Figure 2–16. Each of the first four formants is shown as a resonance curve. A single upsloping curve could represent the contributions from the larynx source, the vocal tract radiation, and a *higher formants correction* (which accounts for formants of higher frequencies that are not individually represented). The acoustic output of the vocal

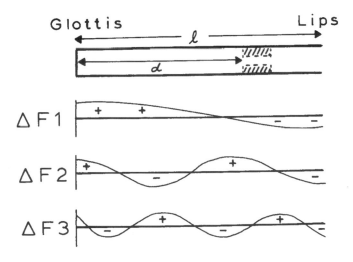

FIGURE 2–15. Effects of local perturbation on the frequencies of the first three formant frequencies, F1, F2 and F3. As the perturbation is moved along the length of the vocal tract, the formants are increased (+) or decreased (-) in frequency as shown for each formant.

tract for the formant configuration shown in Figure 2–16 can be determined by algebraically adding the separate curves. That is, the output spectrum at one frequency, say 1 kHz, is the sum of the magnitudes of the separate curves at that frequency. An example of the result is shown in Figure 2–16.

The first formant is typically the most intense formant, largely because of the interaction with the amplitudes of the other formants. One way of thinking about this is to say that F1 rides on the low-frequency tails of the other formant curves, so that F1 is boosted in amplitude relative to the other formants. Loudness judgments of speech tend to be highly correlated with the amplitude of F1, which is not surprising given that this formant tends to be the strongest.

Note that the vowel spectrum represented in Figs. 2–15 and 2–16 corresponds to the neutral vowel, which has an equal spacing of its formant frequencies. According to perturbation theory described earlier, this neutral vowel may be taken as the starting configuration upon which local perturbations (constrictions) are introduced. Perturbation theory predicts the change in formant frequencies that results from a local constriction. The formant frequency changes, in turn, can be used to predict changes in the formant amplitudes. In other words, the amplitude relations among the formants depend on their frequency relations.

The general principles can be stated quite simply:

1. If the F1 frequency is lowered (raised), then higher formants decrease (increase) in amplitude.

2. If the F1 frequency is lowered (raised), then the F1 amplitude is decreased (increased).

3. If two formants move more closely together in frequency, then both both peaks increase in amplitude.

These principles follow directly from the algebraic additions performed on resonance curves, such as those in Figure 2–17. For example, when the F1 frequency is lowered, the amplitudes of the higher formants are reduced because they then ride on a smaller magnitude of the F1 curve. In similar fashion, F1 will itself lose amplitude because it then rides on lower magnitudes of the other formant tails. Try to imagine the separate formant curves moving relative to one another in the frequency domain and then estimate the effects of these movements on formant amplitude.

Several examples of amplitude relations for English vowels are shown in Figure 2–17. The central conclusion is that formant amplitude relations are determined by formant frequencies. The dependency of resonance amplitudes on

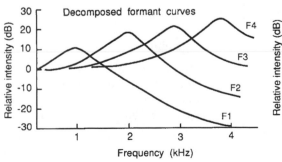
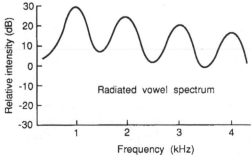

FIGURE 2–16. Decomposed formants (left) and their combination in a radiated vowel spectrum (right).

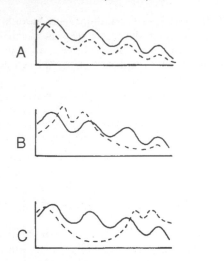

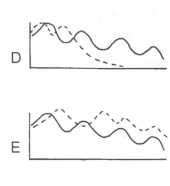

FIGURE 2–17. Effects of selected changes in formant frequency on the amplitude relations of the formants. The solid line in each drawing represents the neutral vowel. (A) As the frequency of F1 is decreased, all formant amplitudes are reduced. (B) As the frequencies of F1 and F2 draw more closely together, their amplitudes are increased. (C) As the frequency of F1 decreases and the frequencies of F2 and F3 come together, there is an overall reduction in the spectrum but a mutual strengthening of F2 and F3. (D) As the frequencies of F1 and F2 are decreased, all formants tend to lose amplitude but there is some mutual strengthening of F1 and F2. (E) As the frequency of F1 increases, all formant amplitudes increase.

resonance frequencies is characteristic of resonators that are connected in series (one after the other). The output of one resonator is the input to the next, so that they interact in determining the relative amplitudes of the resonance peaks in the output spectrum.

Component-Tube Theory

Component-tube or *decoupling* accounts assume that the vocal tract is composed of several different tubes, and that different formants can be identified as originating from one of these component tubes. For example, most vowels can be modeled as having front- and back-cavities, and particular formants can be associated with one cavity or the other, depending on the shape of the cavities. This idea has been discussed by Fant (1960) and Stevens (1998). To determine which component tube is affiliated with a particular formant, it is necessary to deter-

mine the boundary conditions for particular shapes, lengths, and proportions of tubes in the vocal tract. Some general rules are:

1. If one end of a tube is quite narrow, the cavity is modeled as a tube with a closed end, which decouples the tube from the adjoining tube, that is, radical constrictions can decouple a tube from the tubes on either side.

2. If one end of a tube is quite wide, the cavity is considered coupled to the tubes on either side.

3. If both ends of a tube have narrow constrictions, and if the cavity-to-constriction ratio is large, then the tube can be modeled as a Helmholtz resonator.

4. If a tube has a narrow posterior constriction and a wide anterior constriction, the cavity and the anterior constriction can be modeled as a quarter-wavelength tube.

Different combinations of tubes are associated with different calculations of formant frequencies. For mathematical procedures, see Fant (1960) and Stevens (1998). For present purposes, it suffices to make some general observations for vowels, as follows.

Under the appropriate boundary conditions, a Helmholtz resonator can be used to model either the front cavity (the length of the tube anterior to the tongue constriction, plus the lip section orifice) or the back cavity (the length of the tube behind the tongue constriction). For example, in the case of vowel [ɑ], the F1 frequency is sometimes considered as a Helmholtz resonance of the front cavity.

Formants can be associated with standing-wave resonances in any tube that is terminated differently at its two ends. These are calculated as quarter-wavelength resonances ($nc/4l$, where l is the length of the section and $n = 1, 3, 5$, etc.). Formants also can be associated with any tube that has the same terminating conditions at its two ends. These are calculated as half-wavelength resonances ($nc/2l$, where l is the length of the section and $n = 1, 2, 3$, etc.)

Using these ideas, Fant (1960) generated nomograms based on variations in the three control parameters of a four-cavity model of the vocal tract. Badin, Perrier, Boe and Abry, (1990) extended this idea to identify what they called *focal points*, or regions in which formant convergences occur and where formant-cavity affiliations are exchanged. Badin et al. noted that the extreme cardinal vowels [i a u] are focal points.

This theoretical approach is also used in some of the following accounts of vowel acoustics.

Parametric Descriptions of Vowel Articulation

Many efforts have been made to simplify the description of the vocal tract configurations for vowels relative to their acoustic output. Stevens and House (1955) and Fant (1960) described three-parameter models of the vocal tract shape for vowels based on (a) location of the constriction, (b) size of the constriction, and (c) the ratio of mouth opening to length.

Nomograms relating the first three formant frequencies with the three parameters of the Stevens and House model are illustrated in Figure 2–18. This simple description based on three parameters captures significant information about vowel articulation and predicts fairly well the acoustic signal generated by a given vocal tract shape.

Statistical approaches also have been taken to the problem of obtaining simplified descriptions of vowel articulation (Harshman, Ladefoged, & Goldstein, 1977; Liljencrants, 1971; Maeda, 1990). One of the most powerful of these is the use of factor analysis to derive a small set of variables most important for describing vowel articulation. Generally, factor analytic studies indicate that vowel articulation can be described with two tongue factors, a lip factor and perhaps a jaw factor.

Another direction in modeling vowel articulation is to represent the articulatory organs as independently controllable functional blocks, or solid articulatory structures (Coker, 1976; Lindblom & Sundberg, 1971; Rubin, Baer, & Mermelstein, 1981). The model developed by Mermelstein is shown in Figure 2–19. A principal aim of this work is to reduce the number of degrees of freedom in modeling vowel articulation compared to that required for an acoustic tube model of the vocal tract that is quantized into sections of 0.5 or 1.0 cm in length. In addition, such a model has the potential of reflecting the biomechanical properties of the articulators, thereby simulating the natural process of speech.

Source–Tract Interaction for Vowels

It has been assumed to this point that the vibration of the vocal folds (the energy

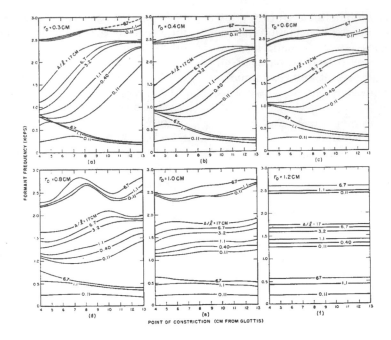

FIGURE 2–18. Nomograms relating the parameters of the Stevens and House model of vowel articulation to the output formant frequencies. The curves show the frequencies of the first three formants as a function of r_0, d_0, and A/1. In each section data are presented for a given degree of constriction (r_0) as indicated, with mouth opening (A/1) as the parameter. Three families of curves corresponding to F1, and F2, and F3 are plotted in each section. The abscissa is d_0, the distance from the glottis to the point of the constriction. Reprinted from K. N. Stevens and A. S. House, (1955) Development of a quantitative description of vowel articulation, *Journal of the Acoustical Society of America*, 27, 484–493. (Reprinted with the permission of the American Institute of Physics.)

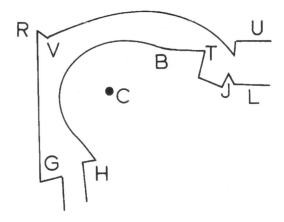

FIGURE 2–19. Components of an articulatory model for speech production. J = jaw, H = hyoid bone, C = center of tongue body, B = point where blade attaches to tongue body, T = tip of tongue, U = upper lip, L = lower lip, V = velum, R = rear–pharyngeal wall, and G = glottal region (periarytenoid area). After Mermelstein, 1973.

source for voiced vowels) is independent of the shaping of the vocal tract (the filter). This assumption typically is made to simplify the description of the source–filter theory of speech production, and it certainly is a useful first approximation in understanding how vowels are produced. In technical terms, the vocal folds are thought to behave as a high-impedance (constant flow or constant current) source. When a source has high impedance, it is relatively unaffected by the load (in this case, the vocal tract filter) placed on it.

However, once this simplifying assumption has served its purpose in introductory discussion, it needs to be discarded—or at least modified—in favor of a more realistic understanding. In reality, the vocal folds are not independent of the tract into which the acoustic energy of voicing is propagated. Rather, the load of the vocal tract can affect how the vocal folds vibrate. For example, Titze and Story (1997) pointed out that the epilarynx (the narrow portion of the pharynx located directly superior to the vocal folds) is shaped in such a way that it enhances the interactions between source and tract. In other (more technical) words, the input impedance of the vocal tract is greatly different from the glottal impedance. Why does this matter? First, it means that vocal vibration may be sensitive to certain shape changes in the vocal tract. Second, it appears that singers can exploit this source-tract interaction to achieve various vocal qualities (Sundberg, 1974, 1977, 1987, 1991; Titze & Story, 1997).

Limitations and Assumptions

Models of natural processes inevitably introduce simplifications. Natural processes, even ordinary ones, are rife with complications and interactions, but many of these may be neglected for the central purpose of modeling, and also the acoustic theory of speech production. Now that the foundations of the theory have been discussed for vowels, it is appropriate to take a moment to note some of the complexities intrinsic to the actual production of vowels by the human vocal tract.

1. The tissues of the vocal tract both absorb and reflect sound energy, but the model developed to this point assumes that the vocal tract is a hard-walled tube. One consequence of this assumption is that it underestimates the losses attributable to the soft tissues of the actual vocal tract. These losses lead to increased formant bandwidths.

2. The human vocal tract is almost constantly changing in its properties (shape and biomechanical features), but the discussion to this point has assumed a time invariance. The simple tube model neglects time-varying complexities.

3. In the natural vocal tract, some sound waves propagate longitudinally (from glottis to lips) but other sound waves propagate in cross modes (from wall to wall in transverse section). Longitudinal propagation pertains to frequencies less than about 5 kHz; transverse propagation occurs for higher frequencies. The models developed so far do not apply with accuracy to these higher frequencies.

4. In human vowel production, the vocal tract is excited by the vibrating vocal folds, which produce an intermittent coupling of the vocal tract to the lungs. The acoustic model simplifies the situation by assuming that the glottis is like a continuously closed end of a tube. This assumption neglects interactions between the respiratory system and the vocal tract. The respiratory system has resonances of its own (Harper, Kraman Pasterkamp, & Wodicka, 2001), and these are activated by vocal fold vibration. When analyzed in detail, speech has not only vocal tract resonances but also resonances associated with the tracheobronchial tree and the lungs.

5. Natural vowels are not produced with a truly periodic voice source and they can involve nonlaminar airflows that result in the generation of noise. The model assumes a periodic vibration of the vocal folds and neglects the possibility of noise components.

6. The human vocal tract is a complex passageway that has both curvature and variable cross-section geometry. The model assumes a straight-tube approximation in which the cross-sectional area is a function of distance along its length.

7. A speaker's vocal tract radiates sound energy into a variable acoustic environment. The model assumes a constant baffle that is approximated by a +6 dB radiation characteristic.

Summary of Linear Source-Filter Theory for Vowels

The quasi-periodic vibration of the vocal folds produces the energy source known as voicing. This source has a harmonic spectrum in which the energy of the harmonic components falls off at the rate of 12dB/octave. This energy activates the resonances (formants) of the vocal tract. The resonances act like a filter, such that the energy in the various harmonics of the source is not transmitted equally. Although there are theoretically an infinite number of formants, we are concerned primarily with the first three—F1, F2, and F3. One reason is that the energy of the source (the laryngeal spectrum) is greatest in the low frequencies that include these first three formants. Further, these three formants are sufficient to account for most phonetic variations for vowels in the world's languages. The higher formants cannot be neglected entirely, and their effects are typically accounted for in a general term called the higher-formants correction. The formants, along with the radiation characteristic, constitute the transfer function of the vocal tract. The radiation

characteristic is a term that accounts for the way in which the vocal tract terminates into the atmosphere. It can be approximated as a 6-dB increase in spectral energy. The source-filter theory usually is introduced with the assumption that the vibration of the vocal folds is completely independent of the shaping of the vocal tract; however, this assumption does not completely conform to reality.

Fricatives

Turbulence and the Reynold's Number

The simplified model for vowels was taken to be a straight pipe. The corresponding simplified model for fricatives is a pipe with a severe constriction (Figure 2–20). The constriction functions as a nozzle. Air exiting from a constriction in a conduit forms a jet. As this jet mixes with the surrounding air, **turbulence** is generated. Turbulence is associated with the generation of eddies that form in the flow in the vicinity of the contraction and expansion of the conduit. The eddies are volume elements of air that perform rotations, or irregular, high-frequency fluctuations in velocity and pressure at a given point in space. For a constriction or obstruction of given dimensions, there is a critical flow velocity above which turbulence noise is generated. The critical flow velocity at which turbulence occurs is given by the **Reynold's number**

$$Re = vh/\nu$$

where v = flow velocity,

ν = kinematic coefficient of viscosity (about 0.15 cm^2 /sec for air), and

h = characteristic dimension (for flow through an orifice, h is on the order of the diameter of the orifice).

As Re increases, an initial region of laminar flow will pass through an unstable region and finally through a condition of full turbulence.

Because volume flow, U(cm^3/sec), is given by

U = vA (A is cross-sectional area),

the Reynold's number can be calculated as

Re = Uh/A $\sqrt{\ }$.

The volume flow U depends on the constriction size and the driving pressure (subglottal pressure), Ps:

U = kA Ps (where k = constant).

Then

Re = Uh / A $\sqrt{\ }$

= kA $\sqrt{Ps}$ h / A $\sqrt{\ }$

= kh $\sqrt{Ps}$ / $\sqrt{\ }$

Turbulence is the source of acoustic energy for various speech sounds, including fricatives, the frication portion of affricates, and the burst of stops. The random pressure fluctuations of the turbulent field generate sound. Volume velocities for fricative consonants lie in the range of 100 to 1000 cm /sec. The critical Reynold's number for speech noise is Re > 1800.

Shadle (1990) concluded from modeling studies that there are at least two major ways in which sound is generated for fricative consonants. The first she termed an *obstacle source*. In this case, sound is generated primarily at a rigid body approximately normal to the flow. For the palatal fricative / ʃ /, the lower teeth seem to form the obstacle. In the case of the alveolar fricative /s/, the obstacle may be the upper teeth. The obstacle source may be likened to a spoiler in a duct. According to Shadle, an obstacle source is associated with a maximum source amplitude for a given flow velocity, by a relatively flat spectrum that falls off with increased frequency, and by a maximum rate of change of sound pressure with volume velocity.

The second source of sound is a *wall source*, which applies to situations in which sound is generated primarily along a relatively rigid wall that runs essentially parallel to the flow. Examples of this kind of sound generation are the non-English fricatives / x γ /. The wall source is associated with a high (but less than maximum) source amplitude for a given flow velocity, by a spectrum that possesses a broad peak, and by a high (but not maximum) rate of change of sound pressure with volume velocity. Shadle suggests that the wall source is really a distributed source, unlike the obstacle source, which can be modeled as a series pressure source located at the obstacle.

Ladefoged and Maddieson (1986) proposed that fricatives could be identified as either obstacle or no-obstacle cases. Obstacle fricatives were considered to be stridents (high-intensity fricatives like [s]), and no-obstacle fricatives as nonstridents (low-intensity fricatives like [θ]). Shadle (1990) cautions against the appealing simplicity of this classification, noting that many factors have to be considered in characterizing sound sources. She points out that there may be a continuum ranging from obstacle to wall source, given that the angle of the configuration relative to the airflow is the critical factor.

Modeling Fricative Production

The major steps in producing a fricative sound are to (1) make a constriction somewhere in the vocal tract, and (2) force air at high velocity through the constriction. Note that these conditions relate to the formula given above for the Reynolds number. When the physical conditions are properly satisfied, turbulent flow is generated in the vicinity of the constriction and also at the teeth in some cases (specifically the cases that Shadle, 1990, called obstacle sources). The turbulent flow is characterized by eddies of particle motion (Figure 2–20) and is the source of turbulence noise. This noise

MODEL OF TURBULENCE NOISE PRODUCTION FOR FRICATIVES

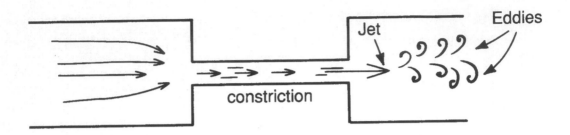

FIGURE 2–20. Model for turbulent noise production in fricatives. The vocal tract has a narrow constriction at some point along its length.

excites the acoustic tube that forms the constriction and also the cavities anterior to the constriction. Under certain conditions, there may be an acoustic coupling to the cavities posterior to the constriction. Figure 2–21 shows a vocal tract configuration for the fricative sound [s], and a two-cavity model for the [s]. The dot near the constriction in both the vocal tract configuration and the two-cavity model represents the location of the noise source.

In the following discussion, a different terminology will be introduced, but the concepts are basically the same as those presented for vowels. The new terms **pole** and **zero** will be used in discussing the transfer function. The term pole is commonly used in engineering and physics to denote a natural frequency of a system. In this book, pole, formant, and resonance are essentially the same concepts, with the major difference being that the term formant refers specifically to poles or resonances of the vocal tract (i.e., formant is a speech term). A zero is a phenomenon that is inverse to a pole. A pole or resonance produces a reinforcement of applied energy. A zero causes a loss of applied energy. In this book, the terms zero, anti-resonance, and **antiformant** are essentially equivalent in meaning, except that the term antiformant is restricted to the vocal tract whereas the

other terms have a more general application in acoustics and other fields.

Like vowels, fricatives can be described mathematically in terms of a transfer function. For fricatives, the function is

$T(f) = [P(f) R(f) Z(f)]$,

where $T(f)$ is the transfer function,

f is frequency,

$P(f)$ is a function that contains the natural frequencies of vocal tract (poles or formants),

$R(f)$ is the radiation characteristic, and

$Z(f)$ is a function containing the zeros (antiformants), which occur at frequencies at which the source is decoupled from the front cavities.

The functions $P[f]$ and $R[f]$ are the same as they would be for a similar vowel sound. The poles are simply the resonance frequencies (what we termed formants for vowels). The pole function $P[f]$ for the fricative are approximately the same as those for a vowel produced with a similar vocal tract shape. Because the poles are natural frequencies of the tract, they do not depend on the location of the source of energy. The radiation function $R[f]$ is as described

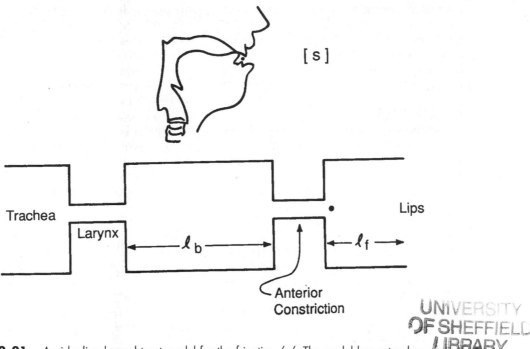

FIGURE 2-21. An idealized vocal tract model for the fricative /s/. The model has a trachea, a laryngeal constriction, a back cavity, an articulatory constriction, and a front cavity.

above for vowels. So far, the concepts are not much different for fricatives than they were for vowels. However, the function Z[f] is new. The function Z[f] represents zeros. Zeros are effectively opposites of poles; they result in a loss of energy transmission. Like poles or formants, zeros have a center frequency and a bandwidth. When a pole and a zero have exactly the same frequency and bandwidth, they cancel each other. Zeros are most easily understood in terms of impedance, or the opposition to sound transmission. An engineer might say that zeros occur at frequencies for which the driving-point impedance of the vocal tract behind the noise source is infinite. In other words, the opposition to energy transmission through the front cavity is so great compared to that in the back cavity that the energy is short-circuited in the back cavity.

What causes zeros to occur in speech production? Basically, zeros arise for two reasons: (1) the vocal tract is bifurcated, or split into two passages (such as an oral pas-sage and a nasal passage), or (2) the vocal tract is radically constricted at some point. It is for the second reason that fricatives involve zeros in their transfer function.

For the average male vocal tract, the poles occur at an average of 1 kHz separa-tion, determined by the length of the vocal tract from glottis to lips. However, because the noise source (articulatory constriction) usually is posterior to the mouth opening, the average spacing of the zeros is greater than 1 kHz. If a long narrow constriction is formed near the mouth opening, some of the poles and zeros tend to move together in pairs, so that their effects cancel. Recall that a pole and zero of the same frequency and bandwidth cancel one another.

Because the average spacing of the zeros is greater than that of the poles, the cancellation is not complete over the fre-quency range. The poles and zeros tend to cancel at frequencies less than the fre-quency for which the constriction length is a quarter wavelength. Above this frequency is a region containing more poles than zeros and in which the poles and zeros are separated. Normally, the first pole is heavily damped and therefore does not affect the output spectrum to a great degree. Another way of stating matters is that cancellation occurs because the coupling between source and back cavities is small. Therefore, the influence of the back cavities can be neglected, and the zeros are determined only by the constriction. This rule breaks down under certain conditions, such as when the back cavity has a tapered shape leading into the constriction. In this condition, the back cavity is not decoupled from the source.

The effect of the front cavity is largely determined by its length (l) in Figure 2–21. When the front cavity is very short, as in the case of the labiodental fricatives [f v], its lowest resonance frequency is too high to offer appreciable shaping of the noise energy. Consequently, the spectrum for these fricatives is flat or diffuse, lacking prominent peaks or valleys. However, as the place of articulation moves backward in the oral cavity, the length of the front cavity increases, and its lowest resonance frequency decreases. In the case of the fricative [s], the lowest resonance frequency is around 4 kHz for a man. This value can be

calculated from the assumption that the front cavity for [s] is about 2 cm in length. Then, using the odd-quarter wavelength relationship discussed at the beginning of this chapter, the first (lowest) resonance of the front cavity should be c/4l or 35,000 cm/sec divided by 4 x 2 cm, or about 4 kHz. Spectral shaping for the [s] is such that prominent regions of noise energy contrast with regions of much weaker energy. The relations between fricative articulation and fricative spectra are shown in Figure 2–22 for labio-dental (or bilabial), lingua-dental, lingua-alveolar, retroflex apical, lingua-palatal and lingua-velar fricatives. The caption for each illustration describes the relationships between the vocal tract configuration and the spectral pattern of each sound. Additional spectral characteristics are described more fully in a later chapter.

As noted earlier, there are conditions in which the back cavity is coupled to the front cavity, in which case the resonances of the back cavity cannot be neglected. The back cavity can be likened to a tube closed at both ends. For this kind of tube, the resonances are given by

$$F_n = (n)(c/2l)$$

$$(e.g., c/2l, c/l, 3c/2l, ...)$$

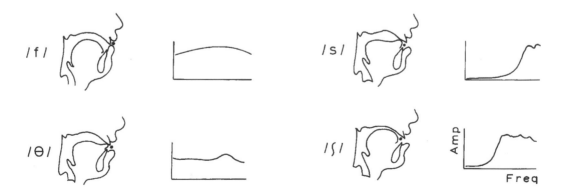

FIGURE 2–22. Articulatory–acoustic relationships for the four fricatives /f/ (fin), / θ / (thin), /s/ (sin), and / ʃ / (shin). The dot indicates the approximate location of the noise source. The length of the front cavity is a major determinant of the resonant shaping of the frication noise.

If the back cavity has a length of 10 cm, then it would have resonances of about 1750 Hz, 3500 Hz, and so on.

We have seen that fricatives can be modeled as a pressure source of either the obstacle or wall type that activates the resonances and anti-resonances of a simple two-cavity model. When the two cavities are uncoupled, then the major filtering effects are exerted by the front cavity, which has resonance frequencies that can be approximated as those of a tube closed at one end and open at the other (i.e., the odd-quarter wavelength relationship, $f_n = (2n-1) c/4l$). When the two cavities are coupled, as is likely to happen if the constriction is gradually tapered, then the back cavity also contributes to the filtering effects. This cavity can be modeled as a tube closed at both ends, thus having resonance frequencies at integer multiples of $c/2l$.

Although fricatives are relatively complex sounds, it appears that a linear source filter model is fairly effective in accounting for the major spectral properties of sustained voiced and unvoiced strident fricatives below 10 kHz. Narayanan and Alwan (2000) reached this conclusion in their development and testing of a hybrid source model for fricative consonants. They also noted that their model based on aeroacoustic principles could be used for the synthesis of fricatives.

Nasals

The nasal sounds include nasalized vowels and the nasal consonants (English /m/, /n/, and /ŋ/). The essential articulatory property of a nasal sound is that the velopharyngeal port is open so that sound energy can pass through both the nasal tract and the oral tract (for nasal vowels) or through only the nasal tract (for nasal consonants). These two vocal tract configurations can be modeled quite simply, as shown in Figure 2–23. Both models involve a side-branch resonator, meaning that one resonator is coupled to another at the velopharyngeal port. In the case of the nasal vowel, both resonators open to atmosphere. In the case of the nasal consonant, the nasal resonator opens to atmosphere while the oral resonator is closed.

For both nasal vowels and consonants, the transfer function consists of poles and zeros. As noted earlier, a bifurcation or splitting of the resonating system introduces zeros into the transfer function. The zeros interact with poles in various ways depending on their frequencies and bandwidths. When a pole and zero have exactly the same frequency and bandwidth, they cancel. When poles and zeros have different frequencies, then they can contribute to a spectrum that reflects their combined influence. Generally, a spectral peak reflects a

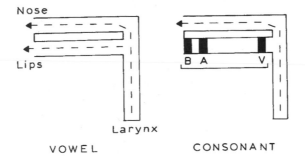

FIGURE 2–23. Simplified vocal tract models for a nasalized vowel and nasalized consonants. The nasalized vowel has open oral and nasal cavities. The nasalized consonant has an oral closure—B(Bilabial); A(Alveolar) or V(Velar)—and an open nasal cavity.

pole and a deep valley reflects a zero. However, this generalization has exceptions and should be used as only a rough rule of thumb in interpreting spectra for sounds known to have poles and zeros in their transfer functions.

As was the case with fricatives, nasals can be understood in part through a consideration of the average spacing of formants and antiformants. It was discussed earlier that the formants for oral sounds such as vowels, depend on the tract length from glottis to lips, or (lp + lo), which has a value of about 17.5 cm for adult males. For this vocal tract length, the formants have an average spacing of about 1 kHz. The formants of the nasal cavity depend on the length of the cavity extending from the uvula to the nares (in Figure 2–24), which is about 12.5 cm in adult males. These formants have an average spacing of c/2ln = 1400 Hz. The antiformants of the nasal cavity also depend on the length of the nasal cavity and have an average spacing of c/2ln = 1400 Hz. Taking these various resonance phenomena together, we see that the combined oral-nasal system has a set of oral formants, a set of nasal formants, and a set of nasal antiformants. Fant described nasalized vowels as being like oral vowels with the effects of nasalization added as a distortion. That is, the nasal formants and antiformants are added to the oral formants of the original nonnasal vowel to yield a complex output spectrum. Additional details on the differences between nonnasal and nasal vowels will be provided later; it is sufficient here to note simply the general model by which nasalization may be understood.

A somewhat more technical explanation is needed to understand the frequencies of the formants and antiformants of nasal sounds. As shown in Figure 2–24, the configuration for a nasal consonant can be considered as three cavities: a pharyngeal cavity, a nasal cavity, and a mouth cavity. Each cavity can be associated with a *susceptance*, its capacity to draw energy. Susceptance is the reciprocal of *reactance*, or opposition to energy. An internal susceptance Bi is defined as the sum of the pharyngeal susceptance, Bp and the nasal

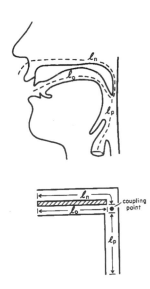

FIGURE 2–24. Illustration of the major dimensions that determine the transfer function for a nasalized vowel: l_n is the length of the nasal cavity; l_o is the length of the oral cavity; and l_p is the length of the pharyngeal cavity.

susceptance Bn. Formants occur when Bi = −Bm. At these frequencies, energy is passed effectively through the system and radiated outside. Antiformants occur when Bm = ∞ (infinity). At these frequencies, the mouth cavity acts as an open circuit, effectively trapping the energy and preventing its radiation through the nasal cavity.

When the oral cavity is closed at some point for a nasal consonant, the frequencies of the antiformants are the frequencies at which the mouth cavity prevents transmission through the nose. Energy at these frequencies does not pass through the nasal cavity. The nasals /m/, /n/, and /ŋ/ are characterized by low (750–1250 Hz), medium (1450–2200 Hz), and high (above 3000 Hz) antiformant positions, respectively. The general rule is that as the place of oral articulation moves back, the frequency of the antiformant increases. A low-frequency formant, the so-called **nasal formant**, occurs at about 250–300 Hz. Higher formants are densely packed, have large bandwidths, and vary with place of articulation. To a first approximation, formants occur at about 250, 1000, 2000, 3000, and 4000 Hz. Specific details on nasal consonants are presented in Chapter 5.

Stops

A **stop** involves a complete closure of the vocal tract and, depending on its phonetic context, a release of the closure and a movement toward another vocal tract configuration. The closure is associated with acoustic silence (although weak voicing energy might be detected if the stop is voiced). During the closure interval, air pressure is impounded in the mouth. Upon release of the constriction, the pressure is abruptly released. The acoustic evidence of this release is a burst or transient. The **burst** is a noise segment similar to the noise segment for a fricative but much briefer. For example, the burst for the alveolar stop [t] as in *tea* is similar to a brief version of the frication segment for the alveolar [s] in *sea*. Par-

ticularly if the stop is followed by a vocalic sound, the burst is followed by another acoustic interval, the transition. During this interval, the vocal tract is adjusted from its closure state to another configuration. Most of the change in vocal tract configuration is accomplished within about 50 msec. In the case of a voiced stop, this transition interval is characterized by a rapidly changing formant pattern. The exact nature of this change is discussed in Chapter 5.

These events in stop production can be modeled, as shown in Figure 2–25, as a vocal tract closure, a burst, and a rapid transition to the configuration of the following sound. Some acoustic features of these three phases are:

1. Vocal tract closure: The primary acoustic correlate is silence, except for voiced stops, for which voicing energy may extend for part or all of the closure interval. When voicing is present, it is associated with low frequency energy in the lower harmonics of the voice source, especially the first harmonic or fundamental frequency. Theoretically, for a hard-walled tube, the F1 frequency is zero during a period of vocal tract closure. However, because the vocal tract is not really hard-walled, the F1 frequency does not actually reach zero but a value close to zero. Consequently, the F1 frequency associated with any severe constriction of the vocal tract is of very low frequency. As the constriction is released, the F1 frequency rises to a value appropriate for the following sound.

2. Burst: The transient noise is shaped spectrally in accord with the resonance properties of the vocal tract. To a first approximation, the noise resembles that of a homorganic fricative. Therefore, the burst for [t] is somewhat like the frication for [s]. As will be discussed in Chapter 6, the burst spectrum reflects place of articulation for the stop.

3. Transition: Because the articulatory movement from a stop to another sound (such as a vowel) usually is completed within about 50 msec, the transition is associated with a brief interval of changing formant pattern. The interpretation of formant-frequency changes is a major topic in acoustic phonetics and is reviewed in Chapter 5.

Affricates

Affricates are similar to stops in having a two-phase production of vocal tract closure followed by a noisy release. However, affricates have a frication segment that is intermediate in duration between the burst for stops and the frication interval for fricatives. The diagram in Figure 2–25 therefore applies to the production of affricates as well as to stops. The basic theory of affricate production is a modification of that presented for stops and fricatives.

Liquids

The liquids in English are the lateral /l/ and the rhotic /r/. They combine features of other sounds discussed so far. Both are similar to vowels in that they have well-defined formant patterns and voiced energy. They are properly called sonorants because their production typically is not associated with significant noise energy.

Rhotic consonants, such as English /r/, are produced with a characteristic lowering of the F3 frequency. The /r/ in English is sometimes described as having either a "bunched" or "retroflex" articulation, but, in fact, the articulation for this sound can be

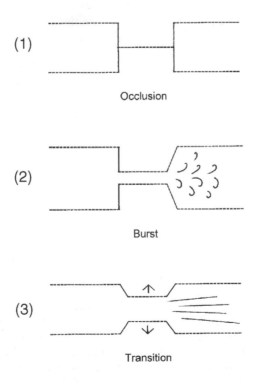

(1) Occlusion

(2) Burst

(3) Transition

FIGURE 2–25. Major events in the production of stop consonants: (1) interval of the vocal tract obstruction; (2) release of obstruction; and (3) articulatory transition into following sound.

quite complex (Westbury, Hashi, & Lindstrom, 1999). At least three major configurations of the phoneme /r/ need to be recognized: (1) tip-up retroflex [r], (2) tip-up bunched [r], and (3) tip-down bunched [r] (Espy-Wilson et al., 2000). The acoustics of /r/ have been modeled primarily through perturbation theory (Johnson, 1997) and decoupling accounts (Stevens, 1998; Alwan, Narayanan, & Haker, 1997). In choosing between these two theoretical approaches, Espy-Wilson et al. (2000) concluded that the decoupling account is preferred. They did not find convincing evidence that speakers exploit points of maximum volume velocity along the vocal tract to accomplish a marked lowering of the F3 frequency. Instead, they interpreted their data to mean that F3 is a front cavity resonance. The evidence that supports this conclusion are (1) eliminating the pharyngeal constriction has minimal effect on F3, and (2) the sublingual space is a crucial factor in determining F3.

Lateral consonants, such as English /l/, have both formants and antiformants and are therefore similar to nasal consonants. Laterals usually involve a splitting of the vocal tract around a midline constriction. The /l/ is produced with a midline apical constriction, which allows sound to radiate through openings at the sides. This midline bifurcation causes the formation of antiformants. The /l/ is acoustically similar to nasals in having a relatively low acoustic energy with a predominantly low-frequency concentration.

The lateral /l/ can be modeled fairly well as a two-cavity (front and back) articulation. The first formant usually has a frequency between 250 and 500 Hz and can be modeled as a Helmholtz resonator. Losses at the oral constriction are considerable and result in large bandwidth of the first formant and an associated reduction of overall spectral amplitude. The second formant can be associated with the half-wavelength resonance of the back cavity. For a detailed analysis, see Narayanan, Alwan, and Haker (1997).

Diphthongs and Glides

Diphthongs and glides (semivowels) are similar to vowels, differing mainly in the presence of a dynamic characteristic, a change in vocal tract configuration. As the articulatory configuration changes, so does the acoustic pattern. Diphthongs and glides are associated with a gradually changing formant structure. The acoustic theory developed earlier for vowels applies in general form to any given configuration in the dynamic complex. For example, the diphthong /aI/ involves a series of vocal tract configurations running from the onglide [a] to the offglide [I].

Nonlinear Theories: Chaos Theory and Fractals

The linear source–filter theory has dominated the acoustic understanding of speech production for the last half century. It should be understood that the linear theory is an approximation, but this approximation has been remarkably successful. A great deal of progress in acoustic analysis and speech synthesis has been based on this theory, but this is not to say that linear source–filter theory as described in this chapter is sufficient to model all acoustic events in speech. Limitations of the theory must be evaluated in various applications. One important limitation is the assumption of independence of source and filter. In reality, source and filter do interact, and the nature of these interactions is an important area of current research. Linearity also may be questionable for some phenomena. Muscle and other tissues are inherently nonlinear, so that as biomechanical properties are modeled, nonlinear solutions may be the rule. It also should be recognized that the one-dimensional (longitudinal) propagation of sound waves in the vocal tract is expected for frequencies below about 5 kHz. At higher frequencies, cross-mode vibrations may occur when the wavelength approaches the cross-dimension of the vocal tract. At a more fundamental level, nonlinear theories of sound production are an important alternative to the standard theoretical model that has been the center-piece of speech acoustics for several decades. This book takes only a brief look at *nonlinear theories of speech production*, which probably will be increasingly important not only for the theoretical understanding of speech but also for the development of various tools for speech analysis and synthesis.

Teager and Teager (1992) argued that sound production in the vocal tract is neither linear nor passive. In fact, they assert that it is not even acoustic. In their view, important nonlinear sources of sound production have been neglected in the standard linear theory. The details of their argument go beyond the scope of this book. It is sufficient to say that nonlinear processes of sound generation are thought to result from the interaction of sheet flows and flow vortices within the vocal tract. Nonlinear approaches are now being applied to various aspects of speech and other sounds, including long-term spectra (Voss & Clark, 1975), irregularities in vocal fold vibration (Baken, 1990), turbulence (Frisch & Orszag, 1990; Narayanan & Alwan, 1995), and the overall characterization of speech (Banbrook, McLaughlin, & Mann, 1999; Sabanal & Nakagawa, 1996).

Chaos theory differs from classical physics in that the latter concentrates on ordered, predictable systems, but the former deals with systems that tend toward disorder. A common example of a disordered system is a rising column of smoke from a chimney. As the smoke rises in the air, it eventually breaks up into complex, seemingly irregular patterns. Chaos theory is well suited to the analysis of dynamic systems composed of many moving elements (e.g., a stream of water molecules, a column of smoke particles rising in the atmosphere, a group of planets orbiting the sun, and, perhaps, the motion of particles in the production of speech). These dynamic systems are said to be *deterministic* (meaning that they follow laws such as those of Newtonian mechanics) but unpredictable (and hence chaotic). These systems often exhibit elements of order that can be observed in a *phase–space graph* (also known as a *phase plot* or *system state space*), which is a diagram that shows the relation of two or more physical features, such as the position and velocity of a moving object. Order can be identified by the appearance of a low-dimensional structure, such as a point, an orbit, or other regular pattern. Although the presence of such structures in the phase-space graph is not sufficient evidence for a chaotic process, it is a first step to determine if chaos is present. Additional analyses are carried out using the *correlation dimension* (symbolized as D_2), which represents a geometric scaling property. A low correlation dimension means that the distribution of points in the phase–space graph can be described by a small number of *attractor dimensions*, that is, an ostensibly complex pattern may in fact be characterized quite simply. To understand the concept of an attractor, let us consider an ordinary physical phenomenon, the heating of water.

Imagine a pan of water placed over a gas burner. If the gas flame is adjusted to provide only a small amount of heating, the heat propagation in the water will be in a state that is called a *conducting regime*. In this state, the heat is conducted through the water, which itself remains motionless. We can tell that the water is being heated simply by touching a finger to it. Suppose we adjust the flame to provide a higher level of heating, enough to set the water into movement. The water has now entered into a *convection regime*, characterized by a boiling action. The transition from conduction to convection regimes is an example of a *bifurcation*, or change in state. The amount of heating is an example of a *bifurcation parameter*. Frequently, a small change in the bifurcation parameter causes a change in the regime of the system under observation. These changes in the system are typically described as *attractors*, see Figure 2–26 for examples of attractors. Attractors represent stable states of a system as observed in a phase–space diagram. The system may pass from one state to another as various conditions change. Turbulence is an example. Recall that the Reynold's number can be used to determine the transition from laminar to turbulent flow. When any of the variables that determine the Reynold's number are changed, a fluid may undergo this transition. It has been shown that the transition is toward an attractor state.

We have seen that attractor dimensions are useful to characterize the distribution of points in the phase–space graph. An additional analysis, *Lyapunov exponents*, is performed to determine the temporal evolution of the trajectories in the phase-space graph. These exponents express the exponential divergence or convergence of trajectories toward an attractor. Lyapunov exponents of positive value are characteristic of chaotic behavior in a dynamic system.

Some aspects of the theory of chaos are closely related to *fractals*, and fractals can make visible the orderliness that hides in chaos. Many complex geometric forms occur naturally: Consider the examples of trees, snowflakes, cumulus clouds, coastlines, and coral formations. Mandelbrot (1982) developed the concept of fractals to address complex geometric forms that may appear on first observation to be highly complex and nonhomogeneous. When a fractal structure is examined with increasing levels of magnification ("zooming" in on smaller and smaller pieces of the structure), additional detail can be seen. However, the structure observed at small scales is similar to that at the large scale. In other words, the fractal structure has a self-similar pattern at various levels of magnification, almost as though the entire structure is generated from a basic template that is repeated at various levels of size. Recognizing the invariant template is the key to fractal analysis. One example of fractal geometry is the turbulence in fluid motion, as discussed earlier in this chapter. Recall that turbulence is a condition in which fluid motion becomes complex, as numerous eddies (rotating volume elements of fluid)

ATTRACTORS

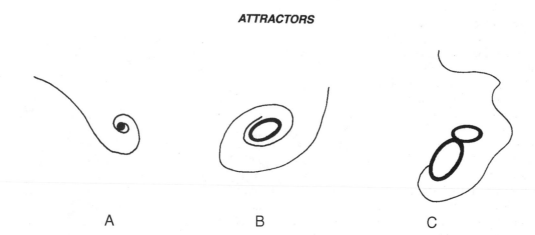

A B C

FIGURE 2–26. Examples of attractors, as they might appear in a phase–space graph. The thick line represents the attractor (a point in A, an elliptical orbit in B, and a more complex figure-8 shape in C). The system is represented by the line in the phase–space graph that eventually converges on the attractor. In this sense, the attractor is a stable state of the system. From *The speech sciences. A volume in the speech sciences* (1st ed.), by Kent, copyright 1998. Reprinted with permission of Delmar, a division of Thomson Learning.

form in the flow pattern. The pattern may appear disorderly and without structure. However, under certain conditions, these patterns contain a certain orderliness in that the turbulent flows are hierarchic patterns of eddies of various sizes (Figure 2–27). At the top of the hierarchy are the largest eddies generated by the forces that drive the flow. These large eddies are themselves unstable and they produce additional, somewhat smaller eddies. These, in turn, become unstable and produce still smaller eddies. This branching process continues until it is braked by molecular viscosity, which imposes a limit to the generation of eddies. The multiply branching effect of eddy formation is called *cascading*.

A fractal that is particularly interesting for the analysis of acoustic events such as speech is the **wavelet transform**. A wavelet is a small piece of waveform that can be expanded or compressed. The idea of the wavelet transform is that complex acoustic patterns can be analyzed into wavelets with various degrees of expansion or compression. Wavelet transforms offer certain advantages in acoustic analysis, and it is likely that they will be increasingly applied to various problems in speech acoustics. More is said about these approaches in Chapter 3.

Linear source–filter theory has been a highly productive theory, but its limitations and assumptions should be carefully evaluated for specific applications. Nonlinear theories may be more appropriate to certain phenomena and the development of these theories should be interesting to observe.

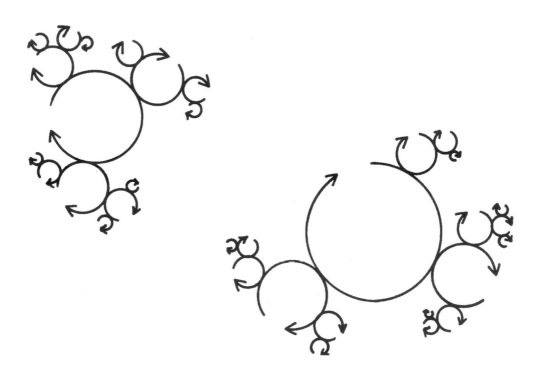

FIGURE 2–27. A schematic illustration of the formation of eddies in turbulent flow. The rotational elements appear as self-similar patterns of progressively smaller size. This is an example of fractal geometry, in which a self-similar pattern is repeated at different scales. From *The speech sciences. A volume in the speech sciences* (1st ed.), by Kent, copyright 1998. Reprinted with permission of Delmar, a division of Thomson Learning.

Summary

The central aim of this chapter is to summarize an important theory known as linear and time-invariant source–filter theory. The crux of this theory is that speech sounds can be understood in terms of a source of energy that is filtered by the vocal tract. This idea is shown in Figure 2–28, which shows the laryngeal source spectrum (with its typical −12 dB/octave fall in energy), the formants (transfer function of the vocal tract), the radiation characteristic (+6 dB/octave), and the output spectrum with conspicuous peaks corresponding to the formants F1, F2, and F3. An understanding of the acoustic theory of speech production prepares the way for a discussion of speech analysis. Knowing the ways in which speech sounds are formed helps to determine appropriate analysis methods and measurements. For example, if a vowel segment is adequately characterized in terms of its formant pattern, then the analysis task is to determine the frequencies and bandwidths of the main formants for that segment. However, if formant pattern is not a sufficient characterization, then some other means of spectral analysis is required to account for vowel acoustics. The acoustic theory also helps in relating acoustic measures for a sound segment to the underlying articulation of that segment. A simple example is the separation between source energy and resonance. The object is to interpret a particular acoustic property with an articulatory correlate. In this sense, the acoustic theory of speech production is central to the analysis of speech. Certainly, one can make acoustic measures of speech without knowing theory, but the interpretation of these measures would be limited at best and misleading at worst. Ideally, measurement and theory are closely coordinated.

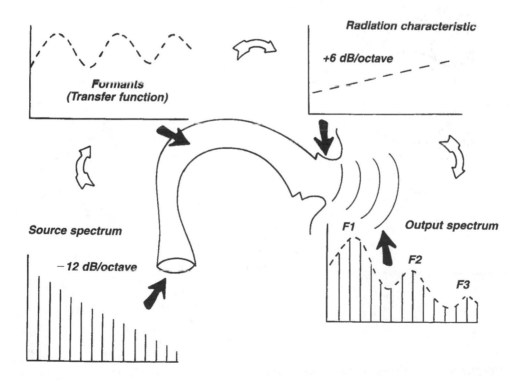

FIGURE 2–28. Diagrammatic summary of the source–filter theory of speech production. From *The speech sciences. A volume in the speech sciences* (1st ed.), by Kent, copyright 1998. Reprinted with permission of Delmar, a division of Thomson Learning.

Introduction to the Acoustic Analysis of Speech

This chapter introduces the basic techniques for the acoustic recording and analysis of speech, beginning with older analog (nondigital) methods and concluding with a discussion of digital signal processing (DSP) techniques. A major objective is to trace the progress that has been made.

A Short History of the Acoustic Analysis of Speech

The power of modern computer methods in analyzing speech can be appreciated by taking a brief historical look at acoustic analysis. The historical review could begin well before the 20th century, but it is sufficient for our purposes to begin with the 1930s and 1940s. Figure 3–1 summarizes the developments since that time up to the present.

The Oscillogram

The first major advance in the acoustic analysis of speech began with *oscillograms* (waveforms, or graphs of amplitude over time) of speech sounds. The sounds selected for analysis were often vowels, because they are relatively easier to analyze than most consonant sounds. The sounds to be analyzed were represented oscillographically as pressure variations over time. This first step was an important advance. Because speech sounds are perishable acoustic events of relatively short duration, representing these sounds in a permanent manner is a technical challenge. With the development of oscillographs based on string galvanometers, it became possible to derive fairly accurate waveforms of sustained vowels. The waveforms indicated certain regularities in these sounds but were not in themselves sufficient to describe some of the important differences

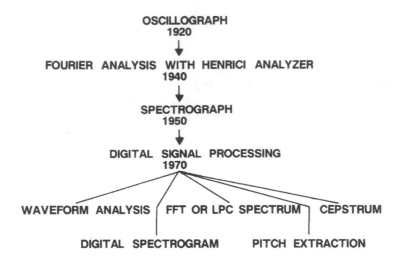

FIGURE 3–1. Some historic developments in the acoustic analysis of speech. The approximate date of each development is noted.

among different vowels. Observation of these differences required the generation of spectral representations, that is, plots of signal energy versus frequency.

The Henrici Analyzer

The advantage of spectral analysis to studying speech is quite like the advantage of spectral analysis to studying light. In optical analysis, light is broken down into components of different wavelengths. In the acoustic analysis of speech, sound is broken down into components of different frequencies. Analysis is a matter of decomposition, or breaking the complex sound pattern into simpler constituents.

One of the earliest tools for spectral analysis was the *Henrici Analyzer*, a mechanical device consisting of five rolling integrating units (glass spheres). The procedure of analysis was as follows:

1. Obtain the oscillogram of the waveform.

2. Select a representative portion, typically in the middle of the wave and enlarge it with a projector.

3. Trace the enlargement on a plain white surface.

4. Trace the enlarged waveform with the Henrici Analyzer.

5. Calculate the values of the amplitude and phase relationships from dial readings associated with the glass spheres.

6. Plot the pressure (in dB) against frequency to obtain spectral (harmonic) analysis.

As the operator traced the acoustic waveform with the analyzer, each sphere integrated a different partial or component of the wave. With each tracing, five harmonic components could be determined. This procedure performs a harmonic analysis, that is, it looks for frequency components within the complex speech signal at integer multiples of a fundamental (lowest) frequency. This method assumes that speech is truly periodic, like the sound of a vibrating guitar string. However, speech is only quasi-periodic. The frequencies that comprise it are not necessarily multiples of the fundamental. As a result, the Henrici Analyzer gave an inaccurate picture of the energy distribution in speech sounds. In addition, the analysis procedure was tedious because the user had to hand-trace the waveforms and read the values representing the frequency components. Nonetheless, the Henrici Analyzer played a significant role in the development of the modern understanding of speech acoustics. It foreshadowed the general approach of spectral analysis of speech. In addition, data derived from this technique contributed to ideas about distinctive energy concentrations in vowel sounds. By careful and diligent work, the users of this device were able to wrest some fundamental principles from the waveform of speech.

Filter Bank Analysis

Another approach to speech analysis was **filtering**. A filter is a frequency-selective transmission system, that is, a filter will pass energy at certain frequencies but not at others. A filter is like an acoustic window that allows some energy to pass while blocking other energy. Figure 3–2 shows the application of a bank of filters to the analysis of speech. The energy of the signal is effectively divided into frequency bands by the filter bank. Each filter passes only the energy in its frequency band. Indicating devices at the output of each filter may be used to display the energy in specific frequency regions. By analogy, a series of screens of different mesh size may be used to separate particle sizes in a pile of gravel. Only the smallest pieces will fall through a sieve with the finest mesh, then slightly larger pieces will fall through a slightly coarser mesh, and so on until the pile has been sorted into several smaller piles according to the size of the particles. Details of filters are discussed later in this chapter. For the present, it is sufficient to say that a filter allows a selective look at the energy in various frequency regions. Much as a prism can divide light into different wavelengths, filters can divide sounds into different frequency components.

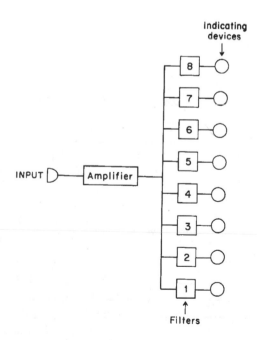

FIGURE 3–2. Schematic diagram of a filter bank for acoustic analysis. The filters numbered 1 through 8 pass successively higher frequency bands. Indicating devices at the output of each filter show the energy present in each band.

Because a filter determines the amount of energy in specific frequency regions, it results in a kind of spectral analysis. The detail of the analysis depends on the number of filters used and their bandwidths. The bandwidth of a filter is the frequency range in which it passes energy. For example, a filter centered at 100 Hz with a bandwidth of 10 Hz would pass only the energy at frequencies between 95 Hz and 105 Hz (105 − 95 = 10 Hz). Usually, much larger bandwidths would be used, so that the entire frequency range of interest (say, 0–5 kHz) could be analyzed with fewer than 25 filters. Using a filter bandwidth of 500 Hz for all filters, a 5-kHz range could be analyzed with 10 filters. Figure 3–3 shows how such an arrangement of filters might analyze different vowels produced by an adult male speaker. In Figure 3–3, we begin to see the real differences among vowel sounds:

the frequencies of the strongest components that make up the complex speech sound. Unlike the Henrici Analyzer, a filter bank makes no assumption that these components are all multiples of the fundamental. Therefore, it gains a wider application to the sounds of speech, including noise.

A practical improvement on the filter bank is a variable band-pass filter (Figure 3–4). The idea is to use an adjustable filter that can act like any of the filters shown in Figure 3–3. The signal to be analyzed is fed repetitively through the variable band-pass filter as its settings are adjusted to different frequency regions. Practically, it is easier to modulate a variable carrier frequency with the signal to be analyzed and use a fixed filter for analysis (a process called *heterodyning*). In this case, the filter is not adjusted but the signal is effectively swept past it.

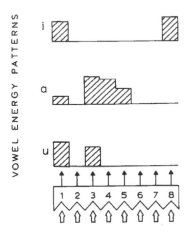

FIGURE 3–3. Hypothetical output of a simple filter bank when the three vowels /i/ (he), /a/ (ha), and /u/ (who) are presented as input. Each vowel has distinctive bands of energy.

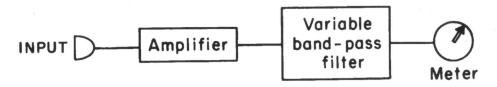

FIGURE 3–4. Acoustic analysis using a variable band-pass filter. The filter is swept across the input signal to indicate the energy at various frequencies.

The Spectrograph

The variable band-pass filter was incorporated in the sound *spectrograph*, a machine developed in the 1940s. The spectrograph provided major advantages to the study of speech. Because it afforded a relatively fast analysis, the spectrograph made it possible for scientists to collect more extensive data. As a result, the pooling of data across subjects became more common. With earlier analysis techniques, data usually were obtained on a very small number of speakers, frequently one. The spectrograph also provided a better delineation of the energy concentrations in speech. Finally, the spectrograph produced a running short-term spectrum, enabling the scientist to visualize how energy concentrations changed in time. The display of the running short-term spectrum is called a **spectrogram**. Because of the strong impact that the spectrograph had on speech research, it is important to understand its essential features. These will be briefly reviewed below. The spectrographic analysis of various types of speech sounds is discussed in detail in later chapters.

A photograph of a spectrograph is shown in Figure 3–5, and its basic operation is illustrated in Figure 3–6. The signal to be analyzed is recorded on a magnetic drum that allows a continuously repeating playback of the signal. The magnetic drum can be likened to a tape loop. The signal then modulates (multiplies) a variable carrier frequency in a process called heterodyning (as mentioned earlier in reference to filter analysis). It is more practical to sweep the signal to be analyzed past a fixed filter than to analyze the original signal with a variable filter. It is for this reason that heterodyning is used. The end result is the same as if the signal were repeatedly played back through a filter that was continuously adjusted to act like a filter bank. In conventional spectrography, two filter bandwidths are used. The wide-band filter has an analyzing bandwidth of 300 Hz, and the narrow-band filter has an analyzing bandwidth of 45 Hz. Some spectrographs have other bandwidth selections, such as 90 Hz and 600 Hz. The selection of analyzing bandwidth is discussed in a later section.

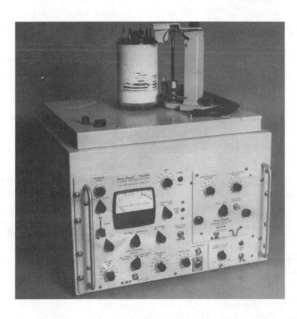

FIGURE 3–5. Photograph of a sound spectrograph produced in about 1980. Courtesy of Kay Elemetrics Corporation.

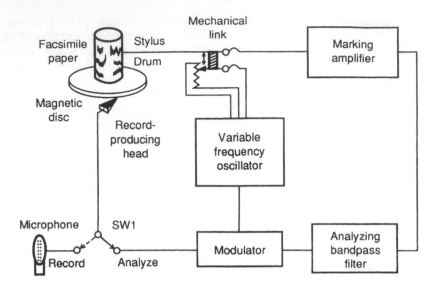

FIGURE 3–6. Schematic drawing of the components of a conventional sound spectrograph.

The output of the analyzing filter is fed to a marking amplifier that provides an increase in the current. At any frequency region in the analysis, the current from the marking amplifier is proportional to the acoustic energy in the signal. The current flows through a stylus that is held in close contact with a piece of special paper that is wrapped around the spectrograph drum. As the drum and attached paper rotate, the stylus gradually moves up the drum in coordination with the analysis frequency. The coordination is accomplished by a mechanical linkage between the moving stylus and a variable oscillator. In this way, the vertical position of the stylus is associated with a particular frequency of analysis. The bottom of stylus travel is the lowest frequency (around 80 Hz) and the top of stylus travel is the highest frequency (around 8 kHz).

The current that flows through the stylus burns the special paper as it turns on the drum to produce a blackened region. The paper is treated so that the burning is limited in extent. In effect, the paper is charred locally as the current passes through it. Therefore, the blackness of the paper corresponds to the energy at that point in the analysis. Although controlled burning to produce a pattern may sound crude compared to modern high-technology visual displays, the idea was quite ingenious. The burning achieved two essential operations: (1) rectification of the electrical signal, so that both positive and negative parts of the waveform were represented in the analysis, and (2) a low-pass filtering (smoothing). The burning process produced an odor rarely described as fragrant, and an accumulation of a fine black soot over the workspace. However, it also yielded spectrograms of high quality.

The complete process, from recording to analysis, involves these steps:

1. The speech sample is transduced by a microphone so that air pressure variations of the acoustic signal are put into the form of voltage variations.

2. The electrical signal is then converted to an electromagnetic signal for storage on the magnetic drum of the spectrograph.

3. The stored magnetic pattern is converted back into an electrical signal for analysis as a spectrogram.

4. The signal is filtered so that the energy in various frequency regions can be determined.

5. The current of the electical signal is amplified and fed to a marking stylus.

6. As the current flows from the stylus through the specially treated paper, a localized burning of the paper occurs. The burning produces a blackening of the paper in proportion to the current flowing through the stylus.

A sample of the finished product, the spectrogram, appears in Figure 3–7. The conventional spectrogram is a three-dimensional display of time, frequency and intensity. Time appears on the horizontal axis, running from left to right. Frequency is plotted on the vertical axis, increasing from bottom to top. Intensity is represented by the blackness of the pattern (the so-called "gray scale"). Figure 3–8 shows spectrograms of three simple acoustic signals. Shown in part A is the spectrogram of a sinusoid ("pure tone"). Because the sinusoid contains energy at a single frequency, the spectrogram displays a single narrow band running horizontally. The location of this band on the frequency (vertical) axis indicates the frequency of the sinusoid. Part B illustrates the spectrogram for a hissing noise. Because the noise contains frequency components at many different frequencies,

most of the spectrogram is blackened to some degree. At about the halfway point on the time (horizontal) axis, the overall blackness increases, corresponding to an increase in the overall intensity of the noise energy. Part C shows a spectrogram for a rapping noise made by knuckles on a table top. Each rap is a brief acoustic event (a transient) having energy over a fairly wide frequency range. Notice that each rap is distinctly represented on the spectrogram. The three spectrograms in Figure 3–8 show the usefulness of this form of analysis in determining how acoustic signals vary in time, frequency composition and intensity.

Speech consists of a variety of sounds. The variations in acoustic properties can occur quite rapidly and it is for this reason that a running spectrum is a desirable form of display and analysis. The spectrogram shows how spectral energy changes over relatively brief intervals of time. The details of this analysis will be considered in Chapters 4 and 5, but it is appropriate to take an early look at the way in which a spectrogram reveals the acoustic features of some speech sounds. Sample spectrograms are shown in Figure 3–9. The spectrogram can depict the very brief energy associated with the explosive release of air in a stop consonant (the point labeled A in Figure 3–9), but the spectrogram also displays the prominent and often lengthy bands of energy that typify vowel productions (point B). When

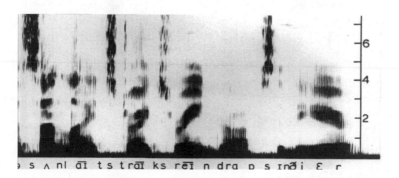

FIGURE 3–7. Sample spectrogram of the utterance, "*The sunlight strikes raindrops in the air.*" A phonetic transcript of the utterance appears at the bottom of the spectrogram.

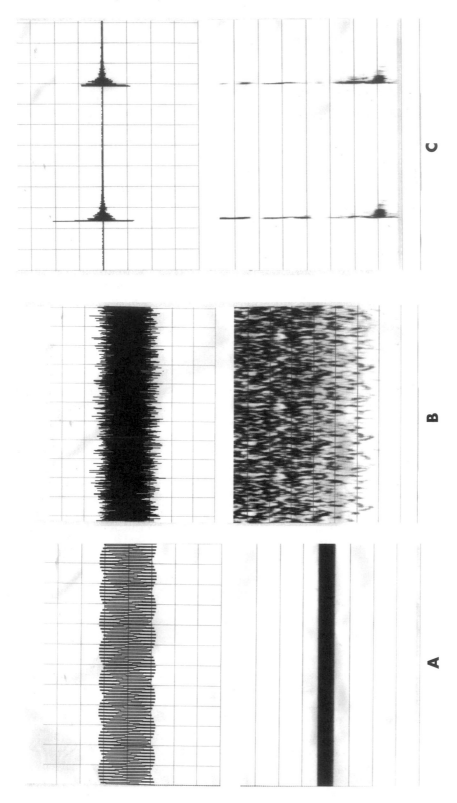

FIGURE 3–8. Sample spectrograms and corresponding waveforms for three types of sounds: (A) a sinusoid or pure tone with a frequency of 4 kHz; (B) a computer-generated noise; and (C) knuckles rapping on a table top.

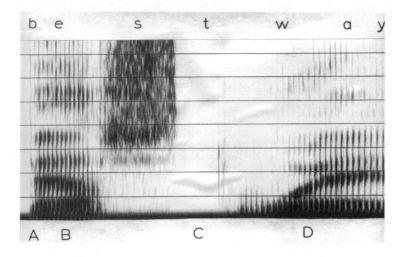

FIGURE 3–9. A spectrogram of the phrase, *best way*, with labeled points corresponding to discussion in text.

no sound is produced, as during the oral closure for a stop consonant, the spectrogram reveals the silence (point C). When the vocal tract changes in its configuration during a gliding sound, the spectrogram portrays the corresponding acoustic change (point D). The spectrogram contained a great deal of acoustic information and it quickly became the standard for speech analysis, despite certain limitations to be considered in a later section. Spectrograms continue to be useful as a fundamental form of speech analysis, although contemporary spectrograms are generated by computers rather than by the device shown schematically in Figure 3–6.

Digital Signal Processing of Speech

The dominance of the vintage spectrograph was seriously challenged only with the introduction of digital computers. The challenge has intensified with the continued refinement of computers (hardware) and analysis programs (software). Some of the developments in the use of digital computers are shown in Figure 3–10. These developments

are taken up later in this chapter and in subsequent chapters. Once the speech signal has been put into a form suitable for storage and analysis by a computer, several different operations can be performed (Read, Buder, & Kent, 1990, 1992). The waveform can be displayed, measured and even edited (for example, deleting one portion and connecting the remaining pieces together to make an entirely new sound). Spectra can be computed using methods such as the Fast Fourier Transform (FFT), Cepstrum, Linear Predictive Coding (LPC), and filtering. It is sufficient to say that algorithms for these analyses have revolutionized the acoustic analysis of speech. Moreover, these analyses are important to many applications in physics, engineering, and biology. Because of its diverse and powerful uses, the FFT has been called the most important numerical algorithm of our lifetime (Strang, 1994). The goal of determining the spectral composition of a signal is common to many science and engineering applications.

The digitized signal can be used to generate spectrograms that are in many ways superior to those made by the spectrographs that occupied speech analysis laboratories beginning in the 1950s. Digital computers

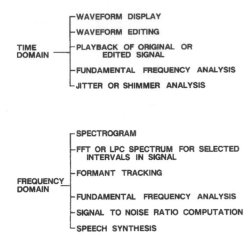

FIGURE 3-10. Some developments in the use of digital methods for speech analysis. These topics will be covered in the following chapters.

can do what the old spectrographs did, but faster, more accurately, and much more cleanly. In addition, computers can perform operations that go far beyond the analysis capabilities of the spectrograph. Many of these capabilities are available even for microcomputers (personal computers). The rapid developments in speech analysis with microcomputers are a major reason for the preparation of this tutorial text. Although speech analysis systems are readily available for microcomputers, many users do not have sufficient background in digital processing to understand the capabilities and limitations of these systems. Both—capabilities and limitations—are significant.

Filtering, sampling and quantization are the basic operations in digitizing a speech signal. Each operation has important consequences for the nature of the signal that is eventually stored in the computer. Consequently, the user of a digital processing system should have a good grasp of these operations. Many speech analysis systems allow the user to specify variables such as filter settings and sampling rate. Careful consideration should be given to these variables whenever a speech signal is digitized. In addition, the user of such systems may encounter a variety of

issues related to amplification, cabling and interfacing. A basic understanding of these issues can help to avoid problems and to ensure that a signal of suitable quality has been obtained.

The basic process in digitization is to convert a continuous (analog) signal to a digital (discrete) representation. The digital representation is a series of numbers. When an analog signal such as an acoustic waveform is digitized, two operations are performed simultaneously. The first is a discretization in time, meaning that the analog waveform is *sampled* at certain time points, usually periodically spaced. The periodic spacing is reflected in the *sampling rate*, which specifies the regularity of the sampling process. A sampling rate of 10 kHz means that the original analog signal is sampled 10,000 times per second. The second operation is a discretization of signal amplitude. This operation, called quantization, represents the continuous amplitude variation of the original signal as a series of levels or steps. Each level is a quantum, and the process of amplitude discretization is therefore one of quantization. Sampling and quantization are the essence of digitization.

The principal steps of the digital processing of speech are shown in Figure 3–11. The original acoustic signal of speech is represented by the function x(t), which is simply the speech waveform as might be obtained directly from a microphone or played back from a tape recorder. The notation x(t) indicates a variable in time, specifically, the amplitude by time variation of the acoustic signal. As noted previously, this waveform is an analog signal and its amplitude varies continuously with time. To store this signal in a modern digital computer, the analog signal must be converted to a series of numbers. The numbers are then stored as a representation of the analog signal. This chapter considers the steps that are taken to convert the analog signal to a digital representation. The process is called **analog-to-digital conversion** and it is typically performed by a an **analog-to-digital converter**, or A/D converter. The reverse operation of *digital-to-analog conversion* is the process by which the series of numbers stored in a computer are converted to an analog signal. This operation is performed by an D/A converter. Typically, systems for the acoustic analysis of speech use both A/D and D/A converters. The A/D converter is used to convert an original analog signal to digital form. The D/A converter then is used to derive analog signals from the

stored digital files, as is required if we wish to hear a digitally stored signal.

Filtering Operations

The first step in digital processing is a **pre-emphasis filtering** in which the high-frequency components of the signal are boosted in amplitude relative to the low-frequency components. Pre-emphasis is desirable, and often necessary, because most of the energy in speech is in the lower frequency range and this energy will dominate the analysis unless some equalization of energy across frequency is attempted. There are two usual ways by which pre-emphasis is accomplished. One is the use of a filter (usually a hardware filter) that provides a 6 dB/octave increase to the speech signal above some breakpoint frequency, f_b, where f_b usually is chosen to be above 100 Hz but less than 1000 Hz. The specification of 6 dB/octave means that for every doubling of frequency (octave) above the breakpoint, the energy increases by 6 dB. For example, a 6 dB boost would be given to energy at 2000 Hz compared to energy at 1000 Hz. The second way to achieve pre-emphasis is by

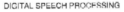

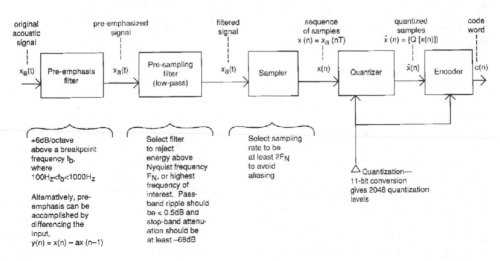

FIGURE 3–11. Major stages in the digital signal processing of speech. See text for discussion.

differencing the input. This operation can be performed by the computer and is expressed by the following formula:

$$y(n) = x(n) - ax(n-1)$$

where x(n) is a sample of the signal at time n,

y(n) is the first-differenced signal,

and a is a constant of multiplication.

Differencing depends on digital operations to be explained later. For the present, it is sufficient to realize that pre-emphasis can be accomplished either by operations on the analog acoustic signal x(t) or by operations on the digitized signal x(n). The two methods yield comparable results. There is a caution to be observed in the use of speech analysis systems. A system that accomplishes pre-emphasis by a differencing computation should not be coupled to a hardware pre-emphasis filter, or the signal will be pre-emphasized twice—once by the hardware filter and again by the differencing operation.

The pre-emphasized signal is then fed to a *pre-sampling filter*. This is a low-pass filter designed to reject energy above the highest frequency of interest. This filtering procedure is based on **Nyquist's Sampling Theorem** (Nyquist, 1928), which states that the number of samples needed to represent a signal is twice the highest frequency of interest in the signal. For example, assume that we are interested in analyzing the speech signal only to 10 kHz. This frequency is the upper limit of analysis and the low-pass filter would be selected to reject energy above this frequency. Filters have various characteristics that define their operation; two of these characteristics to be noted here are the *pass-band ripple* and the *stop-band attenuation*. As shown in Figure 3–12, the pass-band is the band of frequencies in which energy is passed with minimal loss. Many filters have a detectable ripple, or variation in transmission with frequency, within the pass-band. If the ripple is too large, it can distort the analysis of the signal. A useful rule of thumb is that the ripple should be less than 0.5 dB. The stop-band attenuation is a measure of the energy that remains in the region of the filter where energy transmission is minimal. This is the frequency band where energy transmission is most reduced, or filtered out. Filters usually do not succeed in rejecting all the unwanted energy, however, and filters can be compared as to their ability to minimize the energy in the stop-band. For general applications in speech analysis, it is desirable to have a stop-band attenuation of at least −68 dB, meaning that the energy that remains in the stop band after filtering will be at least 68 dB below the energy peak in the pass-band. For the example under consideration, this means that the energy peaks within the pass-band of 0–10 kHz will be at least 68 dB more intense than any energy found within the stop-band.

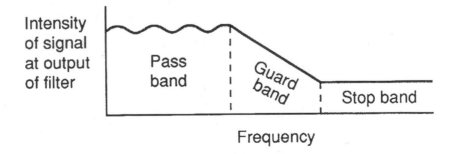

FIGURE 3–12. Frequency response of a low-pass filter. The pass-band is the frequency region in which energy is passed most effectively. The stop-band is the region of maximum opposition (blockage) to signal transmission, and the guard band is an intervening region sometimes called the skirt of the filter.

Sampling

The signal, which is now pre-emphasized and low-pass filtered, is ready for digitization. Digitization really consists of two processes, sampling and quantization. Sampling is the operation by which the analog signal is converted to a series of samples. This conversion can be expressed with the following notation:

$$x(n) = x(NT)$$

where $x(n)$ is a sequence of samples and T is the sampling interval.

The basic process is to convert a continuously varying signal to a series of numbers that can be stored in a digital computer. As shown in Figure 3–13, the term sampling is descriptive of the actual operation. The original analog signal is sampled at regular intervals. The energy between the sampling points is discarded. It may seem strange that this operation occurs with no loss of information. After all, it appears that the original signal, with its infinitely many values along the time axis, is now reduced to a finite number of samples. However, Nyquist's Sampling Theorem states that if the sampling rate is properly selected, the sampled signal contains the same information as the original analog signal. In other words, analog-to-digital conversion can be done without loss of information. This is a fundamental concept in the application of digital computers to the processing of speech or any signal originally in analog form.

How is the sampling rate selected to ensure that information is not lost? The guideline is quite simple: The sampling rate should be at least twice the highest frequency of interest, which we will denote by F_n. In our example, the highest frequency of interest is, $F_n = 10$ kHz. Therefore, the sampling rate should be 2×10 kHz = 20 kHz. If an analog signal that is low-pass filtered at 10 kHz is sampled at a rate of 20 kHz, the digitized signal will be equivalent in information to the original signal. It is important to remember this relation between the pre-sampling filter and the sampling rate of digitization because serious errors can result if this relation is neglected. Now there is nothing really wrong with sampling at a higher rate. For instance, we could sample our 10-kHz low-pass filtered signal at 40 kHz or 4 times the Nyquist frequency. However, this high rate is completely unnecessary and will use twice as much computer memory to represent the sound of interest.

But there *is* something wrong with sampling at a rate lower than twice the highest frequency of interest. When this happens, serious errors can develop in the analysis. These errors are called **aliasing**. The pre-sampling filter is sometimes called an *anti-aliasing filter* in recognition of the need to prevent the errors of aliasing. In common usage, an alias is an assumed or false identity, and this is the essence of the error that can occur in digital processing when the sampling rate is too slow in relation to the frequency range of analysis. By way of illustration, let us consider an example from motion pictures. You probably

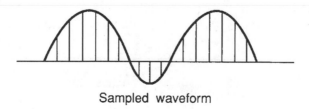

Sampled waveform

FIGURE 3–13. Illustration of sampling of a waveform. Samples are taken at the points marked by vertical lines. Usually, sampling is periodic (recurs at a fixed rate).

have seen movies in which the wheels on a wagon or stage coach appeared to be moving *slowly backward* even as the horses were pulling forward at a considerable speed. The effect is most apparent with wheels that have spokes. Of course, the wheels are not really turning backward, nor is this effect a visual illusion. The apparent slow, backward motion is an example of aliasing—an error in the sampling of the original event. In this case, the sampling rate is determined by the film rate of 30 frames per second, the usual rate in the motion picture industry. The spokes on the rotating wheel of the wagon alter their positions over time, but the relatively slow frame rate of the motion picture camera simply cannot register the actual spoke positions during wheel rotation. As a result, the wheel may appear to be moving slowly in the wrong direction. What you see in the motion picture is an aliased, or false, identification of the actual dynamic event. The problem could be corrected by increasing the frame rate of the motion picture. However, increased frame rate is not important for most of what we see on the screen, so the aliasing of stage coach wheel rotations is simply tolerated as

a minor nuisance. However, aliasing is not just a minor nuisance in digital signal processing. It can cause a seriously erroneous analysis.

Aliasing occurs if frequencies at greater than half the sampling frequency are sampled. For example, if a sampling frequency of 5 kHz is used to digitize signal components at greater than 2.5 kHz, aliasing can occur. The effect of aliasing is illustrated in Figure 3–14. The original signal—the signal to be sampled—is shown at the top of the illustration, and a sampled version of the signal is shown below. At the sampling rate represented by the vertical lines, the signal is undersampled. As a result, the sampling operation yields a false, or aliasing, signal shown at the bottom of the illustration. (Note that at half the sampling frequency, each cycle of a periodic signal is represented by two samples, which is the minimum number of samples that can represent the positive and negative portions of the sinusoidal waveform.)

One kind of aliasing error is the generation of *foldover frequencies* (Figure 3–15). This false frequency information occurs at a frequency given by

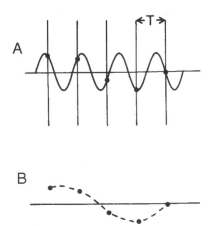

FIGURE 3–14. Graphic representation of aliasing caused by undersampling of a signal. (A) Sampling at a rate of 1/T is the sampling period. (B) Generation of a spurious low-frequency signal, the aliasing signal.

$F_f = S - F$

where F_f is the foldover frequency,

S is the sampling rate, and

F is a frequency higher than half the value of S.

To avoid aliasing, these steps should be followed:

1. Determine the highest frequency of interest in the analysis; this is F_n.

2. Filter the energy above F_n; and

3. Sample the signal at a rate of at least $2F_n$.

Other aliasing products can occur as well, but it is sufficient to note here that the entire problem of aliasing usually can be avoided if the sampling rate is carefully chosen in relation to the frequencies of interest in the original signal and if energy above the highest frequency of interest is filtered out. The major reason for the qualifier *usually* in the preceding sentence is that aliasing can also occur under another condition which results in something called granulation noise. Discussion of this issue will have to be postponed until the following discussion of quantization.

Quantization

Let us review what has happened so far. We began with a continuously variable acoustic signal denoted by x(t). Because this signal cannot be used in its original form by a digital computer, it has to be converted to a digital form—a sequence of numbers (samples). The **sampling** operation essentially chops the analog signal into a number of equal intervals. The size of the interval depends on the sampling rate. The higher the rate, the smaller the interval. For instance, at a sampling rate of 5 kHz, the interval between sampling points is 0.2 msec. At this rate, then, the analog signal is converted to a sequence of 5,000 samples in each second. We now have discrete entries appropriate for use by a digital computer except for one problem—the amplitude or energy level of the samples also must be converted to digital form. Sampling accomplished only part of the digitization operation, namely, the conversion from continuous time to sampled or discrete time.

The remaining operation in digitization is **quantization**. A signal is quantized when the samples determined by the sampling operation are chopped into a discrete number of amplitude levels. The term quantization is descriptive of what is done. A

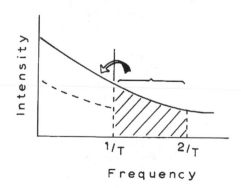

FIGURE 3–15. Graphic representation of aliasing as a foldover frequency. Energy sampled at less than 2/T can appear as low-frequency energy.

quantum is an increment of energy. When an analog signal is quantized, the continuous amplitude variations are converted to discrete values, or increments. The operation is illustrated in Figure 3–16 for various levels of quantization. Notice that if quantization is performed with only a few steps or levels, the quantized signal has a stairstep shape that only roughly resembles the original analog signal. However, as the levels of quantization are increased, the similarity between the quantized signal and the analog signal also increases, that is, the higher the number of quantization levels, the more accurately the quantized signal represents the analog signal. Of course, there is a trade-off against memory demands. As the number of quantization levels increases, so does the need for memory to store the data. As a general rule of thumb, speech should be quantized with at least a 12-bit conversion, which provides 4,096 quantization levels. If too few levels of quantization are used, the signal will have a distortion called quantization noise. Note that with each additional bit of amplitude conversion, there is a doubling of levels of quantization, for example, 8 bits provides 256 levels. 9 bits provides 512 levels, and so on. Conversion at 8 bits, as is sometimes done with low-cost systems, will produce a low-quality signal. For all but the crudest purposes in speech analysis, 8-bit conversion is inadequate. Fortunately, improvements in computers make it easy to obtain excellent quantization, with conversions at 16 or 32 bits being readily available.

The operation of quantization can be expressed fairly simply as a process of discretizing the continuous variations in signal energy that remain after the sampling operation:

$$x[n] = x(n) + e(n)$$

where $x[n]$ is the quantized sample,

$x(n)$ is the unquantized sample, and

$e(n)$ is the error or noise in quantization.

The object is to minimize $e(n)$, that is, to make it small enough that it does not cause problems in analysis or signal quality.

Several choices of quantization are available. Perhaps the simplest is uniform quantization in which the steps or increments are of equal size across the range of signal energy. One disadvantage to this approach is that the speech signal has a

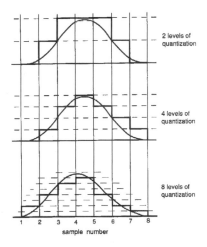

FIGURE 3–16. Illustration of the effects of using different quantization levels to represent a smooth waveform. As the number of levels increases, the fit to the smooth curve improves.

large dynamic range (the range from lowest to highest signal energy in a sample) and speakers vary considerably in their use of this range. If the dynamic range of analysis is adjusted to the most intense portion of a speech sample, the quantization steps for the weaker portions of the sample may be too coarse if a uniform quantization is employed. Therefore, preference may be given to a nonuniform quantization in which the quantization increments are smaller in the low-energy range of the signal. In addition, the signal can be transformed in various ways before quantization is accomplished. For example, one might use a logarithmic transformation of the signal to achieve finer increments for weaker components. However, it should be noted that quantization is inherently a nonlinear operation. Unlike sampling, which is securely based on the sampling theorem, quantization is a very difficult concept mathematically.

After the operations of sampling and quantization, the signal has been digitized as a series of quantized samples. Mathematically, we can express this process as follows:

$$x[n] = \{Q[x(n)]\}$$

where x[n] are the quantized samples corresponding to the

original waveform x(t),

Q is the quantization operation, and

x(n) is the sequence of samples.

The signal is now in a form that can be encoded for storage in the computer. The original time-varying waveform of speech now takes the form of a series of quantized samples. Analog-to-digital conversion is completed.

When the amplitude of the signal is about the same as one quantization increment, the effect of quantization is to produce either a dc signal (a dc shift or change in baseline) or a square wave. The square wave is rich in odd harmonics that can reach far beyond the highest frequency of

interest, F_n. Even the use of an anti-aliasing filter cannot prevent aliasing in this situation, which results in a gritty sound called *granulation noise*. The point to remember is that very low-amplitude signals are vulnerable to the generation of a noise distortion. Quantization level should be chosen carefully if very weak signals are to be processed. Amplification of the signal may be required, and this is considered in a following section. Another important point is that the levels of quantization are distributed over the range of amplitude values (the dynamic range).

Practical Application

As a quick review, let us consider a practical problem in A/D conversion. Suppose that a speech signal is to be analyzed for information that is contained within the frequency range below 3 kHz. Because the total sample of speech is very long, it is important to use as little computer memory as possible to store the signal. What are the appropriate settings for sampling rate, presampling filter and quantization? First, the sampling rate should be at least twice the highest frequency of interest in the analysis, F_n. This highest frequency is 3 kHz, which means that the sampling rate should be at least 6 kHz. Because filter settings sometimes are approximate and because signal energy may be appreciable in the reject band, it is wise to choose a cut-off frequency for the low-pass, pre-sampling filter that is slightly below the sampling rate. Therefore, this filter should have a low-pass characteristic with a cut-off frequency of slightly below 3 kHz, let us say, 2.8 khz. Finally, an 11-bit quantization should provide a sufficiently accurate amplitude conversion, unless there is an interest in small variations in signal amplitude.

Is it ever desirable to *oversample*, that is, to use a sampling rate higher than that derived from the sampling theorem? Yes, it is. First, it may be desirable to oversample when the anti-aliasing filter has a shallow guard band. If the rejection rate of the guard band is shallow, then some undesired signal energy above F_n may be digitized and may result in aliasing. It is usually a good procedure to select a low-pass frequency of the anti-aliasing filter that is less than half the value of the sampling rate. Oversampling also is used to gain temporal resolution. One example is in the determination of vocal fundamental frequency (f_0). Whalen et al. (1990) noted that when a file is sampled at 10 kHz, the accuracy of fundamental frequency determination will be $\pm$ 0.5% for a man with a f_0 of 100 Hz, $\pm$ 1.0% for a woman with a f_0 of 200 Hz, and $\pm$ 2.5% for an infant with an f_0 of 500 Hz. The issue becomes especially important for the determination of irregularities (perturbations) in the voice. One such perturbation is called *jitter*, which is the cycle to cycle variation in the fundamental period. Another perturbation, called *shimmer*, is the cycle to cycle variation in the peak amplitude of the laryngeal waveform. Measurement of these perturbations, or departures from true regularity, can be intolerably imprecise at low sampling rates or low levels of quantization. Oversampling is often used as well in music recording, because it affords a more satisfactory sound quality (a "fuller" or "fatter" sound).

Other Issues in A/D and D/A Conversion

For additional information on A/D and the issues briefly considered below, see Lang (1987) and Gates (1989). What follows are some highly condensed comments on issues related to A/D.

Amplification (Gain)

It is important to know the input range for the A/D converter used in a particular application. Some converters have an input range of - 1 to + 1 volt, but others require an input signal with a different range, for example, -7 to +7 volts, or -10 to +10 volts.

It is desirable to adjust the input signal to this range to take full advantage of the levels of quantization afforded by the A/D. If a signal has a range of only -2 to +2 volts and a converter with $\pm$ 10 volt input range is used, many potential levels of quantization would be lost as the signal is digitized. Because the analog output of instruments such as tape recorders often does not correspond to the signal range of a A/D converter, amplification frequently is needed. Let us take as a simple example the output of a tape deck that provides a signal range of -1 to +1 volt. If this signal is to be fed into an A/D that requires a signal range of -10 to +10 volts, then the tape deck output should be amplified by a factor of ten.

Amplification usually is accomplished by one of two means: (a) using an external amplifier, or (b) using the built-in amplifier provided with some A/Ds. On-board amplifiers come with various features, one of which is programmable gain, or the capability to change the gain in software according to the needs of data conversions. An advantage to an external amplifier is that it can be placed very close to the equipment providing the signal to the A/D. Proximity is particularly important in the case of weak signals. When a weak signal is passed along a long cable, it is vulnerable to noise and further diminution by the resistance of the connecting cable. Noise may arise, for example, because the cable can serve as an antenna, picking up 60 Hz hum from sources such as transformers and fluorescent lights. Signal diminution is possible because the wire in cables, even though it is a conductor, presents some resistance to the flow of electrical energy. The resistance is proportional to the length of the wire. The rule is simple: keep the connection between the signal instrument and the A/D as short as practical.

Cabling

Connecting instruments together may seem a trivial matter but this is in fact a very important consideration. Incorrect choices or faulty procedures can greatly impair the performance of a speech analysis system. One factor to consider is the type of cable that is used to make the connections. The cost of a cable increases with its ability to keep noise out of the signal. The least expensive are single wires and flat cables. The major difference between these two pertains to the number of connections that must be made. When many connections are made with single wires, the result can be a confusing jumble. Flat cables reduce the confusion because they may contain several wires. For applications involving a high-frequency signal or a signal with a low signal-to-noise ratio, single wires or flat cables are not the connections of choice. It is preferable to use one of the following: twisted-pair, coaxial, or triaxial cable. These connections protect the signal from environmental contamination. Finally, as noted above, it is always desirable to keep cable lengths to a minimum.

Interface

Cables require connectors so that signals may be passed from one device to another. For digital signals, the problem of interface arises. *Interface* refers to the communication scheme that allows devices to exchange signals. There are two main types of interface—serial and parallel. There are large number of issues that arise in interfacing, most of which are not directly relevant to the applications in this book. Readers who need information in this area might consult Lang (1987) or general references for the particular computer systems involved.

Some General Considerations in Acoustic Analysis of Speech

We now consider the two broad domains of acoustic analysis: time domain and frequency domain. Although these domains are related by mathematical transforms, such as the Fourier transform, they are not necessarily equal for various purposes in acoustic analysis. Each has certain advantages and disadvantages in examining speech sounds.

The advantages of **waveform** (time-domain) representation are as follows.

1. The waveform can be a faithful representation of the original sound and, therefore, a good reference to ensure quality of reproduction and analysis.

2. Typically, the waveform can be obtained simply and inexpensively.

3. The waveform is a sensitive record of temporal variations in the signal and is, therefore, of particular value when subtle temporal factors are to be observed. Many frequency-domain techniques lose some of the temporal information in the signal.

4. With a waveform of a signal, it is often easy to detect distortion events (e.g., peak clipping which results when the high-amplitude excursions are cut off) or the presence of a contaminating signal (e.g., background noise).

Among the disadvantages of a waveform (time-domain) representation are the following:

1. The waveform can be expensive to store because the speech signal typically has a large bandwidth and, therefore, has a high storage requirement. Modern computers with their vast storage capacities have reduced the seriousness of this problem.

2. Waveforms generally are difficult to interpret and summarize. Even experts can find it difficult to guess which speech sound is represented by a particular waveform. For example, the waveforms of vowels sounds do not permit an easy identification of their phonetic quality.

3. The waveform is sensitive to phase variations that may not be important to

the ultimate analysis objective and may be ignored by the ear.

The advantages of **spectral** (frequency-domain) representation include:

1. The spectrum can permit relatively easy and economical characterization of many important features (e.g., formant frequencies of vowels, energy regions of aperiodic sounds).

2. The spectrum is insensitive to phase variations that can be neglected in typical applications of speech analysis.

3. The spectrum can be used to characterize steady-state events or, with proper sampling, dynamic events such as transitions.

4. The running spectrum, as in a spectrogram, offers segmentation capabilities that are difficult to achieve in a waveform.

The disadvantages of spectral (frequency-domain) representation are:

1. Sometimes it is difficult to detect distortion events in a spectrum or to notice the addition of noise.

2. Analyses performed with some standard methods may not reflect psychophysical processing, for example, nonlinearities.

3. Analyses may disguise or obscure some properties of interest.

4. Spectral analyses can be expensive to perform in terms of time and resources (hardware or computation).

5. Spectral analyses can be insensitive to some temporal variations in the signal.

"Modern analytic techniques" mean digital techniques, that is, computing with samples of speech represented as numbers. Analog devices, which deal with continuous data, are still used in amplifying, recording, and playback, but rarely in analysis. Instruments for speech analysis are now basically of two types: "dedicated" devices specifically designed for speech, such as digital spectrographs, and general-purpose computers running programs for analyzing speech. The similarities are more basic than the differences: both are, in fact, digital computers, operating on speech which has been sampled as described in this chapter. They perform similar computations and typically produce similar monitor displays, which the user may choose to print.

The difference is that in the dedicated device, the hardware and the analysis programs have been selected and optimized to work together in analyzing speech, and the programs have been written (semi-permanently) into the machine's memory. As a result, the dedicated device may operate faster or display results more perspicuously, but in principle, a general-purpose computer can be programmed to do the same analyses. Instructions for using a dedicated device deal solely with analyzing speech, whereas the user of a general-purpose computer typically confronts at least two manuals: one for the basic machine and one for the speech-analysis program.

Typically, a disadvantage of a dedicated device is that the user cannot modify or add to its programs. By contrast, for some micro- and minicomputers, users may choose from several programs available for various combinations of analyses. Some programs even make it relatively easy for a user to add her own analyses. Some programs are in the public domain, such as those developed with government support, and can be obtained for a small copying fee. Because of the fundamental similarities between dedicated and general use computers, we will not usually need to distinguish between them in discussing analytic techniques. With either type, it is up to the user to determine that a particular analysis is appropriate to his purposes and his data. A sophisticated user also starts with some known data in order to check whether the analyses are performed accurately.

Waveform Display

In the beginning of this chapter, we began our brief history of acoustic analysis with the oscillograph, which traced on paper the changes in voltage from a microphone, representing the changes in air pressure which pass from speaker to listener. Displaying such a sound pressure waveform is one basic function of most devices for speech analysis. From such a display, one can determine duration and relative amplitude. One can judge periodicity, and from the duration of periods one can estimate fundamental frequency. Typically, one can select portions of the waveform for closer inspection and for editing. We will review each of these functions below. Figure 3–17 shows the waveform of one utterance of "we" as displayed by a program named CSpeech running on a personal computer.

Measuring Duration

Note the left and right cursors in Figure 3–17: the user set them around "we," using both visual and auditory cues. The next word in the utterance was "show," and the thicker waveform beyond the right cursor results from the noise of the [ʃ]. By moving the cursors and playing back the sound between them, the user could judge at what point the sound quality changed from

vowel to fricative. The sampling rate at which the sound was recorded was 22 kHz (22,000 samples per second). Thus, the time between samples was 0.045 ms, that is, 45 μs (microseconds), the potential time resolution of a recording at that rate. CSpeech reports (line 1 of the display) that the time between the cursors is 263.273 ms, so the user might conclude that the syllable "we" was precisely that long.

However, there are two hidden limitations. The main one is the difficulty of judging exactly where a speech segment begins and ends. In this case, is the left cursor precisely at the beginning of the vowel? How much difference would it make if the user decided that the vowel begins later, where the waveform becomes periodic or where it first exceeds some voltage (amplitude) threshold? Should the right cursor be moved inward to the last regular period of the vowel? Such questions become critical in attempting to make reliable measurements, especially of different types of speech sounds or sounds in different contexts. To say that the potential resolution is 0.045 ms is misleading, because no one can locate boundaries of speech units that precisely. Articulation takes time, so speech sounds begin and end gradually. The second limitation is that while the potential resolution is 0.045 ms, the smallest cursor movement may be larger than that, depending on the duration of sound

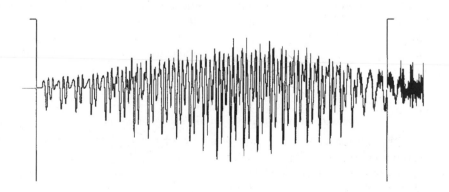

FIGURE 3–17. Speech waveform of the beginning of *"We show speech."* Cursors mark *"we."*

displayed. In this case, one cursor movement was 0.4 ms, so that was the effective resolution. If we had displayed several seconds of speech, the resolution would have been coarser. For both these reasons, we cannot always take (or offer) duration measurements at face value.

Resolution is an issue in the amplitude dimension as well. "Twelve-bit quantization" means that the input voltage is represented by a number which can take on 4,096 different values. Thus, if the input voltage ranges from +10 volts to -10 volts, that 20-volt range will be divided into 4,096 steps, or 5 mv (millivolts) per step. That resolution is normally adequate for speech analysis, but you should know the resolution of your equipment. Some inexpensive sampling devices use only 8-bit resolution (256 different values), which makes a considerable difference in the quality of the recorded speech and in subsequent analysis. The greater the resolution, the stronger the signal, as compared with the noise introduced by the quantization process. Table 3–1 shows the relationship between amplitude resolution (in bits, steps, and millivolts) and this signal-to-quantization noise ratio, for a few commonly used levels of resolution.

Bear in mind that this signal-to-noise ratio is a theoretical maximum for a signal of constant energy, which speech never is. In Table 3–1, it looks as if even 8-bit resolution equals the signal-to-noise ratio of an ordinary cassette tape recorder, but several other factors operate to reduce the actual ratio and to introduce other kinds of noise. To name just one example, if the sampling hardware is set for a 20-volt range of input,

but the actual input spans only two volts (+1 to -1), which many preamplifiers provide, the amplitude resolution is only one-tenth of the potential, and noise will be much louder in relation to the signal.

Editing

Because we can select portions of digitized speech (usually with cursors on a screen) and play them back, we can edit speech. For example, suppose that you have recorded an utterance of "team." You can hear that the [t] is aspirated ([tʰ]), and for a perception experiment, you would like to remove the aspiration and play the result. Figure 3–18 shows such an utterance, with the cursors marking the aspiration. In "the old days" (about 30 years ago), you would have cut the recording tape with a razor blade and spliced it back together. Today, we have an electronic equivalent: cutting at the cursors and rejoining the digitized sound. The precise way in which you do this depends on the program or device; some have a "splice" command, some require you to transfer segments to another channel or to label and list the segments to be spliced. In any case, the operation will be cleaner, faster, and more accurate than tape splicing, mainly because you can locate the cutting points more accurately by viewing the waveform and listening to the portions before, after, and between the cursors.

However, some tips from expert tape splicers still apply. Most basically, no splice will be completely natural because of coarticulation. If you cut a consonant from a vowel, the vowel will still contain transi-

TABLE 3–1.
Amplitude resolution and signal-to-noise ratio.

Bits	Steps	Step size (if 20v range)	Signal-to-Noise Ratio
8	256	78 mv	41 dB
12	4096	5 mv	65 dB
16	65536	0.3 mv	89 dB

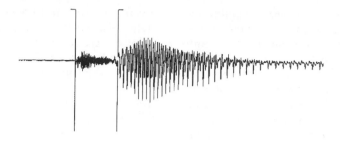

FIGURE 3–18. Speech waveform of *team*, with the cursors marking the aspiration of the [t^h].

tions which suggest that consonant, or at least its place of articulation. Vowels before nasals will be nasalized, those before /r/ will be rhotacized, and those before voiceless consonants will be shortened. Almost all speech sounds contain effects of their contexts. Second, a splice where the waveform is strongly positive or negative will probably produce a popping noise (an acoustic transient). Skilled splicers make their cuts at moments when the waveform is at or near the zero line, or at least join two ends at the same amplitude. Fortunately, with electronic tape splicing you can easily experiment with different splices.

Measuring Amplitude

The speech waveform also provides information about relative amplitude. The top channel in Figure 3–19 shows the waveforms of "import," the noun with stress on "im," and "import," the verb with stress on

"port." One can see that the amplitude of the first syllable ("im" with primary stress) is greater than that of the third, and that the amplitude of the fourth syllable ("port" with primary stress) is greater than that of the second.

Such comparisons of the raw waveform can be difficult, however, because the viewer must somehow combine the negative (downward) half of the waveform with the positive half. Both represent changes in air pressure which move the eardrum of a listener. Channel 2 in Figure 3–19 shows the same waveform rectified, that is, with negative pressures changed to positive—the effect is that the lower half of the waveform in channel 1 has been "folded up." This makes it easier to compare not only the overall amplitude of syllables but also the shape of amplitude change during each syllable. We can infer, for example, that within each "im" (syllables 1 and 3), the greater amplitude is in the first half of the syllable, that is, the vowel rather than the nasal.

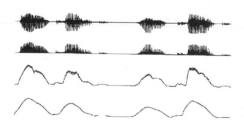

FIGURE 3–19. Speech waveform of *IMport* (noun) *imPORT* (verb), with three representations of amplitude. Channel 2 is the waveform rectified; channels 3 and 4 are rms amplitude contours, calculated with a 20 ms and an 80 ms sliding window, respectively.

The waveform in channel 2 still has all the jaggedness of the original, however. To obtain a smooth amplitude curve, we must somehow average the signal over time. In effect, we did that informally, "by eye," when we assessed the shape of each syllable. Such smoothing can be done arithmetically, and one way is known as rms amplitude, for "root-mean-square" averaging. The name identifies three of the steps, in reverse order. To calculate rms amplitude:

- Select a **"window"** length, the number of samples of speech to be averaged;
- Square the value of each sample in the first window, thus eliminating negative numbers and exaggerating differences;
- Calculate the arithmetic mean, or average, of the squared values in the window;
- Take the square root of the resulting mean, bringing it back to the original scale;
- Move on to the next window, that is, the next set of samples.

The waveform in channel 3 of Figure 3–19 is the rms amplitude of the original waveform, calculated with a 20 ms "sliding" window, that is, one that advanced by just one sample with each rms calculation. Now much of the jaggedness is gone, and the average has been calculated precisely.

To create an even smoother curve, we lengthen the window, averaging over longer stretches. The rms amplitude curve in channel 4 is exactly like that in channel 3 except that it was calculated with an 80 ms window. However, note that the window length has an effect: if we were trying to locate the exact peak of each syllable, we would get slightly different answers from channels 3 and 4.

Amplitude and English Stress

This discussion of Figure 3–19 may leave the impression that syllable stress, or prominence, in English is signaled mainly by amplitude. Indeed that is also our intuition. Most speakers of English would report that the main difference between the noun "import" and the verb "import" is in which syllable is louder. However, duration is also a factor. In Figure 3–19, the second (stressed) syllable of the verb is longer than that of the noun. In fact, duration is actually a more consistent cue to stress than amplitude is; in Figure 3–19, the "im" syllables are atypical, in that they do not differ in length. Notice also that we do not compare "im" with "port" with respect to stress; because they are made up of different speech sounds, they are inherently different in both amplitude and duration.

Measuring Fundamental Frequency

One can easily "see" that some parts of the waveform are periodic, that is, they consist of similar patterns of change repeated over time. For example, in Figure 3–17 ("we"), most of the waveform between the cursors is periodic. The largest patterns (longest periods) result from the vibrations of the vocal folds and correspond to the frequency which we perceive as pitch; as those patterns become more frequent, the perceived pitch increases. Because we are very good at recognizing visual patterns, it seems easy for us to judge periodicity in a waveform display. To program a computer to make the same judgments turns out to be quite difficult. However, even human judgments are usually unclear about where periodicity begins and ends. At the right side of Figure 3–17, for instance, just where does the vowel *stop* being periodic? Similarly, after the left cursor in Figure 3–17, the sound is rapidly changing in amplitude and quality; that is the nature of /w/. Is there an aperiodic portion at the beginning? Answers to such questions are partly arbitrary because the vocal folds move and change their modes of vibration gradually. Precisely because we can now see the effects of vocal fold activity (and of articulation) on an expanded time scale, we realize that speech does not change instantaneously. Technically, speech is only quasi-periodic, because it is constantly changing in frequency and quality.

Within these limitations, we can use a waveform display to measure the duration of periods and, therefore, the fundamental frequency of voiced speech. Figure 3–20 displays a vowel, with the cursors surrounding ten periods. The interval between the cursors is 95.9 ms ("Length ="; line one), so the average duration of one period is 9.59 ms. Since duration and frequency are inverses, the fundamental frequency, on average, is 104 Hz ($[1/9.59] \times 1000$), or ten times the frequency shown at the end of line one. Averaging over ten or twenty periods in this way is usually desirable for two reasons. First, the error, or uncertainty, in setting the cursors is reduced by a factor of ten, and second, we usually want to know the average pitch in some region of the waveform, not the absolute frequency of one particular vocal period. Of course, this method of measuring fundamental frequency can be tedious if you have many measurements to make. The next-to-last section of this chapter will discuss several other methods, but there are no perfect ones.

Filters

Basic terms

We saw in Chapter 2 that a filter is a system that passes (or enhances) some frequencies but attenuates others. Filtering also was mentioned early in this chapter, as in the use of a bank of filters to perform a spectral analysis of speech. Now it is time to take a more detailed look at filtering.

Because a filter offers a frequency-selective transmission of energy, it has a *response curve* that varies across the frequency spectrum. As shown in Figure 3–21, a filter's response curve will have one or more *pass-bands*, and one or more *stop-bands*. The filter may be a high-pass or a low-pass filter (if the pass band is above or below the stop band), or in the general case, as in Figure 3–21, it may be a *band-pass* filter, with stop bands on both sides. The frequency at which the filter's response starts to change is called the *corner frequency*. Because the change actually occurs over a range of frequencies, the corner frequency is only nominal, however. If the change in response is abrupt, the filter is said to have sharp cut-offs or steep skirts. Real filters do not have perfectly flat response in the pass-band or the stop-band; instead, they have some ripple in their response, as in Figure 3–21. Figure 3–21 turned upside-down would be the response curve of a *band reject* filter, with a stop-band in the middle and pass-bands on either side. A band reject filter with a narrow stop band is called a *notch filter*.

Uses of Filters in Speech Science

Two common applications were introduced in this chapter: pre-emphasis and anti-aliasing. A pre-emphasis filter for speech is a

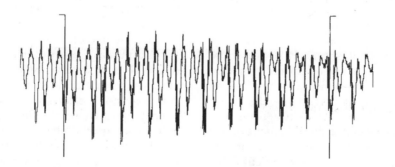

FIGURE 3–20. Speech waveform of *we*, with the cursors marking 10 glottal periods. The duration of that portion is 95.8 ms, so the average f_0 is 104 Hz.

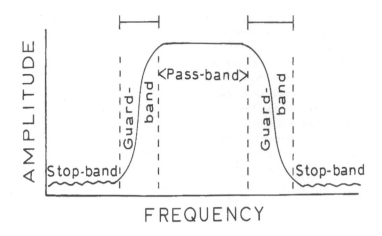

FIGURE 3–21. Response curve of a band-pass filter, identifying the pass-band, stop-bands, and guard bands.

high-pass filter, usually with a response that increases at 6 dB per octave above a corner frequency of a few hundred hertz. Such a filter enhances higher frequencies, which are of lower amplitude in speech, on average. In fact, as speech radiates from the lips, it is attenuated by 6 dB per octave, so pre-emphasis at that rate simply restores the signal actually generated in the vocal tract.

An anti-aliasing (pre-sampling) filter is a low-pass filter which sharply attenuates frequencies above half the sampling rate. As explained in Chapter 3, such a filter is necessary for digital recording and analysis but not for analog processes, such as a conventional tape recording.

Another use of filtering is to focus an analysis on a frequency range of interest. For example, suppose that you wish to study two types of [s] sounds, such as those in Korean. All [s] tokens consist primarily of high-frequency sound, and they are low in amplitude compared to vowels. If you simply plot a sound-pressure waveform with an amplitude scale wide enough for vowels, *all* tokens of [s] will be of low amplitude, and you will have difficulty discerning any differences. However, if you first apply a high-pass filter, the amplitude

of high-frequency sounds such as [s] will be relatively greater, and differences among them will be easier to see. Other analyses, such as spectrograms, are also typically more revealing if the frequency range of interest has been made more prominent by filtering.

Another use for filters is in the study of perception. For example, suppose that you work for a telephone company, evaluating possible improvements to the transmission systems. Such systems now transmit a bandwidth of only about 300 to 3000 Hz; in effect, they are band-pass filters. Suppose that some projected improvement to the system would widen that bandwidth to 5000 Hz. You might undertake a series of perceptual studies to determine whether the effect on people's perception is worth the increase in cost.

A fifth major use for filters in the study of speech is in spectrographic and spectral analysis. As noted early in this chapter, a spectrograph breaks speech into its frequency components by filtering it, with either analog or digital filters. The bandwidth of these filters makes a crucial difference to the resulting spectrogram. Some examples of this difference are shown later in this chapter.

These are only some examples of how filters are used in the study of speech. A central part of speech science is concerned with the frequencies that make up speech, and whenever one focuses on a certain range of frequencies, one is using filters. Filtering is also an essential part of producing speech, as we saw in Chapter 2.

Analog versus Digital Filters

Filters can be constructed in two forms: analog and digital. An analog filter is an electronic circuit, tuned to respond to a certain range of frequencies—in short, it is a resonator. Such a circuit is made up of resistors, capacitors, and inductors. By adjusting the values of these components, we can modify the response curve of our filter, affecting bandwidth, corner frequencies, and ripple. (For examples, see Baken, 1987, pp. 21–26.)

A digital filter, on the other hand, contains no such physical components; it is a rule, an equation, applied to a sequence of samples of speech. The simple example introduced earlier in this chapter was that of differencing, subtracting from each sample some proportion of the preceding sample:

$$y(n) = x(n) - ax(n-1)$$

where $x(n)$ is a sample in the original signal at time n

$y(n)$ is the corresponding sample of the differenced signal

and a is a constant multiplier, usually between 0.9 and 1.0.

In other words, we step backwards through a digitized signal, sample by sample, subtracting from each sample some large proportion of its predecessor, so that the resulting samples represent mainly the changes. Why does such an operation act as a high-pass filter? Basically because differences from sample to sample are high-frequency variation, assuming that the sampling rate is high. These variations are relatively well-preserved by differencing, but low-frequency (slow) variation is attenuated at each step. In fact, when a = 0.9, differencing yields a response curve close to a 6 dB per octave pre-emphasis.

Of course, there are other kinds of digital filters. In fact, any function of frequency may be considered a filter. Of particular interest in speech science are filters based on linear predictive coding (LPC), discussed below. The parameters of LPC analysis represent formant frequencies and bandwidths, so one can filter a signal by altering those parameters.

The Time/Frequency Tradeoff

Whether analog or digital, filters share a crucial property with all other resonators, namely, that there is a tradeoff between frequency resolution and time resolution. One aspect of this tradeoff is fairly obvious: a wideband filter will "smear" a range of frequencies by responding to any frequency within its bandwidth. As shown in Figure 3–22, a filter with a 300 Hz bandwidth centered on 450 Hz will respond efficiently to any frequency between 300 and 600 Hz; it will fail to distinguish between them. Conversely, a filter with a 60 Hz bandwidth (narrow-band), also centered on 450 Hz, will respond efficiently only to frequencies between 420 and 480 Hz, giving us finer-grained information about frequency.

What is less obvious is that the reverse is true for the filters' response over time. The wideband filter responds *quickly* to signals within its frequency range, while the narrow-band filter responds more *slowly*. That is why a narrow-band spectrogram (that is, one produced with narrow-band filters) provides fine-grained frequency information but smears it over time, obliterating brief events, while a wide-band spectrogram smears information across frequency but displays brief events more clearly. Figure 3–23 illustrates this difference for a segment of the vowel [i]. The wide-band analysis (top part of Figure 3–23), by virtue of its time resolution,

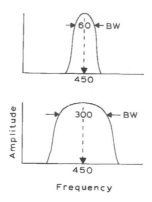

FIGURE 3–22. Response curves of wide-band (lower curve) and narrow-band (upper curve) band-pass filters.

shows the vertical striations associated with glottal pulses, whereas the narrow-band analysis (bottom part of the figure), because of its frequency resolution, displays the harmonics of the laryngeal source. The trade-off between frequency and time resolution is an example of the *principle of indeterminacy* in physics. As applied to speech analysis, it means that we cannot achieve both precise frequency resolution and precise time resolution in the same analysis (at least not with the conventional methods described in this chapter). Because wide-band and narrow-band analyses are complementary in this respect, it can be desirable to use both types to determine the acoustic properties of a particular speech sample. Figure 3–24 shows the use of both analyses for the phrase *talk today.* Notice that the vertical striations associated with glottal pulses and the noise bursts associated with the consonants *t* and *d* are well-defined in time in the wide-band analysis (top part of Figure 3–24). However, the harmonics of the voice source are evident only in the narrow-band analysis (bottom part of the figure).

In an analog filter the bandwidth is the range of frequencies to which the tuned circuit resonates. A digital filter does not literally resonate. How then can it have a bandwidth? A digital filter cannot filter one sample (one number), of course; it can find variation (i.e., frequencies) only in a series of samples. The counterpart to bandwidth in a digital filter is the number of samples (often called "points") which the filter takes as a unit of analysis. A small difference in frequency takes a long time to manifest itself: for instance, two frequencies that are only 10 Hz apart take 1/10 s (second) to differ by a full cycle, but differences of 100 Hz show up ten times faster. If our filter operates on a long interval (many samples), it can detect small differences in frequency, but its response will change only after that interval—slow response in time. In other words, we have exactly the same tradeoff between time and frequency resolution in digital filtering that we had with hardware filters. Either way, if you want to respond to small differences in frequency, you have to operate on long intervals of time, or if you want to work with short intervals of time, you can see only large differences in frequency. Neither resonators nor equations can be highly selective in both time and frequency, because time and frequency are inversely related.

Whenever we filter a signal, we lose some information about changes over time. In fact, this effect can be quantified: the *time constant* of a filter (analog or digital) is the time required for its response to decay to

glottal pulse

wide band (handwritten)

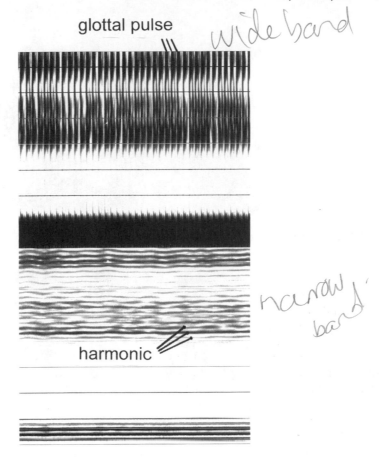

narrow band (handwritten)

harmonic

FIGURE 3–23. Wide-band (top) and narrow-band (bottom) analyses of the same speech sample (a segment of a sustained vowel [i] as in *he*) to illustrate differences in frequency and time resolution between the two analysis filters. Note that vocal fold vibration is analyzed as glottal pulses (vertical striations) in the wide-band analysis and as harmonics (thin horizontal bands) in the narrow-band analysis.

about 37% of its peak value. More precisely, the proportion is $1/e$, where e is the base of the natural logarithms. It is the filter's response to its highest *pole*, its most resonant frequency, which is measured. Some computer programs allow you to construct filters that meet various specifications; the time constant is one such variable, along with corner frequencies and bandwidth. Sometimes the time constant for a digital filter is stated in terms of number of samples. For example, a time constant of 100 samples at a 10 kHz sampling rate means that the response decays to $1/e$ in 10 ms.

Such a filter would distort the most rapid changes in speech, such as stop bursts and vowel transitions.

Although filters have many practical applications in the study of speech, perhaps their greatest importance is as models of the vocal tract, because as we saw in Chapter 2, the vocal tract is a complex and changing filter. Given excitation from the vibrating vocal folds or a fricative constriction, the vocal tract enhances some frequencies while suppressing others. It can be described as a set of resonators, each with a center frequency and a bandwidth. This

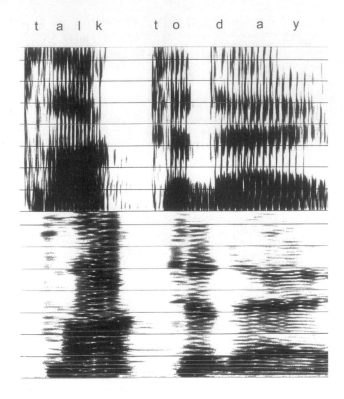

FIGURE 3–24. Wide-band (top) and narrow-band (bottom) analyses of the phrase *talk today*. Notice the difference in time and frequency resolution between the two types of analysis.

view of speech has permitted speech science to apply the known properties of filters to the analysis of speech production.

Types of Filters

There are some classic types of filters which illustrate the tradeoffs that a filter designer must make. These types were originally analog filters, but they can be mimicked by digital filters.

- *Butterworth filter:* maximally flat, that is, minimal ripple in either pass-band or stop band. The tradeoff is gradual transitions between stop and pass bands.
- *Chebychev filter:* sharper transitions than Butterworth, but ripple in the pass-band.
- *Chebychev II filter:* the opposite; ripple in the stop band, but flat pass-band.

- *Elliptic filter:* ripple in both the pass and the stop bands, but sharpest transitions between bands ("steep skirts").

As these descriptions illustrate, in addition to the tradeoff between frequency and time resolution, there is a tradeoff between ripple and sharp transitions. The choice depends on the application. For example, sharp transitions are not desirable in pre-emphasis, but they are essential in anti-aliasing; any frequency components above half the sampling rate will add distortion to a digitized signal.

Spectral Analysis

The discussion to this point covers the procedures by which a signal is stored in a digital computer and displayed as a waveform for the purpose of making temporal and amplitude measurements. We turn now to some of the most important applications in acoustic analysis–spectral analysis. For this purpose, it is necessary to select a portion of the waveform (or more accurately, a sequence of digital values that represents the waveform). This selected interval is called a **frame** and is illustrated in Figure 3–25. The duration of the interval selected for analysis is called the *frame length* and is typically on the order of 20–30 ms (long enough to include two or three glottal periods) but shorter or longer values may be appropriate for certain analysis purposes. Analysis of a speech sample of any length requires the use of several successive frames (the frame "walks" along the waveform, so that a constant interval is selected for analysis at various regions of the signal). The *frame interval* defines the degree of overlap across successive frames. If the overlap is too large, unnecessary computation is performed. If the overlap is too small, then the analysis might miss rapid changes in the signal. The energy in a frame

is weighted according to a window. As discussed earlier, the window is a weighting function that minimizes signal amplitude at the edges of the window. The analysis frame and window define a portion of the signal that will be analyzed with a short-term transform of some kind.

The whole process, beginning with the original signal and proceeding through filtering, A/D conversion, frame selection, windowing, and application of a short-term transform, is shown in Figure 3–26. The short-term transforms include various types of spectral analysis as well as other functions such as autocorrelation. All of them operate on the signal contained in the analysis frame. We now discuss these short-term analyses.

Fourier Analysis

Fourier analysis takes its name from the mathematician Jean Baptiste Joseph Fourier, who was made a baron by Napoleon in 1808 for his government service, not his

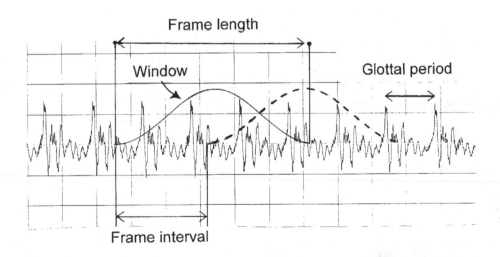

FIGURE 3–25. Illustration of short-term analysis of a speech waveform, showing frame length, frame window, and window shape. The analysis is performed on the portion of waveform contained in the frame. This interval is shaped by a window or weighting function. The analysis frames are repeated at points determined by the frame interval. For many short-term analyses, it is desirable to include at least two glottal periods within the analysis frame.

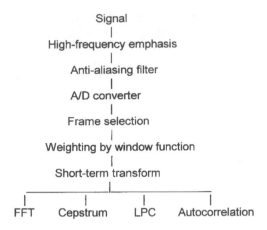

Signal
|
High-frequency emphasis
|
Anti-aliasing filter
|
A/D converter
|
Frame selection
|
Weighting by window function
|
Short-term transform

| | | | |
FFT   Cepstrum   LPC   Autocorrelation

FIGURE 3–26. Diagram of the major steps in digital short-term analysis, beginning with the operations of analog-to-digital conversion and proceeding through frame selection, windowing, and calculation of a particular short-term transform, four of which are discussed in this chapter.

mathematics. Fourier showed that periodic waveforms, no matter how complex, can be analyzed as the sum of an infinite series of sinusoidal components, varying in amplitude and phase. Each component is an integer multiple of the fundamental. This proof is essential to speech science, because we often deal with complex periodic waveforms whose strongest component frequencies are the resonances of the vocal tract and are essential to production and recognition. Thus, Fourier analysis can tell us a great deal about speech sounds. Essentially, it transforms a periodic amplitude by time waveform into a frequency waveform, known as a spectrum, a graph of the amplitude of the various frequency components.

However, as usual in applying mathematics to the physical world, there are a few "catches." First, Fourier's theorem applies to periodic waves, whereas speech sounds are only quasi-periodic, as we have seen. For instance, any sound which dies out is not truly periodic. Second, Fourier was talking about continuous waveforms, whereas in digital analysis we are dealing with discrete samples from such a waveform. Third, carrying out Fourier's analysis as he developed it is computationally difficult, even though we settle for a finite num-

ber of components. However, it turns out that there are solutions to all these problems. We can adapt Fourier analysis to a quasi-periodic waveform by *windowing* (gradually increasing and decreasing the amplitude of the signal, rather than turning it on and off abruptly). There are **Discrete Fourier Transforms (DFTs)** which apply to sampled data, and one type of DFT is a **Fast Fourier Transform (FFT)**, which desktop computers can do rapidly.

Even before the computational improvements, Fourier's theorem was essential, because it guaranteed that a complex waveform *had* component frequencies which a bank of filters, for example, could find. As we saw earlier, that was in fact the form that analysis took in analog devices. Now digital analysis consists of an FFT of samples from a waveform. It yields a spectrum showing the amplitude of each harmonic of the fundamental. (Theoretically, it ought to indicate the relative *phase* of each component, too, but phase is not nearly as important as frequency and amplitude for specifying speech sounds.)

Figure 3–27 shows such a spectrum for a portion of the vowel [i] in "we." The horizontal axis is frequency, from 0 to 5000 Hz (the filter cut-off). The vertical axis is

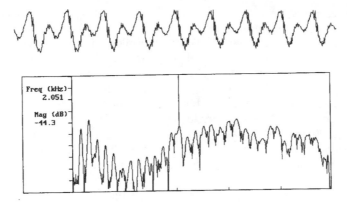

FIGURE 3–27. Speech waveform and Fourier spectrum of [i]. The cursor in the spectrum points to the 13th harmonic, which is near the peak of F2.

amplitude, from a zero dB reference level at the top down to -80 dB at the bottom. Each peak in the graph is a harmonic (integer multiple) of the fundamental. The cursor (vertical line) points to the thirteenth harmonic, which is a local maximum because it is near a resonant frequency of the vocal tract articulating this vowel: the second formant. As the side panel indicates, the frequency of this harmonic is 2051 Hz, and its amplitude is 44 dB below the reference level. The first formant is near the second harmonic, at approximately 300 Hz. This wide separation between first and second formants is a distinguishing characteristic of the vowel /i/. Fourier analysis makes it possible for us to identify such essential properties of speech sounds.

Linear Prediction

Fourier analysis is basic to the study of speech, but it is not the only way of determining a spectrum nor the best for all purposes. A more recently developed method of analysis is **linear prediction** or **linear predictive coding** (LPC) (Atal & Hananer, 1971; Atal & Schroeder, 1970). LPC comes from two sources: the branch of statistics known as time-series analysis, which aims to identify regularities in time-varying

data, and the branch of engineering concerned with transmitting signals. Time-series analysis applies not only to speech but also to birthrates, electroencephalograms, sunspots, and stock market prices—any stream of data over time.

A classic problem in transmitting signals is that the capacity of any channel is limited. Intercontinental telephone channels via satellite, for example, are expensive, and so engineers try to find ways of compressing the signals. One way is linear predictive coding. LPC builds upon the fact that any sample in digitized speech is partly predictable from its immediate predecessors; speech does not vary wildly from sample to sample. Linear prediction is just the hypothesis that any sample is a *linear* function of those that precede it. Expressed as an equation, this hypothesis is:

$$x(n) = a_1[x(n\text{-}1)] + a_2[x(n\text{-}2)] + \dots - e(n)$$

which means: the sample at time n [x(n)] is equal to the preceding sample [x(n-1)] times some weight [a_1] plus the one before that times some weight plus more weighted samples minus some error [e(n)]. To the extent that this prediction is accurate, one can transmit not the individual samples but the weights and errors. This appears to have complicated our transmission, not simplified it; the simplification is that the weights do not change as rapidly as the samples themselves. That is, if we sample a signal 10,000 times per second, we have a new sample every 100 μs. But while the signal remains in one pattern (e.g., a steady-state vowel), the LPC weights tend to remain the same. It turns out that they need to be updated only every 10 or 20 ms in order to transmit intelligible speech, a saving of about one-hundredfold. Of course, the prediction is not completely accurate, so the transmitted speech is not perfect. One variable is the number of preceding samples included in the prediction, usually on the order of 10 to 20 for speech analysis.

As discussed so far, linear predictive coding is a model of the sequence of samples that make up a signal, a representation of the signal over *time*. However, a set of linear prediction coefficients has an equally valid interpretation in terms of *frequency*. It is the frequency response of a digital filter derived from those coefficients. (The derivation is beyond the scope of this book; for an overview, see Makhoul, 1975.) In its frequency interpretation, the weighted terms in the equation represent the frequencies and amplitudes of the resonances of the vocal tract, and the error term, known as the *residual*, represents that which remains unaccounted for. If the model of the resonances is a good one, what remains is just the input: the excitation of the vocal tract by the signal at the glottis. Thus, the LPC model as a whole represents exactly what we want to know.

Linear predictive analysis, like a Fourier transform, relates a representation in time to one in frequency. A key difference is that a Fourier spectrum represents harmonics of the fundamental, while an LPC spectrum represents formant frequencies and amplitudes (resonances). Which is better depends partly on your purposes. In the Fourier spectrum, formant frequencies can only be inferred from the frequencies of high-amplitude harmonics, a problem which becomes severe for speech with a high fundamental frequency. Monsen and Engebretson (1983) compared LP analysis with spectrographic measurement, using experienced readers of spectrograms. For samples with f_0 between 100 and 300 Hz, those readers could measure the center frequency of F1 and F2 to within ±60 Hz; spectrographic measurements were less accurate for F3. Both methods proved much less accurate when the fundamental frequency exceeded 350 Hz. The choice also depends on the sample; Fourier analysis assumes that there is a harmonic (periodic) structure; the LP analysis does not. However, the LP analysis makes assumptions of its own: most LP analyses today are models of resonances only, not anti-resonances. However, the vocal tract does introduce anti-resonances, especially in the production of nasal and lateral speech sounds. For this reason, linear predictive analysis (at least an "all-pole" model) is not a good choice for analyzing such sounds.

For sounds which fit both models, we would like to see both representations of the spectrum. Figure 3–28 shows a linear predictive spectrum superimposed on the Fourier spectrum of Figure 3–27 (same vowel, same axes). The LP spectrum shows no harmonics; it is a *spectrum envelope*. Note that in general it fits the peaks of the Fourier spectrum well. In this case, the two analyses yield highly similar spectra, partly because the speech being analyzed fits both models: it is voiced (periodic) and non-nasalized. However, note also that from the Fourier analysis alone, one would have difficulty in inferring the precise frequency of F2, measured as 2012 Hz on the LPC spectrum. From the Fourier spectrum, an expert can infer that F2 is centered between the 12th and 13th harmonics, but it is difficult to interpolate exactly where. In the Fourier spectrum, f_0 is the difference in frequency between two harmonics. In the LP spectrum, there is no indication of fundamental frequency, although f_0 can be derived from LP analysis because the glottal source should be the main component of the error term. (Although it is unusual to do so, harmonics can be seen in a LPC spectrum if the number of LP coefficients is increased substantially; this is an illustration of the principle that the sensitivity of the LP analysis to spectral variation depends on the number of coefficients).

Real-time Spectrographs

Digital spectrographs now on the market carry out Fourier and other analyses and display a spectrogram in real time. "Real time" simply means the duration of the signal itself; a real-time analysis is one conducted as the signal arrives, with no delay. (Make an allowance for the hyperbole of advertising, however.) In this section, we will use the Kay DSP 5500 Sona-Graph™ as our example. (For those who like technical details, the Kay actually uses three microprocessors: one to manage the display and respond to commands from the user, and two which are specially designed to analyze signals like speech.)

From the user's point of view, perhaps the principal advantage of current spectrographs is that the analysis is always displayed first on a monitor, like that of a computer. The user then chooses whether or not to print that display. Previously, the printer was the only display, so a user had to wait a minute or two for each analysis to be printed—even if it turned out to be a poor one. The monitor display saves a great deal of time and money. Another difference is the great flexibility in selecting analyses and displays. One chooses from menus of analysis types, frequency ranges, time scales, effective bandwidths, and other parameters. Most of these choices are not new. Previously, one could select a frequency range and print a waveform or an amplitude contour above a spectrogram, for example; but the range of possible combinations is now much greater. A third major difference is in measurement. One measures time or frequency by moving cursors on the screen, which is easier, faster, and more accurate than measuring a printed spectrogram. One prints spectrograms to document one's work, not to make measurements. In short, the main advantages are in the way one interacts with the device, not in the nature of the analysis itself.

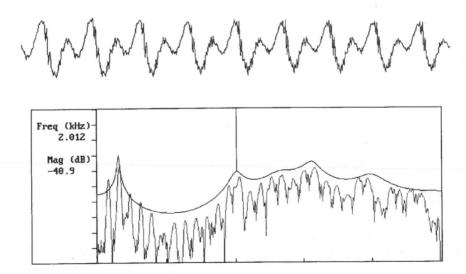

FIGURE 3–28. The same waveform as in Figure 3–27, but with an LPC spectrum overlaid on the Fourier spectrum. The cursor points to the peak of F2.

Figures 3–29 and 3–30 show one of the many possible combinations: Figure 3–29 is the documentation and Figure 3–30 the graphic display. In Figure 3–30, the spectrogram has the traditional three dimensions; it represents the utterance, "We show speech" (not the same utterance as in earlier figures). Above the spectrogram is a power spectrum (left) and a waveform (right) for the interval bounded by the vertical cursors in the spectrogram, that is, the steady-state portion of [i] of "we." The frequency cursors on the spectrum mark the first and second formants of this vowel, at 260 Hz and 1980 Hz. (Only the lower frequency cursor appears on the spectrogram.) We can answer several questions from these two displays:

- *How long is the portion of vowel between the two time cursors?*
  117 ms. In the text, under cursor readings, see ^T, the difference between the two time cursors.
- *How many periods are there in that portion of vowel?*
  About 15. In the spectrogram, count the vertical striations between the two time cursors.
- *What formant transitions precede the vowel?*

```
        KAY ELEMETRICS CORP. MODEL 5500
           SIGNAL ANALYSIS WORKSTATION
UW PHONETICS LABORATORY
Date: JANUARY   22 1989    Time:  2:17:29 PM
Analysis by:

INPUT SETTINGS      Channel 1          Channel 2
Source              LEFT CONNECTORS    LEFT CONNECTORS
Frequency Range     DC - 8 KHz.        DC - 8 KHz.
Input Shaping       HI-SHAPE           FLAT
Buffer Size         4.0 SECONDS        4.0 SECONDS

ANALYSIS SETTINGS   Lower Screen       Upper Screen
Signal Analyzed     CHANNEL 1          CHANNEL 2
Analysis Format     SPECTROGRAPHIC     POWER AT CURSORS
Transform Size      100 pts. ( 300 Hz) 1024 pts. ( 29 Hz)
Time Axis           50ms    (1sec)     12.5ms   (250ms)
Frequency Axis      FULL SCALE         FULL SCALE
Analysis Window     HAMMING            HAMMING
Averaging Set Up    NO AVERAGING       NO AVERAGING

DISPLAY SETTINGS    Lower Screen       Upper Screen
Time Divisions      .05000 Sec.        .01250 Sec.
Freq. Divisions     500.0 Hz.          500.0 Hz.
Dynamic Range       42 dB              72 dB
Analysis Atten.     20 dB              0 dB
Set Up Options Set to:  #00

CURSOR READINGS:
FC1:   260.0 Hz. , FC2:  1980. Hz.  , ^F:  1720. Hz.
FC1: -33 dB,   FC2: -49 dB,   ^F: 16 dB
^R1:  2.728 Sec.          ^R2:  2.845 Sec.
^T:  .1172 Sec.
PITCH    TC1:      Hz.  TC2:     Hz.
AMPLITUDE TC1:     dB   TC2:     dB

SUBJECT MATTER
            "We show spee(ch)"
```

FIGURE 3–29. The textual printout which accompanies Figure 3–30. Both were produced by the Kay Elemetrics model 5500 digital spectrograph.

In the spectrogram, trace F2, for example, in the vowel of *show*, between the two fricatives.

- *What is the effective bandwidth of the analysis?*
  300 Hz in the spectrogram [wide band] and 29 Hz in the spectrum [narrow band]. In the text, under Analysis Settings, see Transform size.
- *Were the high frequencies boosted before the analysis?*
  Yes for the spectrogram; no for the spectrum. In the text, under Input Settings, see Input Shaping.
- *What analysis window was applied to the sample?*
  A "Hamming" window, a particular gradual onset and offset. In the text, under Analysis Settings, see Analysis Window.
- *At what rate was the speech sampled?*
  Not answered in the display. With this spectrograph, the effective sampling rate is always 2.56 times the highest frequency displayed (8 kHz), so it was 20.48 kHz.

For many purposes, a wide-band spectrogram and narrow-band spectrum, as in Figure 3–30, is a good combination. After all, the special value of a spectrogram is to show us the dynamic changes in speech over time, so time resolution is often important. However, one can just as easily select other combinations on a digital spectrograph. For versatility, speed, and convergence of information, it seems hard to beat today's digital spectrographs. Some offer both Fourier and LPC analysis, with the ability to alter LPC parameters and resynthesize utterances, as well as to pass data to and from computers. Basic research on speech will develop even better analysis models.

We have now discussed two common short-term transforms, the FFT and LPC.

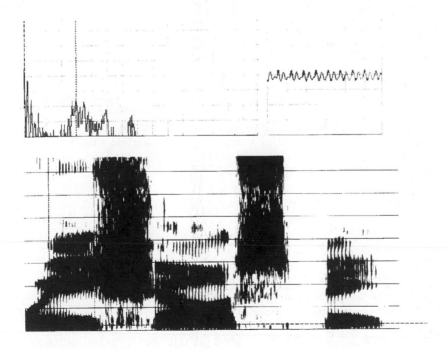

FIGURE 3–30. Spectrogram of "*We show speech,*" produced by an adult male. The two windows above the spectrogram show a Fourier spectrum of the vowel of *we* and the waveform at the beginning of that vowel.

These are useful for general analysis purposes, such as estimating formant structure of a sound. Two additional short-term transforms, **cepstrum** and **autocorrelation**, typically are used to extract the fundamental frequency and they are discussed in the next section along with other means of determining the fundamental frequency of the voice.

Determining Fundamental Frequency

One of the principal goals of speech analysis is to determine f_0, which listeners generally perceive as pitch. An earlier section of this chapter touched on the problem of extracting f_0. It was noted that there is no perfect means of making this measurement. It may be surprising, but the estimation of f_0 is by no means a simple matter, especially when the object is to make the estimation for different speakers and different speech samples. A variety of procedures have been introduced (Hess, 1982, 1992), and what follows is only a sampling of possibilities.

By Hand and by Eye

Because f_0 is the reciprocal of the fundamental period, one way of estimating f_0 is to measure successive fundamental periods. On a sound pressure waveform display such as Figure 3–17, one can measure the duration of periods and thus determine f_0, either period-by-period or as an average over time. This method can be quite accurate, but it is slow, and more important, it is not precisely reliable (repeatable). Because it depends on placing the cursors around perceived patterns, two researchers may get different results from the same data. Filtering out higher frequencies may make the fundamental periods easier to identify, but the basic problems of speed and reliability remain.

Similarly, one can measure the frequency of the fundamental on a Fourier spectrum or a spectrogram with methods discussed below. These are the frequency-domain counterparts of measuring duration by hand, and they suffer from the same defects, plus that of poor resolution in some cases. Researchers have developed many devices and programs for tracking fundamental frequency automatically, seeking one which is fast, accurate, and reliable. So far, no method has all these virtues, especially across varied speech samples.

Spectrographic Methods

A spectrogram displays the frequency components of speech over time, and one component is the fundamental frequency. Displaying f_0 on a spectrogram goes back to early publications about the spectrograph (Koenig, Dunn, & Lacy, 1946). However, the fundamental is shown quite differently in wide-band and narrow-band spectrograms. Consider again the wide-band spectrogram in Figure 3–30, specifically the vowel [i] of "we," between the cursors. We would expect to find the fundamental frequency displayed like a formant: as a dark horizontal line but at a low frequency, and indeed there is a dark line at the bottom of the spectrogram of this vowel. However, the digital filter which produced this spectrogram had a bandwidth of 300 Hz, that is, it resonated to excitation over that range of frequency. In this case, that filter responded to both the fundamental and its second harmonic at the same time; they have been smeared together. Worse yet, this vowel has a low first formant (F1), which also affects that lowest 300 Hz bandwidth. Thus the dark bar at the bottom of the spectrogram includes these three sources of sound; we cannot identify f_0 within it.

However, the fundamental *is* reflected in the voiced segments of Figure 3–30; note the vertical bars in the three vowels of "We show speech." Since darkness on a spectrogram represents the amplitude of the spectrum, a dark vertical striation represents a moment of relatively great amplitude across a range of frequencies. In fact, each of these striations represents the resonating of the air in the vocal tract in response to a glottal pulse. (The resonation actually starts at each closure of the glottis.) These striations gradually become farther apart in the vowel of "speech," indicating the falling pitch at the end of this utterance. In the vowel of "we," there are fifteen striations between the cursors: fifteen glottal pulses. The time between the cursors (^T in Figure 3–29) is 0.117 seconds. The number of pulses divided by the time in seconds yields the number of pulses per second. In this case 15/0.117 = 128 Hz, the average pitch during this vowel.

This method of determining fundamental frequency has the same problems of speed and reliability as measuring glottal periods in the time domain. It is only as precise as our ability to count the vertical bars and to place the cursors at their edges, the boundaries of glottal periods. In this

case, we could have achieved greater precision by expanding the time scale, separating the striations further. We can best obtain an average f_0 over time, spreading the measurement error over several periods. Fortunately, an average is often just what we want.

Narrow-band Spectrograms

We cannot see the fundamental directly in Figure 3–30 because the analyzing filter has too great a bandwidth, so let us narrow the bandwidth. Figure 3–31 shows two spectrograms of "Yes" spoken with a rise-fall intonation. The upper one is a *narrow-band* spectrogram. Having separated each span of 59 Hz, we can now see the fundamental and its harmonics as equally-spaced horizontal lines within the broader formants. The rising-falling pattern is especially clear

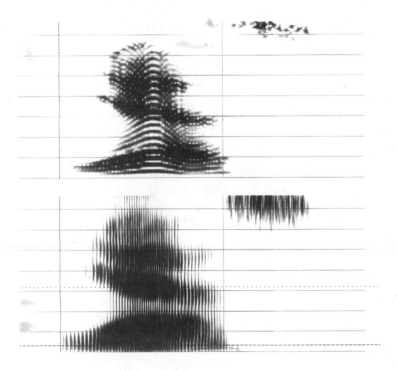

FIGURE 3–31. A wide-band (lower) and narrow-band spectrogram of *yes*, spoken with a rise–fall intonation. The analysis bandwidths are 300 Hz and 59 Hz, respectively.

— narrow band
good for pitch over time

in the mid-frequency harmonics. A narrow-band spectrogram is particularly good for seeing a pattern of pitch change over time.

We can quantify f_0 from this display by measuring the frequency of the fundamental or one of its harmonics, each an integer multiple of the fundamental. If possible, we choose one of the harmonics, such as the tenth. In Figure 3–31, the lowest bar is the fundamental, with a peak at 160 Hz, and its tenth harmonic has a peak at 1600 Hz, just above the fourth horizontal grid line (1500 Hz). We measure its frequency (by moving a horizontal cursor) and divide by 10 to obtain f_0. Our measurement errors are also divided by ten, so they will be one-tenth as large as if we measured f_0 itself. Being multiples of the fundamental, the harmonics change more rapidly: H10 changes 10 times as much as f_0 in the same period of time. If we look only at the harmonics, changes in pitch appear more dramatic than they really are, but after we divide, the measurements are correct.

For measuring f_0 or one of its low harmonics, the higher frequencies are irrele-vant. One can change the frequency scale displayed on a spectrograph in order to "zoom in" on the relevant lower frequencies. Figure 3–32 shows the same word and the same intonation pattern as in Figure 3–31, but limited to 0–250 Hz and with an even narrower-bandwidth analysis. With the fundamental (and parts of the second harmonic) filling the screen, we can both visualize and measure the change more precisely.

The digital spectrograph on which these figures were created also has a program for computing and plotting fundamental frequency. In Figure 3–33 a wide-band spectrogram of "yes" is in the bottom half, while a sound-pressure waveform is centered in the top half. Under the waveform are three intersecting lines. The dashed line that is lowest during the vowel but rises high during the fricative is a count of zero crossings (the number of times that the waveform crosses the zero point). The dotted line that falls almost to zero during the fricative is amplitude. The dashed line that appears only during the loudest part of

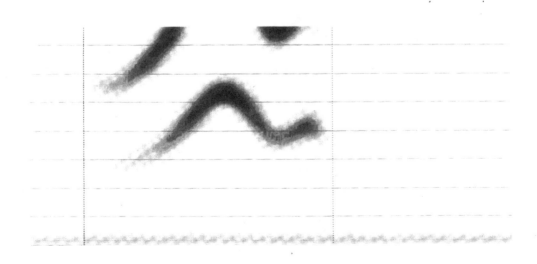

FIGURE 3–32.   A narrow-band spectrogram of the same intonation contour as shown in Figure 3–31, but for the frequency range from 0 to 250 Hz only. The result shows the contour of f_0 and parts of the second harmonic.

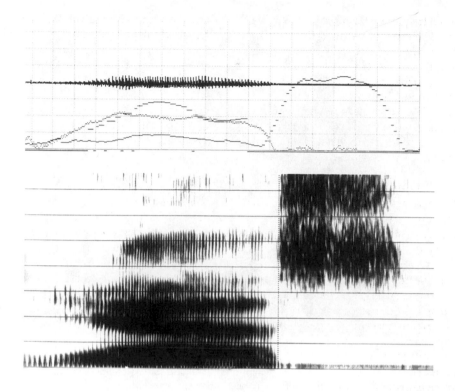

FIGURE 3–33. The "combination" display of the Kay 5500 spectrograph. The lower channel is a wideband spectrogram of "*yes*," spoken with rise–fall-rise intonation. The upper channel shows the speech waveform above traces which represent zero crossings, amplitude, and fundamental frequency. These traces are distinguished by color on the monitor of the spectrograph.

the vowel (rising, falling, and finally rising a bit) is the fundamental frequency.

Dedicated Devices

Some stand-alone devices graph fundamental frequency and amplitude in "real time" (that is, as fast as the speech is produced). Two well known ones are the Kay Visi-Pitch™ and the Voice Identification PM Pitch Analyzer™, both of which measure f_0 period-by-period. Such devices are speedy, portable, and relatively easy to use, but they are not entirely accurate. A typical error is to double the true f_0; this error is often easy to detect, because it produces a few points that are substantially out of line with the rest. Precisely because these

devices are independent, it can be difficult to align and integrate their displays with those from a spectrograph or a computer. Figure 3–34 shows the pitch and amplitude contours of an utterance as displayed by a PM Pitch Analyzer.

Computational Methods

In addition to using spectrographs and other devices designed specifically to analyze speech, researchers are now programming ordinary computers to track fundamental frequency in a speech signal. There are many types of such programs, for the simple reason that none of them is perfect. Like the dedicated devices, these programs make characteristic errors, such as

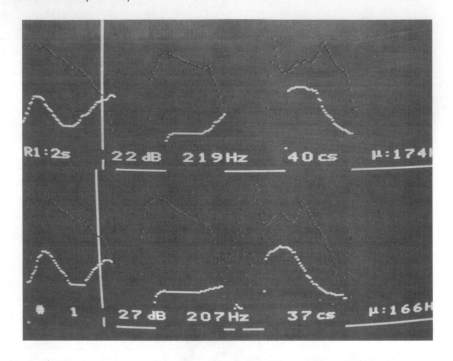

FIGURE 3–34. Fundamental frequency (white) and amplitude (black) contours on the display of a Voice Identification PM Pitch Analyzer. The numbers represent amplitude, f_0, and time at the points marked by the cursors.

confusing F1 with f_0, doubling the frequency of f_0, finding a fundamental frequency in unvoiced parts of the signal, or failing to find it in voiced portions. In this section, we will survey just three approaches, as examples: cepstral analysis, autocorrelation analysis, and pattern recognition, a more general alternative.

Cepstral Analysis

A method of f_0 analysis developed since the mid-1960s is known as **cepstral** analysis, pronounced /ˈkɛpstrəl/. This technique starts with a speech signal and applies a Fourier transform to yield a spectrum such as that in Figure 3–27. The harmonics displayed in such spectra are periodic, that is, they recur at a regular interval. In fact, that interval is the fundamental frequency, as the harmonics are at multiples of the fun-

damental. We could measure that interval by hand, moving the cursor to each harmonic. In Figure 3–27, we would find that the harmonics are 127 Hz apart: f_0 is at 127 Hz, H2 at 254 (as shown), H3 at 381, and so on. Cepstral analysis is primarily a way of recovering that interval precisely and automatically.

Consider the spectrum in Figure 3–27. Its units (amplitude vs. frequency) are different from those of Figure 3–17 (pressure vs. time), but it is certainly a periodic waveform, so the Fourier theorem is applicable. To separate the frequency components of the pressure waveform in Figure 3–17, we applied a Fourier transform, producing Figure 3–27, its spectrum. If we now apply a Fourier transform again to the periodic waveform in Figure 3–27, we will separate *its* components, of which the main one is the fundamental period. (Actually, we apply the Fourier transform to a *log power spectrum*, that is, a spectrum of the logarithms of the squared and summed complex numbers that make up a basic Fourier spectrum.) The result of such a transformation (on a different sample) is shown in Figure 3–35, and sure enough, there is a spike at one component.

We suspect that this component corresponds to the fundamental period, but what are the units of Figure 3–35? A Fourier transformation moves between the time domain (a time axis) and the frequency domain (a frequency axis). By applying the same transformation again, cepstral analysis reverses that: we start with a time axis (the sound pressure waveform), transform to a frequency axis (the Fourier spectrum), and then transform back to a time axis (the cepstrum). Thus, the horizontal axis of Figure 3–35 is measured in milliseconds. The spike is at about 8.5 ms, the period of a fundamental frequency of 118 Hz.

To indicate that these units are those of cepstral analysis, they have been given their own names (Noll, 1967). "**Cepstrum**" is just "spectrum" with the first syllable read backwards (because cepstral analysis reverses a spectrum, in a sense). The corresponding time unit is "**quefrency**," that is, "frequency" with the first two syllables reversed (because it is the Fourier inverse of the frequency axis of a spectrum). Other units in cepstral analysis are named similarly: "harmonics" become "**rahmonics**," which are the low-quefrency components in Figure 3–35. The names may be an excess of cleverness, but the result is clear: the quefrency peak in Figure 3–35 represents the fundamental period in the original speech.

Cepstral analysis requires quite a lot of computing: taking the Fourier transform of a log power Fourier spectrum of the original signal, to obtain just one f_0 measurement. However, with Fast Fourier Transforms and more powerful but inexpensive computers, it has become practical to perform cepstral analysis of longer stretches of speech data, plotting the changes in fundamental period over time automatically and accurately. Moreover, improvements in the computational algorithm have made cepstral analyses more robust in the face of noise. Ahmadi and Spanias (1999) describe a modified cepstrum-based method that performed very well on a large voice database. Although

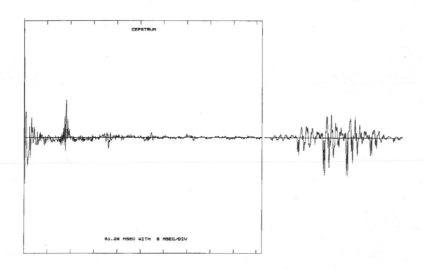

FIGURE 3–35. Cepstrum in box and the windowed waveform on which it was calculated. The peak is at the fundamental period.

this discussion emphasizes the use of the cepstrum for determining f_0, there are other applications of this transform that make it of considerable interest in modern speech science and speech technology.

Autocorrelation

Two series of numbers are said to be highly correlated if they increase and decrease together. Such a series of numbers might be the hourly temperatures for yesterday and today, for example. If the temperature followed the same pattern of increases and decreases from hour to hour, the two lists of numbers would be highly correlated, even if yesterday was, say, much colder than today. When we sample a speech signal digitally, we get a series of numbers, each one representing the amplitude of the sound pressure waveform at a particular moment, as graphed in the upper channel of Figure 3–36.

To say that this waveform is periodic is to say that there is a repeated pattern of increases and decreases. If we were to compute the correlation between this waveform and an exact copy of the waveform (thus *auto*correlation), the two copies would, of course, be perfectly correlated. But what if we computed the correlation of this signal with a slightly delayed copy of itself, as between the top and middle channels in Figure 3–36? The correlation would be highest when the delay, known as the *lag*, was close to one pitch period, as between the top and bottom channels in Figure 3–36. If we compute the correlations at lags which range over probable pitch periods (say, from 20 ms to 3 ms, corresponding to 50 to 300 Hz in f_0), we would see peaks in the correlations at the actual pitch period (and its multiples). This is the essential idea of autocorrelation pitch analysis. It works because in voiced speech, formant structure does not change drastically within a few milliseconds, so that successive periods resemble each other. In unvoiced sounds such as [f] or [s], on the other hand, the quality does change rapidly because of the aperiodic noise source, so autocorrelation

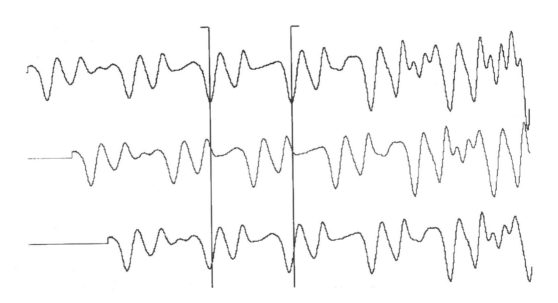

FIGURE 3–36. Vowel waveform (top channel) with two lagged copies of itself. The cursors mark one fundamental period in the top channel and approximately one period in the lower channels.

over a short term will normally yield no regular peaks. Of course, even voiced speech is only *quasi*-periodic; it does change somewhat in quality (and pitch) from period to period. Relatively slow change does not disturb autocorrelation analysis, however, because of the remaining overall similarity from period to period.

Unfortunately, autocorrelation in this simple form applied to a "raw" speech signal does not work particularly well. The formants also affect the location of correlation peaks, so that a common error is to find, not the glottal period, but the glottal period plus the period of the first or second formant. Research since the 1960s has been devoted to preprocessing the signal to reduce the influence of the formants. A simple method is low-pass filtering to effectively eliminate formants at frequencies higher than the highest expected f_0. Much more sophisticated techniques, beyond the scope of this introduction, are also used. To mention one improvement, autocorrelation functions are calculated for a particular time point using multiple lengths of the analysis windows and then weighting the candidates of the pitch period obtained from the different windows (Takagi, Seiyama, & Miyasaka, 2000). In addition, the autocorrelation function can be computed on different versions of the signal, such as the center-clipped signal or the inverse filtered signal. Any adaptation must confront two basic problems: formant structure does change over time (sometimes rapidly), which disrupts autocorrelation analysis by changing the shape of the waveform, and the frequency of F1 is in some instances lower than f_0, so that simply filtering the signal will not always work. Despite these difficulties, autocorrelation is one of the more reliable methods of determining fundamental frequency, and a number of procedures can be considered.

Pattern Recognition

All these relatively elaborate methods have limitations. We are tempted to return to the basic observation with which we started: that the periodicity of voiced speech is evident in repeated patterns in the sound-pressure waveform. Consider, for example, Figure 3–37: its four channels display the waveforms of [i], [æ], [ɔ], and [u], the vowels of "bead," "bad," "baud," and "booed," respectively. In each, we see a shape that is repeated from five to seven times across the screen; that shape varies from vowel to vowel. Can we not somehow find such periods automatically from the waveform alone, without first finding a spectrum, a cepstrum, or an autocorrelation? Can computers learn to recognize the pattern that our "eye" sees at once?

This is a case of pattern recognition, a process which is central to research in artificial intelligence. We begin to see the difficulty when we try to state an explicit procedure, such as: "Put the cursors at two successive peaks," (or "two successive valleys"). There are many peaks and valleys in a speech waveform; how do we state which ones? If we said, "two peaks that *match*," we would have to state a criterion for *matching*, which is exactly the difficulty. If we said, "two successive *major* peaks," we would have to distinguish the "major" ones without relying circularly on the notion we are trying to explicate—that of "pattern."

Most approaches to this problem first simplify the waveform. One way is to low-pass filter at several hundred hertz, higher than any likely fundamental frequency, unless our speaker is an infant. That removes many of the local peaks by removing the effects of higher formants. Figure 3–38 displays a vowel waveform (top channel) and that same waveform filtered at 850 Hz (middle channel). An alternative simplification is to "peak-clip" the waveform, leaving only the peaks or valleys, as in the bottom channel of Figure 3–38. (Just reduce all values to zero unless they exceed a certain threshold.) Another simplification is to ask the human operator for an estimate. If the program knows that the right answer lies in the vicinity of 100 Hz, it can rule out peaks which are much too close or too far apart.

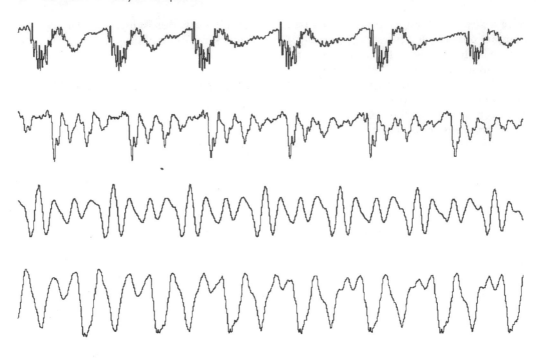

FIGURE 3–37. Speech waveforms of [i], [æ], [ɔ], and [u] (top to bottom channels). In each waveform, one can see five to six fundamental periods.

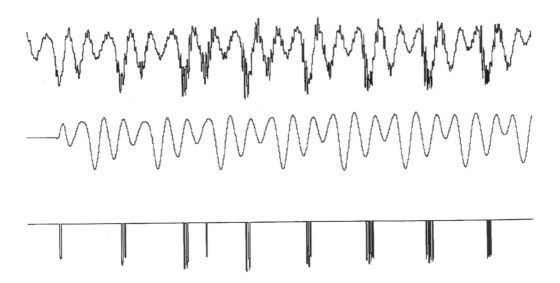

FIGURE 3–38. Top channel: speech waveform of the vowel [i]. Middle channel: the same waveform low-pass filtered at 850 Hz. Bottom channel: the same waveform amplitude-clipped, so that only negative peaks remain.

The analysis then proceeds to identify candidate peaks, zero crossings, or valleys. Because this process is by no means foolproof, there are various elaborations. Ideally, these methods find the period (and thereby the frequency) of *each* glottal period. That can be an advantage over autocorrelation or frequency-domain analysis, which must deal with at least several periods. Even when this analysis succeeds, however, it is not doing what a human being does. We do not look for just peaks, valleys, and zero crossings; we recognize a similarity in overall shape from period to period.

Comparisons of Different Methods

The most reliable approaches to tracking fundamental frequency today are those which use more than one method and then select a median (central) or modal (most frequent) value. Of course, these multiple analyses require more computing, but they offset the weaknesses of one method with the strengths of another. Different methods tend to fail in different situations, so the right answer is likely to be prominent within a set computed in several ways.

However, it is still relevant to ask if some algorithms are superior to others for certain purposes or conditions. Parsa and Jamieson (1999) compared seven algorithms designed to yield high precision estimates of f_0. They used different kinds of signals, including varying f_0, varying levels of noise, varying shimmer, and varying jitter, and they also compared the different algorithms for analyzing both normal and pathologic voices. They concluded that the waveform matching function (a pattern recognition procedure) is preferred for voice perturbation measures of both normal and pathologic samples. This method was quite robust in the face of both shimmer and jitter, but it was affected by signal-to-noise ratios lower than 15 dB. The Parsa and Jamieson article is a good reference to

consult when making a decision about algorithms for extracting f_0.

Recovering the Glottal Waveform

Sensing the Motion of the Glottis

One way to improve the accuracy of almost any method of tracking fundamental frequency is to start with the waveform at the glottis rather than at the lips. Plotting the glottal waveform is of value also in testing the source–filter view of speech production and in studying abnormalities of the vocal folds and in voicing. Phoneticians have observed the glottal waveform directly by passing tiny microphones down toward their glottises. This technique is not only uncomfortable but dangerous; if the fine wires holding the microphone should break, it may drop all the way into the lungs. There are now ways to pick up the glottal waveform externally. One is the *electroglottograph* (EGG), which tracks the motion of the vocal folds by passing radio-frequency waves through the larynx and measuring changes in impedance caused by the opening and closing of the folds. EGG can be used to determine a number of properties of vocal fold vibration (Abberton, Howard, & Fourcin, 1989; Childers, Hicks, Moore, Eskenazi, & Lalwani, 1990; Hertegard & Gauffin, 1995). A promising new technique is electromagnetic glottography (Titze et al., 2000). Even a simple and inexpensive *accelerometer*, a small contact microphone in effect, can measure the motion of the surface of the throat as it is pushed in and out by the pressure above or below the glottis. Figure 3–39 shows the sound pressure waveform of a vowel [a] (top channel) and the simultaneous motion of the throat as transduced by an accelerometer taped to the front of the throat below the larynx (middle channel). Fundamental frequency can be observed and measured more reliably in the latter by most methods.

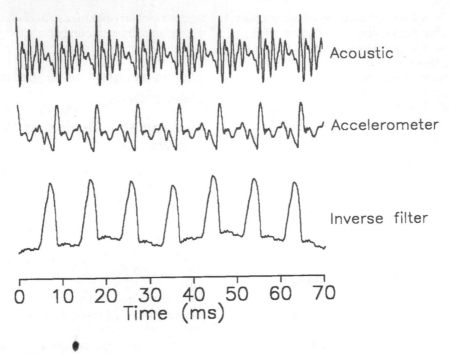

FIGURE 3–39.   Top channel: speech waveform of the vowel [a]. Middle channel: output of accelerometer placed on the outside of the throat, just below the larynx. Lower channel: the waveform in the top channel after LPC analysis and inverse filtering to estimate the glottal airflow waveform.

Inverse Filtering

Another approach is based on the source-filter view of speech presented in Chapter 3. Recall that in this view, the spectrum of sound at the glottis is filtered by the transfer function of the vocal tract and the lips. In other words, the speech signal that radiates from our lips has a spectrum which is just that transfer function applied to the spectrum produced at the glottis. If we could undo the effect of the transfer function, we would recover the glottal spectrum, where the fundamental frequency is quite obvious, because the action of the vocal folds is by far the greatest perturbation in the flow of air at that point.

From X-ray films we know quite a lot about the shape of the vocal tract and therefore its transfer function in the normal production of most speech sounds (in English and some other languages, at least). If we compute a transfer function appropriate to a given steady-state stretch of speech, take its inverse, apply that inverse to the spectrum of the radiated speech, and then compute the waveform corresponding to that spectrum, we do indeed get a waveform which corresponds closely to the pressure waveform at the glottis. The bottom channel in Figure 3–39 shows the underlying glottal waveform as estimated by inverse filtering of the vowel waveform in the top channel. Note that when the glottis closes (where this trace falls sharply), pressure *below* the glottis rises, as shown in the middle channel. Again, measuring fundamental frequency or computing its contour over time is relatively easy in the estimated glottal waveform, because the effects of the transfer function, the resonances, are gone.

As you might expect, inverse filtering is computationally demanding, and it is still being developed. It requires a signal with accurate reproduction of low frequencies. You cannot apply inverse filtering to tape recordings from ordinary microphones, let alone from telephones, for instance. However, inverse filtering can provide noninvasive evidence of glottal and laryngeal abnormalities as well as help track fundamental frequency.

Looking to the Future: Chaos Theory, Fractals, and Wavelets

Although these analytic tools are not commonly used today—and are not generally available with commercial systems for the analysis of speech—they may well be major choices in the future. Therefore, it is appropriate to comment briefly on these analyses. These approaches are based on the idea that speech is a nonlinear process, which is a very different view taken so far in this chapter. The standard form of the source-filter theory discussed in Chapter 2 is that speech is produced by a biologic system that is linear and time invariant. However, as noted in the final section of that chapter, some writers advocate a nonlinear approach to theory and analysis. Chaos theory has swept through virtually all sciences, physical, biologic, and social.

Only selected examples of these analyses are considered here. Banbrook, McLaughlin, and Mann (1999) explored the analysis of sustained vowels with a range of invariant geometric features developed to analyze chaotic systems. They concluded that although voiced speech could be characterized by a small number of dimensions, it is not necessarily chaotic. Sabanal and Nakagawa (1996) also reported that fractal properties are an effective way to analyze speech sounds, including both vowels and consonants if time-dependent fractal dimensions are used in the analyses.

Recording Speech: Basic Requirements

This chapter concludes with a brief description of what is usually the beginning of speech analysis—the essentials of speech recording. This reverse chronology is justified by the fact that issues in recording of speech reflect some of the topics addressed in the discussion of speech analysis. Ultimately, analyses of speech are limited by the quality of the recordings of speech signals. All too often, poor quality of recording limits or even precludes some potentially interesting analyses.

The design of a laboratory for acoustic recordings and acoustic analysis should consider several issues, including the recording environment, the recording equipment and medium, storage requirements, and expectations for types and amount of analysis. Each of these is considered briefly. Also see Gopal (1995).

Recording Environment

A first step that can be critically important to the success of any attempts to record speech signals is to evaluate the recording environment and remedy any problems that might be noted. Background noise from several sources can contaminate speech recordings. Some sources are: fluorescent lighting; paging systems; nearby bathrooms, corridors, and elevators; playgrounds or parks; heavily traveled roadways; and electronic equipment (including personal computers). Environmental noise can severely limit the accuracy of acoustic analysis, especially for the perturbation measures of jitter and shimmer (Ingrisano, Perry, & Jepson, 1998) When it is not possible to eliminate sources of undesirable noise, it may be feasible to make recordings at times when the noise is reduced in intensity or is less likely to occur (such as early mornings or evenings). If nothing can be done to eliminate a noise in the recording environment, then filtering may be considered as a way of eliminating the undesired acoustic energy.

Even if extraneous sources of sound are not present, other problems can occur. One of these is *reverberation*, or sound reflected within the recording room. For some applications, reverberation can be a considerable problem (Bachety, 1998). Reverberation can be especially troublesome for rooms that have hard parallel surfaces (a typical situation in most buildings). Sound waves are bounced back and forth in rooms of this kind, causing a condition known as *"slap echo"* that is especially disruptive for high frequencies. Another reflection problem, called *"near-field reflections"* results when a recording microphone is located close to a hard surface. Therefore, it is often better to place a microphone near the center of a room rather than close to a wall.

Recording Equipment and Medium

Several different types of microphones are available. Although some users prefer a full-size microphone mounted on a table top or a microphone stand, there is good reason to consider a *miniature head-mounted condenser microphone*. Modern microphones of this type can ensure high-quality recordings even when the speaker changes head or body position. Winholtz and Titze (1997) reported on a microphone of this type that is well suited to general recording needs. These microphones and their head mounts are light and usually can be worn comfortably for long periods if necessary.

Type of recorder and medium are joint decisions. Among the choices are: (1) *analog tape recorders* with either reel-to-reel tapes or cassette tapes; (2) a *digital audio tape (DAT) recorder*; (3) a *CD-ROM*, or (4) a *digital disk*. For most purposes, a DAT recorder will provide satisfactory results. DAT recorders are available with different sampling rates, but most users should be satisfied with a sampling rate of 44.1 kHz and either 16- or 32-bit conversion. A 16-bit conversion permits 65,536 levels of amplitude to be represented in the digitized speech sample. DAT recorders have controls that are highly similar to those on analog tape recorders. Therefore, most users adapt quickly to the digital technology.

For recordings of high quality, sampling rates should be higher than 8 kHz. Bettagere and Fucci (1999) reported that listener-rated quality was superior for digitized speech sampled at 16 kHz compared to analog tape-recorded speech. When a sampling rate of 8 kHz was used for digitized speech, the quality was essentially equal to that of analog tape-recorded speech.

Ideally, recordings of speech would last indefinitely. However, recordings deteriorate with time, especially in environments with high temperatures and humidities. Both analog and digital tapes are metal particle tapes that are subject to eventual deterioration (Speliotis & Peter, 1991). For magnetic media generally, deterioration can be detected within 5 to 8 years after recordings are made (Leek, 1995). It should not be assumed that DAT affords a relatively permanent storage of recorded information. Although control of temperature and humidity will extend the accuracy of the recorded information, errors ultimately will contaminate the quality of the recorded data. A permanent acoustic archive would have to be based on other recording media, but these are not typically used in general-purpose speech recordings.

Conclusion

In this chapter we have presented some of the current techniques for analyzing speech. These techniques are continuously changing; in both spectral and fundamental frequency analysis, new mathematical approaches and new ways of displaying the signal and its components have been appearing regularly. The excitement of speech science today is not only in new understanding of speech and new practical applications of that understanding, but also in new ways to gain understanding. Similarly, the motivation for all this development has at least three sources: the basic desire to understand a central human activity, the desire to develop better therapy for speech that has somehow gone wrong, and considerable commercial interest in speech synthesis and speech recognition. In particular, the difficulty of programming machines to recognize speech has forced us to recognize that what we thought we knew about speech even five years ago was incomplete.

One example can illustrate the unsolved problems: a child, a woman, and a man can each say the same sentence with the same intonation, and each can recognize that they have done so. Therefore, the three utterances must have something in common. Yet all of the techniques surveyed in this chapter cannot define what that commonality is, at least not in such a general way that we can design a machine which can recognize words in context spoken by any normal speaker. Notice that if we could do so, we would have a general transcriber, a hearing machine for the deaf, and other devices that respond to complex spoken commands. All these practical goals and many others help to energize speech science today.

As a result of that energy, the ideas in this chapter, even more than those in some others, are subject to change. That is part of the excitement of contemporary speech analysis.

Summary

This chapter began with a brief review of the history of the acoustic analysis of speech. The history is largely one of analog instrumentation. The dominant equipment today is digital. Anyone who would use modern methods of acoustic analysis, therefore, should understand the basic principles of digital signal processing. This chapter discussed basic operations of digitization and selected analyses that are used in the digital signal processing of speech. Particular attention has been given to a number of different analysis methods that provide information on the temporal and spectral properties of speech sounds. Forthcoming chapters summarize the results of these analyses for various aspects of speech (vowels and diphthongs in Chapter 4, consonants in Chapter 5, speaker variables in Chapter 6, and suprasegmental properties in Chapter 7).

The Acoustic Characteristics of Vowels and Diphthongs

4

CHAPTER

Part I: Vowels

General Issues in Vowel Production and Perception

In some respects, the vowels are the simplest sounds to analyze and describe acoustically. At least in the traditional understanding, vowels are associated with a steady-state articulatory configuration and a steady-state acoustic pattern. Supposedly, then, a vowel can be indefinitely prolonged as an articulatory or acoustic phenomenon. In this view, it is not necessary to consider the time dimension beyond choosing an instant that is taken as representative of the vowel production. Theoretically, one could take a single glottal pulse as defining the vowel because this pulse would reflect the vocal tract resonances associated with a particular vowel. In addition, vowels often have been characterized with a very simple set of acoustic descriptors, namely, the frequencies of the first three formants, as shown in Figure 4–1. A given vowel could therefore be represented as a single point in a three-dimensional space defined by the F1, F2, and F3 frequencies.

Assuming that a vowel is adequately represented by just one time sample and by the frequencies of its first three formants, about all that is needed to characterize the vowels in American English is a three-dimensional chart showing the formant-frequency values of each vowel. In fact, an even simpler representation often is used—the two-dimensional vowel chart that shows the frequencies of only the first two formants F1 and F2. The F1–F2 chart, like the one shown in Figure 4–2, is perhaps the most widely used and best known acoustic description of a class of speech sounds. Almost every introductory textbook that touches on the acoustic properties of speech includes this chart in some form. In the following sections, we consider the degree to which such a simplified description suffices for the acoustic description of vowels.

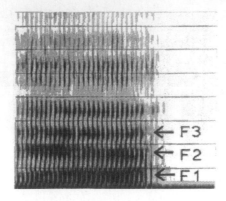

FIGURE 4–1. Spectrogram of the vowel æ, with arrows pointing to the first three formants F1, F2, and F3. The thin lines in the horizontal grid represent frequency intervals of 1kHz.

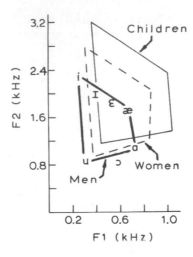

FIGURE 4–2. F1–F2 chart showing the vowel quadrilaterals for men (labeled with phonetic symbols), women, and children.

Simple Target Model

The classic view of vowels and their perception may be termed the *simple target model*. This model assumes that the vowel exists in a canonical form that is invariant across phonetic contexts and is sufficiently defined by a static vocal-tract shape or by a point in the F1–F2 plane (or, alternatively, by a point in the 3-dimensional F1–F2–F3 space). This model is implicitly assumed in many introductory (and some not-so-introductory) accounts of vowels. This model is not without limitations or difficulties. First, as becomes immediately evident in any F1-F2 chart that includes data for speakers who differ in age and sex, vowels that are heard to be phonetically equivalent by listeners very often have marked differences in their formant frequency values. A classical portrayal of the acoustic diversity for a given vowel is reproduced in Figure 4–3, which shows the F1 and F2 frequencies for several vowels produced by a sample of 76 speakers including men, women, and children. As explained in Chapter 2, these differences are to be expected from acoustic theory in that the resonance frequencies of a pipe are determined in part by the length of the pipe. The longer the pipe, the lower are the resonance frequencies. Obviously, a F1–F2 chart like that shown in Figure 4–3 does not give clear support for the simple vowel target model. This model can work only if some form of speaker normalization is applied. Speaker normalization for vowels refers to a process which eliminates, or corrects for, interspeaker differences in vowel formant frequencies. The process typically involves a scaling transform. Normalization is not a trivial problem, and continuing efforts are being made to identify a reliable solution, especially with the rapid development of machine speech recognition. This problem is considered in more detail later in this chapter and in Chapter 6.

Temporal or dynamic variations are another difficulty for the simple vowel target model. One limitation is the model's inability to account for the phenomenon of target undershoot (Lindblom, 1963). This phenomenon is illustrated in Figure 4–4, which shows the formant patterns for a vowel produced in isolation and the "same" vowel produced in a CVC syllable. Note that the F2 frequency achieved in the CVC syllable does not reach the "target" value determined from the isolated vowel. It appears that the vowel in the CVC syllable undershoots the target. In fact, X-ray data on vowel articulation and acoustic data for vowels confirm that such undershoot effects are abundant in speech. Therefore, the F1-F2 points for a speaker's productions of the same vowel in different contexts will display a range of values. The simple vowel target model must account for this variation. One possible solution is to propose that listeners compensate for the acoustic undershoot by a perceptual overshoot that essentially corrects for the acoustic discrepancy (Lindblom, 1963).

A close acoustic analysis of vowels reveals that they differ not only in the formant frequency values of their steady-state portions but in several other respects as well. For example, Lehiste and Peterson (1961) found that vowels differ from one another in the following ways:

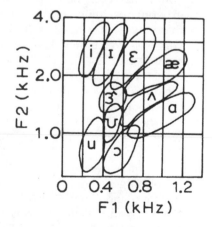
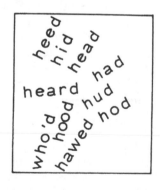

FIGURE 4–3. (Left) F1–F2 chart showing vowel ellipses that enclose the majority of the F1 and F2 frequencies reported by Peterson and Barney (1952) for vowels produced by men, women, and children. F2 frequency scale is logarithmic. (Right) Key words for vowels are positioned so as to correspond to the F1–F2 ellipses at the left.

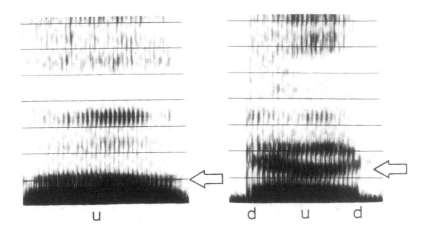

FIGURE 4–4. Spectrographic illustration of vowel undershoot. A sustained, isolated production of vowel /u/ at the left is taken as a target pattern. The production of the same vowel in the syllable /dud/ at the right shows a higher F2 frequency for /u/ than occurs in the target pattern. This difference is called *undershoot* and reflects the effects of phonetic context.

1. Vowels have inherent differences in duration. Long or tense vowels have greater durations than short or lax vowels, and vowels produced with a relatively open jaw position (the "low" or "open" vowels) are longer than vowels produced with a relatively close jaw position (the "high" or "close" vowels).

2. When vowels are produced in context with other sounds, they differ in their formant trajectories. For example, tense vowels tend to have proportionately short offglides (vowel-to-consonant transitions) and long steady states. Lax vowels, on the other hand, tend to have proportionately long offglides and short steady states.

Work by DiBenedetto (1989a and b) also casts doubt on the suitability of the simple target model. She reported that a target defined by the time at which F1 reaches its maximum frequency is not an invariant attribute of the vowel. Rather, the temporal pattern of F1 had to be taken into account to determine an invariant correlate of vowel articulation. Her research showed that lower vowels are associated with higher F1 onset frequencies and F1 maxima near the onset of the vocalic portion of a syllable. These results indicate that a single F1 property, such as F1 maximum frequency, is not sufficient to make distinctions of vowel height.

These temporal or dynamic differences are not addressed by the simple target model. That such differences are relevant to vowels has been demonstrated in several experiments. In one of these, it was shown that vowels in context could be identified very well even if only their transitional segments were presented (the steady state segments were edited out). In fact, vowel identification was about equally accurate when only the transitions were presented or when only the steady state segments were presented (Jenkins, Strange, & Edman, 1983).

Another test of the adequacy of the simple target model was performed by Hillenbrand and Gayvert (1993), who synthesized steady state vowels using the fundamental frequency and formant frequency data reported by Peterson and Barney (1952). The synthesized tokens were presented to listeners for vowel identification. If the simple target model is correct, then very high rates of identification would be expected, because the essential acoustic information is available to the listeners. But, Hillenbrand and Gayvert reported an identification error rate of 27.3%, more than four times the 5.6% error rate that Peterson and Barney obtained for their listeners who identified vowels produced naturally. Hillenbrand and Gayvert explained this large difference in error rate in terms of the dynamic cues that aid vowel identification.

Elaborated Target Models

In recognition of these limitations of the simple target model, some writers have proposed other models that can be called elaborated target models. Most of these account primarily for the problem of speaker normalization. A usual solution is to transform the acoustic measurements of vowel formants to a perceptual or psychophysical space. Such a space may have dimensions scaled in mels or Barks (these transformations are defined in Appendix C). The idea behind these efforts is that the auditory system accomplishes a normalization of the acoustic data. Therefore, a transform similar to that supposedly applied by the auditory system will solve the normalization problem. The Bark transform is considered later in this chapter.

Dynamic Specification Model

Strange (1987) believed that neither the simple target model nor the elaborated target model could adequately account for vowel perception. She proposed instead a dynamic specification model in which temporal or dynamic information, as well as steady state information, is used to identify vowels. Included in this information is the nature of the formant transitions into and out of a vowel steady state and the duration of the steady state. Obviously, a simple F1-F2 chart cannot adequately represent a vowel sound according to this theory. What is needed is a representation that includes temporally defined spectral information. That is, vowels should not be conceptualized as formant steady states but rather as formant histories.

Vowel Identification: Templates versus Constructed Patterns

The foregoing discussion introduced the problem of vowel normalization. We can phrase the basic question quite simply: If speakers differ in the acoustic properties of their vowels, then how is it that a listener knows which vowel a given speaker is trying to produce?

One answer to this question, as given by Joos (1948), is that a listener actively constructs idiosyncratic vowel patterns for each speaker. These patterns, or reference frames, can be developed on the basis of a small number of utterances from that person. According to the reference frame hypothesis, the general acoustic context of a vowel provides the essential information from which the listener can construct a referential vowel space for a given speaker. One possibility is to estimate vocal tract length from the average F3 frequency (Claes, Dologlou, Tenbosch, & Vancompernolle, 1998). Then, vowels produced by that speaker are interpreted within the vowel space. A variant of this idea is that listeners construct the referential vowel space on the basis of a speaker's vowel [i] (as in *he*). This vowel has special distinctive properties that make it a good "calibration" vowel (Matthei & Roeper, 1983). A weakness of this concept is that listeners cannot always wait for a speaker to produce vowel [i]. The warning, "Look out for that car," as it might be yelled by a passerby who notices a recklessly driven car, does not contain the handy calibration vowel. The endangered listener who waits for vowel [i] may well wait into eternity.

An alternative idea is that listeners acquire vowel templates based on their long-term experiences with the speech of various persons. These templates are like acoustic averages determined for men, women, and children (Bergem, Pols, & Koopmans-van Beinum, 1988). When listeners try to identify a vowel, they match the unknown vowel with an appropriate template vowel that is an average for men, women, or children. The appropriate template is selected on the basis of the pitch and timbre of the unknown vowel. Bergem et al. (1988) argue that the template theory is supported by the fact that listeners can identify with considerable accuracy even single vowels (without context) produced by any speaker (men, women, or children).

Acoustic Description of Vowels

With these models as a backdrop, we now consider the acoustic specification of vowels. The candidate parameters for the acoustic description are formant pattern, spectrum, duration, and fundamental frequency. A further choice is the scale used for expression of frequency measurements. As noted in Chapter 3, linear scales of frequency traditionally have been assumed for speech analysis. However, it is well known that the human auditory system does not analyze frequency in a linear fashion. Therefore, it has been suggested that speech analysis should be performed in a way that models the analysis done by the human ear. The selection of appropriate nonlinear frequency scales is a major issue in the acoustic analysis of speech, and this topic will recur in this book. Appendix C describes some of the more commonly used frequency transforms.

Vowel Formant Pattern

Much of the experience with synthetic speech lends support to formant pattern as a primary cue for vowel perception. When vowels have been synthesized using the formant frequencies estimated from natural speech, the results have been generally satisfactory (Fry, Abramson, Eimas, & Liberman, 1962; but note the high error rates reported

by Hillenbrand & Gayvert, 1993). Indeed, the bulk of current work on speech synthesis relies on a formant specification of vowels and a formant-based strategy is one of the most common forms of speech synthesis (Chapter 8). Formant frequencies derived from analyses of natural speech are used to specify the formant pattern of synthetic vowels. The overall success of this approach might be taken to favor formant descriptions, though not necessarily a description based only on static assumptions.

Tables 4–1 and 4–2 list the average fundamental frequency and the first three formant frequencies for several vowels produced by men and women, respectively. The data from Peterson and Barney (1955) are possibly the most frequently cited values in acoustic phonetics and therefore, they qualify as classic. Their vowel samples were recorded from 76 speakers (men, women, and children) and were analyzed both acoustically and perceptually. This vowel study was one of the first to examine the acoustic properties of speech sounds in a large sample of speakers. The more recent data from Hillenbrand, Getty, Clark, and Wheeler (1995) represent a replication and extension of the Peterson and Barney study. Values are reported for several other studies, including: Zahorian and Jagharghi (1993); Hagiwara (1995); Yang (1996); Childers and Wu (1991), Assmann and Katz (2000), and Lee, Potamianos, and Narayanan (1999). The means and standard deviations calculated for F1, F2, and F3 frequencies give an average set of values for each vowel and an index of the variation across studies. Note that these statistics are based on only six of the reported studies in Tables 4–1 and 4–2 that appear to be most comparable in their overall formant-frequency patterns. For males (Table 4–1), the standard deviations for F1 are generally less than about 50 Hz. For F2 and F3, the standard deviations are larger than for F1. The values for F2 generally are less than 130 Hz, with the exception of /u/. Generally, the standard deviations for F2 are larger than those for F3. For females, (Table 4–2), the standard deviations for F1 are, with two exceptions, less than 100 Hz. The standard deviations for F2 and F3 tend to be larger than those for F1, and the values typically are larger for F3 than for F2. Possibly, the F2 frequency is more sensitive to dialectal and idiolectal variation than is the F3 frequency, which could explain the greater variation in F2 than F3 frequencies.

TABLE 4–1

Mean data on fundamental frequency and the first three formant frequencies for vowels of American English produced by adult male speakers. The data are from (1) Peterson and Barney (1952), (2) Hillenbrand et al. (1995); (3) Zahorian and Jagharghi (1993); (4) Hagiwara (1995), (5) Yang (1996), (6) Childers and Wu (1991), (7) Assman and Katz (2000), and (8) Lee, Potamianos and Narayanan (1999). Means (M) and standard deviations (sd) are shown for F1, F2, and F3 when a sufficient number of values are present; these statistics are based only on the data from studies 1 through 6.

		i	ɪ	e	ɛ	æ	ɑ	ɔ	o	ʊ	u	ʌ	ɝ
f_0	1	136	135	—	130	127	124	129	–-	137	141	130	133
	2	138	13?	129	127	123	123	121	129	133	143	133	130
	5	136	130	128	132	126	125	128	129	135	135	127	130
	6	132	130	—	124	123	120	120	—	126	130	120	122
	7	110	108	111	102	101	103	101	112	112	131	102	105
	8	132	136	—	129	123	135	127		149	144	130	134
F1	1	270	390	—	530	660	730	570	—	440	300	640	490
	2	342	427	476	580	588	768	652	497	469	378	623	474
	3	272	410	—	550	656	749	637	456	439	324	—	445
	4	291	418	403	529	685	–-	—	437	441	323	574	429
	5	286	409	469	531	687	638	663	498	446	333	592	490
	6	303	439	—	542	645	673	615	—	487	342	591	477
	7	300	445	497	534	694	754	654	523	426	353	638	523
	8	292	458	—	590	669	723	601	—	501	342	610	471
	M	294	416	449	544	654	712	627	472	454	333	604	468
	sd	26	17	—	20	36	54	37	30	20	26	27	25
F2	1	2290	1990	—	1840	1720	1090	840	—	1020	870	1190	1350
	2	2322	2034	2089	1799	1952	1333	997	910	1122	997	1200	1379
	3	2209	1859	–—	1740	1748	1192	1004	1176	1234	1396	—	1286
	4	2338	1808	2059	1670	1600	–-	1248	1188	1366	1417	1415	1362
	5	2317	2012	2082	1900	1743	1051	1026	1127	1331	1393	1331	1363
	6	2172	1837	—	1690	1622	1098	990	—	1168	1067	1194	1276
	7	2345	1974	1982	1855	1809	1214	1081	1182	1376	1373	1455	1457
	8	2266	1851	—	1707	1725	1204	929	—	1269	1181	1288	1265
	M	2275	1923	2077	1773	1731	1153	1018	1100	1206	1190	1266	1336
	sd	68	99	—	89	125	113	131	130	130	241	102	44
F3	1	3010	2550	—	2480	2410	2440	2410	—	2240	2240	2390	1690
	2	3000	2684	2691	2605	2601	2522	2538	2459	2434	2343	2550	1710
	3	2971	2600	—	2535	2345	2501	2400	2307	2349	2352	—	1656
	4	2920	2588	2690	2528	2524	–-	2441	2430	2446	2399	2496	1683
	5	3033	2671	2636	2561	2497	2318	2527	2375	2380	2282	2494	1787

(continued)

TABLE 4–1 (continued)

	Vowel											
	i	I	e	ɛ	æ	ɑ	ɔ	o	U	u	ʌ	3^
6	2851	2482	—	2456	2357	2457	2465	—	2307	2219	2401	1707
7	3003	2654	2557	2643	2580	2468	2564	2390	2364	2321	2539	1686
8	2930	2588	—	2549	2532	2496	2599	—	2466	2411	2557	1612
M	2964	2596	2672	2528	2456	2448	2464	2393	2359	2306	2466	1706
sd	68	76	—54	102	80	58	67	78	70	68	44	

TABLE 4–2

Mean data on fundamental frequency and the first three formant frequencies for vowels of American English produced by adult female speakers. The data are from (1) Peterson and Barney (1952), (2) Hillenbrand et al. (1995); (3) Zahorian and Jagharghi (1993); (4) Hagiwara (1995); (5) Yang (1996), (6) Childers and Wu (1991), (7) Assmann and Katz (2000) and (8) Lee, Potamianos, and Narayanan (1999). Means (M) and standard deviations (sd) are shown for F1, F2, and F3 when a sufficient number of values represent; these statistics are based only on the data from studies 1 through 6.

		Vowel											
		i	I	e	ɛ	æ	ɑ	ɔ	o	U	u	ʌ	3^
f_0	1	235	232	—	223	210	212	216	—	232	231	221	218
	2	227	224	219	214	215	215	210	217	230	235	218	217
	5	221	216	209	211	209	205	206	207	214	228	206	211
	6	233	228	—	219	216	214	216	—	220	222	215	217
	7	216	207	209	204	199	208	194	201	207	217	199	201
F1	1	310	430	—	610	860	850	590	—	470	370	760	500
	2	437	483	536	731	669	936	781	555	519	459	753	523
	3	338	486	—	745	922	981	793	532	528	400	—	542
	4	362	467	440	806	1017	—-	947	516	486	395	847	477
	5	390	466	521	631	825	782	777	528	491	417	701	523
	6	378	512	—	661	842	838	745	—	522	409	724	558
	7	429	522	572	586	836	688	816	636	516	430	767	640
	8	360	532	—	694	787	894	726	—	595	412	740	543
	M	369	474	—	697	855	877	772	532	503	408	757	520
	sd	44	27	—	76	115	80	114	14	24	30	56	29
F2	1	2790	2480	—	2330	2050	1220	920	—	1160	950	1400	1640
	2	2761	2365	2530	2058	2349	1551	1136	1035	1225	1105	1426	1588
	3	2837	2284	—	2123	2089	1440	1176	1419	1437	1617	—	1532
	4	2897	2400	2655	2152	1810	—	1390	1392	1665	1700	1753	1558
	5	2826	2373	2536	2244	2059	1287	1140	1206	1486	1511	1641	1550
	6	2586	2197	—	2013	1933	1246	1190	—	1386	1361	1445	1504
	7	2588	2161	2309	2144	2051	1273	1203	1470	1685	1755	1751	1508
	8	2757	2183	—	2057	2078	1459	1079	—	1522	1388	1609	1481
	M	2822	2350	—	2153	2048	1349	1159	1393	1395	1374	1533	1562
	sd	52	98	—	118	180	142	150	183	204	295	156	47

(continued)

		Vowel										
	i	I	e	ɛ	æ	ɑ	ɔ	o	U	u	ʌ	3ʌ
F3 1	3310	3070	—	2990	2850	2810	2710	—	2680	2670	2780	1960
2	3372	3053	3047	2979	2972	2815	2824	2828	2827	2735	2933	1929
3	3456	3093	—	3041	2981	2847	2860	2789	2848	2766	—	1992
4	3495	3187	3252	3064	2826	—	2725	2903	2926	2866	2988	1995
5	3416	3014	2991	2968	2928	2563	2895	2836	2836	2796	2901	1927
6	3286	2996	—	2956	2982	2945	2853	—	2792	2730	2863	2024
7	3256	2965	2990	2929	2875	2966	2947	2634	2734	2636	2887	1870
8	3291	3064	—	3005	2916	2950	2986	—	2887	2804	2957	1884
M	3389	3069	—	3000	2923	2796	2811	2839	2818	2760	2893	1971
sd	82	68	—	43	69	141	76	47	81	67	78	39

The values in the formant-frequency tables should not be taken prescriptively, but rather as averages around which considerable variation can occur. Generally, the formant-frequency values from the Peterson and Barney study agree reasonably well with those from the more recent studies. However, for both men and women, the F2 frequencies tend to be lower for back vowels in the Peterson and Barney study than in the other studies. The F2 values for [u] vary markedly. Dialectal differences may account for these variations. Caution should be observed in applying the data from any of the five studies to speakers who may have different dialects from those represented in the investigations. Hagiwara's (1997) data for 15 southern Californian English-speaking monolinguals differ in some potentially important respects from the results in the study by Hillenbrand et al. In particular, the F1–F2 results for /ae/ in Hillenbrand et al. are raised to such an extent that the F1–F2 vowel space is more of a triangle than a quadrilateral. But Hagiwara's data show a quadrilateral shape similar to the shape that represents the Peterson and Barney data. As Hagiwara pointed out, American English "is an amorphous entity at best, and ... there are considerable regional (and also social) differences, particularly in urban centers" (p. 658).

A rough rule of thumb in relating the vowel formant frequencies to vowel articulation is that F1 varies mostly with tongue height and F2 varies mostly with tongue advancement (that is, with variation in the antero–posterior position of the tongue). Figure 4–5 shows stylized formant patterns that illustrate this acoustic-articulatory relation. Caution should be followed in the use of this rule, because there are exceptions. However, multidimensional scaling experiments confirm the general accuracy of the rule. Rakerd and Verbrugge (1985) reported the following significant correlations between perceptual dimensions and acoustic parameters of vowels: Dimension D1 (interpreted as advancement) with F2 and F3 frequency; Dimension D2 (interpreted as height) with F1 frequency, and Dimension D3 (interpreted as tenseness) with duration. In general, low vowels have a high F1 frequency and high vowels have a low F1 frequency. Back vowels have a low F2 and typically a small F2-F1 difference, whereas front vowels have a relatively higher F2 frequency and a large F2–F1 difference. It appears, then, that a vowel's formant pattern can be used to identify a vowel and even to establish relationships between acoustic and perceptual parameters. For example, the differences in F2 frequency described above for the Peterson–Barney (1952) and the Hillenbrand et al. (1995) vowel data appear to indicate that back vowels were produced with a more fronted articulation by the subjects in the Hillenbrand et al. investigation. Perhaps this result means that back vowels in contemporary American English are shifting toward the front of the mouth.

As already noted, it is not entirely certain that formants are the best (most accurate and most efficient) description of vowels. Some experiments using synthesized vowels cast doubt on the role of formants. Of particular interest are experiments that have studied two-formant models of vowels. These studies have explored listeners' identifications of various combinations of F1 and F2 patterns. Carlson, Fant, and Granstrom (1975) reported a study in which F1 was held at values appropriate for natural speech but F2 was varied experimentally. Sometimes the experimental F2′ (the prime is used to distinguish this formant from an actual for-

mant in natural speech) varied over a range of values, including frequency values beyond those expected for F2 in natural speech. A graphic summary of the results is given in Figure 4–6. The open rectangular bar shows the frequency value of F2′ that gave the most satisfactory acoustic result for each vowel. For the back vowels, F2′ approximates the value for F2 in natural speech. However, for the front vowels, a very different result can be seen. F2′ for vowels [e] and [ae] falls about midway between the natural F2 and F3. For vowel [i], F2′ falls close to the natural F4.

These results are hard to reconcile with a simple formant model of vowel perception. Different approaches have been taken to predict F2′ from acoustic measures of

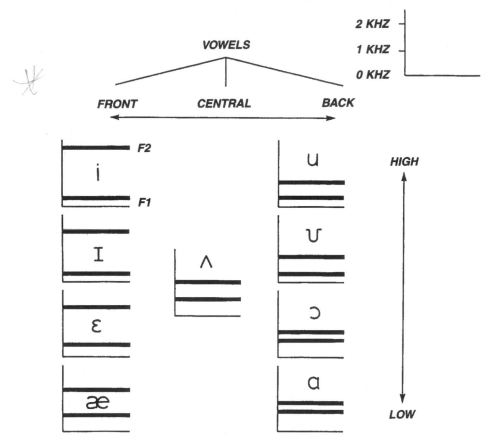

FIGURE 4–5. Stylized spectrograms showing the relationship between F1 and F2 formant frequencies and tongue position in the oral cavity.

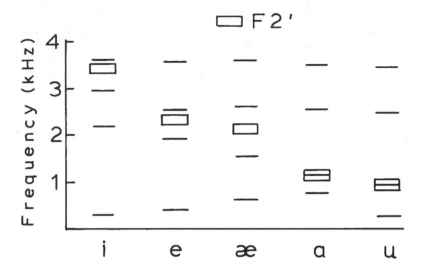

FIGURE 4–6. Stylized spectrograms to show effective second formant frequencies (F2′) compared to natural second formant frequencies for five vowels. See text for explanation. Redrawn with permission from R. Carlson, G. Fant, and B. Granstrom (1975). Two-formant models, pitch and vowel perception. In G. Fant and M.A.A. Tatham (Eds.), *Auditory analysis and perception of speech* (pp. 55-82). London: Academic Press. Copyright 1975.

vowel formants (Bladon, 1983; Bladon & Fant, 1978; Paliwal, Lindsay, & Ainsworth, 1983). Bladon (1983) concluded from an evaluation of these approaches that the best explanation may rest in an auditory spectral integration of vowel formant energy within a broad bandwidth of about 3.5 Bark. (The Bark is a nonlinear transformation of frequency and is defined in Appendix C). As vowel formant energy moves into and out of this integrating bandwidth, nonlinearities in perceived vowel quality would result. The 3.5 Bark integration also has been indicated in other experiments on the perception of vowels and vowel-like sounds (Chistovich & Lublinskaja, 1979; Chistovich, Sheikin, & Lublinskaja, 1979). If nothing else, these experiments and attempted explanations tell us that the phonetic quality of a given vowel can be associated with more than one specific formant pattern.

As mentioned earlier, various nonlinear transforms of frequency have been proposed for the analysis of speech. The Bark transform is one of the most influential of

the nonlinear scales because this transform is thought to be a good approximation to the actual frequency analysis performed by the ear. Bark-transformed formant frequencies are sometimes used in preference to linear formant-frequency values. In an important paper, Syrdal and Gopal (1986) reported on the accuracy of vowel classification achieved with the Bark transform. They concluded that Bark differences were especially useful in classification. Bark differences represent the difference between two Bark-transformed formant-frequency values, as presented in Table 4–3. This table shows that a given vowel can be classified with respect to Bark difference values.

Another nonlinear scale is the equivalent-rectangular-bandwidth-rate (ERB-rate scale) which was introduced by Patterson (1976) and defined analytically by Moore and Glasberg (1983), Glasberg and Moore (1990) and Greenwood (1990). The major difference between the ERB-rate scale and the Bark scale is that, at frequencies below 500 Hz, the Bark scale is linear but the ERB-rate

TABLE 4–3

Classification of vowels of American English based on critical distance features in five Bark difference dimensions. Adapted from A. K. Syrdal and H. S. Gopal (1986). A perceptual model of vowel recognition based on the auditory representation of American English vowels. *Journal of the Acoustical Society of America, 79,* 1086–1100. (Reprinted with permission by the American Institute of Physics.) Copyright 1986.

Vowel	$F1-f_0$ < 1 Bark	$F2-F1$ < 3 Bark	$F3-F2$ < 3 Bark	$F4-F2$ < 3 Bark	$F4-F3$ < 1 Bark
/i/	+	−	+	+	+
/ɪ/	+	−	+	−	+
/ɛ/	−	−	+	−	+
/æ/	−	−	+	−	+
/3^/		−	+	−	−
/∧/	−	−	−	−	+
/a/	−	+	−	−	+
/ɔ/		+	−	−	+
/U/	+	−	−	−	+
/u/	+	−	−	−	+

scale gives values that fall between a linear and logarithmic transform. At these low frequencies, the ERB-rate scale gives a better frequency resolution (smaller bandwidths) than the Bark scale. The differences between the ERB-rate and Bark scales may be more important for speech intonation than for vowel formant analysis (Hermes & van Gestel, 1991). The advantage of the ERB-scale is that it outperforms the Bark scale at low frequencies but is comparable to the Bark scale at high frequencies. Hence, the ERB-scale offers the same advantages as the Bark scale for formant-frequency analysis but offers superior analysis for intonation.

As Chapter 7 discusses in some detail, vowel sounds are important carriers of intonation, and it is, therefore, desirable that the acoustic analysis of vowels can extract intonational information as well as formant-frequency information. The acoustic analysis of speech often must extract more than one type of information. Because vowels have a "double duty" as phonetic segments and as carriers of prosodic and extralinguistic information (such as emotion), an adequate account of acoustic analysis may include several acoustic measures. This chapter focuses on the phonetic or segmental aspects.

Suprasegmental aspects are taken up in Chapter 7, but some preliminary comments are included here.

Studies have been done to determine the relationship between vowel formant frequencies and the optimal octaves in vowel perception. If a certain number of vowel formants, say the first three, is the principal determinant of vowel quality, then filtering experiments should show that the optimal octaves for vowel perception are located so as to contain these energy regions. The results of these filtering experiments are a little more complicated than that. Miner and Danhauer (1977) reported the following optimal octaves for the three vowels [i], [u] and [a].

[i]: 1250-2500 Hz; 2500-5000 Hz; 5,000-10,000 Hz (all of which approached the identification levels of the control (unfiltered) vowel.

[u]: 80-160 Hz and 160-315 Hz (which closely approximated the identification levels of the control vowel.

[a]: 630-1250 Hz and 1250-2500 Hz (the first of which was more effective than the second).

The Miner and Danhauer data indicate that the optimal octaves for vowel perception are not necessarily in the vicinity of the vowel second formant. In fact, only vowel [a] conforms to the prediction that F2 is critical for vowel identification. Interestingly, for vowel [i], three non-overlapping bands were about equally effective for vowel identification (though not equal in listeners' judgments of distortion).

Although questions remain about the choice of formant pattern as the best acoustic description of vowels, many applications have satisfactorily used this approach. As will be discussed in more detail later, modern speech synthesis (speech production by machine) often relies on formant-frequency specifications of sounds to produce machine-generated speech (so-called formant synthesizers). One advantage of the description of vowels by formant pattern is economy. In most cases, it is necessary to specify only the first three formants to acheive a good result. In addition, the formant patterns of vowels frequently are continuous with the formant patterns of neighboring consonants. Another advantage of formant description is that the formants typically are easily observed in acoustic analyses of speech. Indeed, in one approach to speech synthesis, salient acoustic properties, such as formant patterns, are traced from displays of natural speech and used as input specifications for synthesis. The synthesized pattern is thus a facsimile of the original natural speech.

The discussion so far as been restricted to American English. Acoustic data on the vowels in various languages, although not abundant, allow a further examination of the role of formant frequencies in the phonetic specification of vowels. Before turning to some data for individual languages, it is appropriate to take a broad perspective on the issue of vowel system inventories. A good starting point is an analysis of the vowels in a large database collected for 317 languages. This database is known by the abbreviation UPSID, which stands for the UCLA Phonological Segment Inventory Database (Maddieson, 1984). Schwartz, Boe, Vallee, and Abry (1997) examined this database to discover "major trends" in the vowel inventories of this sample of languages. Figure 4–7 shows the grid in which the 37 vowel symbols in UPSID are represented. Among the major conclusions reached by Schwartz et al. are the following that have particular relevance to the present discussion:

1. Languages first select vowels from a primary vowel system that has a high frequency of occurrence across languages and in which duration is the typical diacritic (modification). The primary system consists of 3 to 9 vowels, but 5- to 7-vowel systems are particularly favored. Among the vowels in this system, the most frequently occurring are the 3 corner vowels /i/, /a/, and /u/.

2. When languages have more than about 9 vowels, they tend to select additional vowels beyond the primary set by exploiting a new dimension. These additional vowels are termed a secondary vowel system and generally consist of 1 to 7 vowels (with 5 being preferred).

3. The vowels in both primary and secondary systems are concentrated at the periphery of the vowel grid (i.e., the sides of the vowel quadrilateral), and there is a tendency for a balance between front and back vowels. When this balance does not occur, front vowels usually outnumber back vowels.

4. The preferred nonperipheral vowel is the schwa, the occurrence of which does not seem to interact with other vowels in a particular system. That is, schwa is a "parallel" vowel whose occurrence may be motivated by intrinsic principles such as vowel reduction.

Further insights into the selection of vowels in particular languages come from a

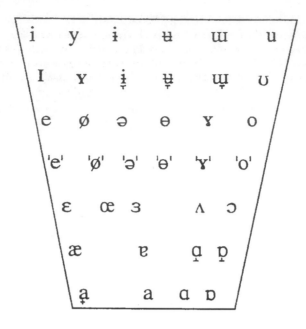

FIGURE 4–7. Grid for representing the 37 vowels symbols in UPSID. Reprinted from J. L. Schwartz, L.-J. Boe, N. Vallee, and C. Abry (1997). *Major trends in vowel system inventories. Journal of Phonetics, 25,* 236. Reprinted with permission of Academic Press. Copyright 1997.

consideration of psychoacoustic properties (Iivonen, 1994, 1995). It has been thought for a long time that vowels are selected in accord with principles of maximal contrast. That is, referring to the grid in Figure 4–7, if a language has only 3 vowels, 2 of which are /i/ and /u/, then /a/ is far more likely to be selected than, say, /I/ or /o/. Maximally contrastive vowels are expected to be more easily discriminated perceptually, thereby reducing the probability of confusions and reduced intelligibility.

Now we turn to examples of formant frequencies in different languages. If one makes the assumption that an /i/ is an /i/ is an /i/, regardless of the language in which it appears, then a single set of acoustic data (adjusted for age and sex variations) would suffice for each vowel phoneme in the International Phonetic Alphabet. Is this simplifying assumption safe to make? Sample values are given in Tables 4–4 (Hebrew), 4–5 (Spanish), 4–6 (Japanese), 4–7 (Estonian), 4–8 (Swedish),

4–9 (Greek), 4–10 (Dutch), 4–11 (British English), 4–12 (Korean), and 4–13 (Hindi). A cautionary note is important: these tables are based on data from different numbers of subjects (who may vary in physical characteristics such as length of the vocal tract, and in sociolinguistic characteristics such as regional dialect) and from different procedures of recording and analysis. Direct comparisons should be made with these thoughts in mind.

As an example of the kind of cross-language question one might ask about vowels, consider: Is the vowel /i/ in Swedish identical to the vowel /i/ in American English (or any other language) as far as formant frequencies are concerned? The answer cannot be given with great confidence at this point, but it appears that the formant-frequency values for vowels represented by the same IPA symbol are to some degree tuned to individual languages (Andrianopoulos, Darrow, & Chen, in press; Bradlow, 1995; Krull & Lindblom,

TABLE 4–4
Formant frequencies of five modern Hebrew vowels produced by one adult male speaker — L-male (Laufer, 1975), six male speakers — A-male (Aronson, Rosenhouse, Rosenhouse, & Podoshin, 1996; and six female speakers — A-female (Aronson et al., 1996). Aronson et al. reported results for both LPC and FFT analysis; the LPC values are given in this table.

		F1	F2	F3	F4
Vowel					
[i]					
	L-male	310	2560	2990	3710
	A-male	300	2670	3320	4015
	A-female	325	2715	3130	4170
[e]					
	L-male	510	1990	2610	3455
	A-male	470	1185*	2470	4350
	A-female	540	2325	3075	4220
[a]					
	L-male	760	1240	2720	3670
	A-male	710	1232	2720	3650
	A-female	880	1530	2995	3870
[o]					
	L-male	510	975	2760	3440
	A-male	442	866	2268	3252
	A-female	523	984	2965	3530
[u]					
	L-male	310	835	2820	3480
	A-male	320	784	2576	3615
	A-female	384	886	2945	3670

* Reported value from LPC analysis is decidedly higher than the value of 1875 Hz obtained from FFT analysis. The FFT value probably is the better choice.

TABLE 4–5
Formant frequencies of the Spanish vowels produced in CVCV utterances by four adult male speakers of Madrid Spanish. Reprinted from A. R. Bradlow (1995). *A comparative acoustic study of English and Spanish vowels. Journal of the Acoustical Society of America, 97,* 1916-1924. (Reprinted with permission of the American Institute of Physics). Copyright 1995. Values shown are means (with standard deviations in parentheses).

	F1	F2
Vowel		
[i]	286 (6)	2147 (131)
[e]	458 (42)	1814 (131)
[a]	638 (36)	1353 (84)
[o]	460 (19)	1019 (99)
[u]	322 (20)	992 (121)

TABLE 4–6

Formant frequencies of the 5 Japanese vowels as produced by one adult male speaker. Reprinted from T. Hirahara and H. Kato (1992). The effect of F_0 on vowel identification. In Y. Tohkura, E. Vatikiotis-Bateson, and Y. Sagisaka (Eds.), *Speech perception, production and linguistic structure,* (pp. 89-112). Amsterdam: IOS Press. (Reprinted with permission of ATR Auditory and Visual Perception Research Laboratories, Kyoto, Japan). Copyright 1992.

	F1	F2	F3	F4
Vowel				
[i]	281	2281	3187	4281
[e]	469	2031	2687	3375
[a]	750	1187	2594	3781
[o]	468	781	2656	3281
[u]	312	1219	2469	3406

TABLE 4–7

Formant frequencies for Estonian vowels produced by an adult male speaker. Reprinted from A. Eek and E. Meister (1994), Acoustics and perception of Estonian vowel types, *PERILUS*, No. XVIII, pp.55-90. Reprinted with permission of the Department of Linguistics, Stockholm University.) Copyright 1994.

	F1	F2	F3	F4
Vowel				
[i]	254	1881	2980	3402
[e]	356	1810	2532	3198
[ae]	661	1332	2227	3148
[y]	254	1780	2156	3178
[ø]	376	1546	2044	3051
[u]	274	549	1831	3036
[o]	396	630	1968	3036
[a]	610	946	2441	3031
[ə]	386	1088	1912	3056

TABLE 4–8

Formant frequencies of ten Swedish vowels; average values for 24 adult male speakers producing isolated long vowels. Reprinted from G. Fant (1973), *Speech Sounds and Features* (p. 96), MIT Press. (Reprinted with permission of the MIT Press, Cambridge, Massachusetts.) Copyright 1973.

	F1	F2	F3	F4
Vowel				
[i:]	255	2190	3150	3730
[e:]	345	2250	2850	3540
[ɛ:]	505	1935	2540	3370
[ae:]	625	1720	2500	3440
[y:]	260	2060	2675	3310
[ʉ:]	285	1640	2250	3250
[ø:]	380	1730	2290	3225
[u:]	290	595	2330	3260
[o:]	390	690	2415	3160
[a:]	600	925	2540	3320

TABLE 4–9

Formant frequencies of five Greek vowels (stressed, focused position at slow tempo). Speakers were five young men who spoke standard (Athenian) Greek. Reprinted from M. Fourakis, A. Botinis, and M. Katsaiti (1999) Acoustic characteristics of Greek vowels, *Phonetica, 56*; 28-43. (Reprinted with permission, S. Karger AG, Basel). Copyright 1999.

	F1	F2
Vowel		
[i]	340	2046
[e]	491	1788
[a]	738	1350
[o]	508	1020
[u]	349	996

TABLE 4–10

Formant frequencies of 12 Dutch vowels; means for 50 male speakers (Pols, Tromp, & Plomp, 1973). Reprinted from L. C. W. Pols, H. R. C. Tromp, and R. Plomp (1973), Frequency analysis of Dutch vowels from 50 male speaker. *Journal of the Acoustical Society of America, 53*, 1093-1101. (Reprinted with permission of the American Institute of Physics.) Copyright 1973.

	F1	F2	F3
vowel			
[i]	294	2208	2766
[I]	388	2003	2571
[e]	407	2017	2553
[E]	583	1725	2471
[a]	795	1301	2565
[ah]	679	1051	2619
[c]	523	866	2692
[o]	487	911	2481
[u]	339	810	2323
[y]	305	1730	2208
[oe]	438	1498	2354
[ø]	443	1497	2260

1992). Some variation in formant frequencies is readily evident by comparing the different values for /i/ for male speakers in Tables 4–5 through 4–13. F1 values for this vowel (310, 286, 281, 254, 255, 340, 294, 300, 341, and 385 Hz) cover a frequency range of 131 Hz. F2 values (2560, 2147, 2281, 1881, 2190, 2046, 2208, 2300, 2219, and 2480 Hz) cover a range of nearly 700 Hz. Other vowels that are nominally the same in the IPA exhibit a similar variability across languages. Vowels classified as /u/ have a F1 frequency range of more than 300 Hz and a F2 frequency range of nearly 800 Hz. Possibly, there are at least three major types of /u/, with one type having a very low F2 frequency (below 600 Hz), a second having a F2 frequency in the range of about 800 to 1000 Hz, and a third with a F2 frequency higher than 1200 Hz.

Because the data compiled in Tables 4–5 through 4–13 pertain to very small

TABLE 4–11
Formant frequencies of British English vowels. Based on data in J. C. Wells, *A study of formants of the pure vowels of British English*. Unpublished M.A. thesis, University of London, 1962.

	F1	F2
Vowel		
[i:]	300	2300
[I]	360	2100
[e]	570	1970
[ɑ:]	680	1100
[o]	600	900
[o:]	450	740
[U]	380	950
[u]	300	940
[ʌ]	720	1240
[3]	580	1380

TABLE 4–12
Formant frequencies of 10 Korean vowels. Means for 30 male (M) and 30 female (F) speakers (Yang, 1996). Reprinted from B. Yang (1996), A comparative study of American English and Korean vowels produced by male and female speakers. *Journal of Phonetics, 24, 245–261.* (Reprinted with permission of Academic Press.) Copyright 1996.

		F1	F2	F3
Vowel				
[i]	M	341	2219	3047
	F	344	2814	3471
[ɨ]	M	405	1488	2497
	F	447	1703	2997
[e]	M	490	1968	2644
	F	650	2377	3068
[ɛ]	M	591	1849	2597
	F	677	2285	3063
[a]	M	738	1372	2573
	F	986	1794	2957
[o]	M	448	945	2674
	F	499	1029	3068
[ø]	M	459	1817	2468
		602	2195	3013
[u]	M	369	981	2565
	F	422	1021	3024
[y]	M	338	2114	2729
	F	373	2704	3222
[ʌ]	M	608	1121	2683
	F	765	1371	3009

[handwritten marginal note: females higher frequencies or pitch]

TABLE 4–13

Formant frequencies of ten Hindi vowels in C₁VC₂ words. Means for two male speakers calculated from data reported by Khan, Gupta, and Rizvi (1994).

	F1	F2	F3
Vowel			
[ʌ]	585	1290	2005
[a]	665	1155	2140
[I]	430	2125	2860
[i]	385	2480	3310
[U]	505	1255	2000
[u]	580	1340	2215
[e]	530	2230	3195
[ɛ]	610	2440	3450
[o]	535	1190	2025
[ɔ]	595	1260	2155

numbers of speakers, caution should be exercised in drawing any major conclusions. Still, it is striking that the formant-frequency data are as disparate as they are. By comparison, the F1 and F2 values reported for several studies of American English in Tables 4–1 and 4–2 generally agree fairly well, with the acknowledged exception of some back vowels. Taking vowel /i/ for example, the F1 and F2 frequencies for the male speakers in Table 4–1 have a mean of 294 Hz (sd = 26 Hz) and 2275 Hz (sd = 68 Hz), respectively. If it is true that vowels are tuned to a particular language, then the IPA symbols are only a general indication of acoustic similarity among sounds from different languages.

There may not be a single, universal formant-frequency specification for any given vowel, although there may be a statistical preference (a mode) for a particular set of values. The origin of cross-language differences is not clear, but—assuming that these differences are actual and not simply variability resulting from procedural differences—one possibility is that different languages have different **base-of-articulations** (Honikman, 1964; Bradlow, 1995). The base-of-articulation of a language is an articulatory setting that reflects the settings of the most frequently occurring segments and segment combinations in the language. For example, perhaps back vowels in German

are generally more extreme (lower in F2) than in many other languages, including English. Presumably, base-of-articulation could be predicted from data on frequency of occurrence. However, it appears that few experimental tests of this hypothesis have been conducted. A related problem is vowel normalization for cross-language data. Ideally, a particular strategy for vowel normalization could be applied across the vowel data from different languages. However, Disner (1980) cautioned that "comparisons of the normalized vowels of one language with the (separately) normalized vowels of another language are not valid if the vowel systems are different" (p. 2253).

The question of vowel formant patterns also can be approached from the perspective of difference limens (DLs) (also sometimes called just noticeable differences, or JNDs) for the perception of formant frequency. That is, how sensitive are listeners to small changes in the frequency of one or more formants? Early data on this topic indicated that DLs for formant frequencies were on the order of 3-5% of the formant frequency (Flanagan, 1955; Mermelstein, 1978; Nord & Sventelious, 1979), although DLs as large as 13% also have been reported (Nakagawa, Saito, & Yoshino, 1982). More recent studies report DLs on the order of 1-2% of the formant frequency (Hawkes, 1994; Kewley-Port, & Watson, 1994;

Kewley-Port & Zheng, 1999). One reason for the different results is that the smaller DLs were obtained in studies that employed a listening task that minimized the uncertainty between successive stimuli. A general conclusion on the matter is that listeners can detect a change as small as 1% of the formant frequency for vowels in American English (e.g., about 20 Hz for the F2 of vowel /i/ produced by an adult male) but as large as 13% of the formant frequency for vowels in Japanese (Nakagawa et al., 1982). It may be tentatively concluded that the DLs for formant frequency are determined in part by the number of vowels in the subject's language. If this is correct, then DLs are determined in large part by experience, with the smallest DLs expected for languages with many vowels. By this reasoning, native speakers of Danish (a vowel-rich language) should have exceptionally small DLs whereas speakers of some Hawaiian dialects (with as few as 3 vowels) should have large DLs. It would be of interest to know if native speakers of a 3-vowel language acquired smaller DLs for formant frequencies if they subsequently learned a 15-vowel language. Kewley-Port and Zheng (1999) reported that for speakers of American English, the resolution of vowel formants under fairly ordinary listening conditions (vowels in sentences) was about 0.28 Barks, compared to a distance of 0.56 Barks between the closest vowels in the language.

It is pertinent here to consider the reliability of the acoustic analysis of vowel formants. There is no doubt that the reliability of formant-frequency measurement varies with the quality of the speech being analyzed, the experience of the person performing the analysis, and the method of analysis. Surprisingly few systematic studies of formant-frequency measurement have been reported, but Monsen and Engebretson (1983) can be taken as a benchmark. They determined the reliability of formant measurement with both LPC and spectrography. With high-quality recordings of normal speech, the first three formant frequencies were estimated to within ±60 Hz with LPC analysis. With spectrography, the same accuracy applied to measurements of F1 and F2 frequency, but the error in the measurement of F3 frequency was on the order of ±110 Hz. A major point to be made is that the error in formant-frequency measurement by acoustic analysis may be as large as, if not larger than, the DL for formant frequency in ideal listening conditions.

Finally, as discussed briefly in Chapter 3 and in more detail in Chapter 6, the acoustic analysis of vowel formants is limited by the f_0 associated with a particular vowel production. This is not simply a problem of acoustic analysis, because the same general issue applies to the auditory analysis of vowels. The problem arises because, in the analysis of voiced vowels, the transfer function is sampled at multiples of f_0, so that the short-term spectrum reflects the fine spectral structure of the voice harmonics, and not simply the formants. The peaks in the short-term spectrum are located at harmonics of f_0. The same problem affects auditory analysis because cochlear excitation patterns for low frequencies resolve harmonics. One solution is to model vowel analysis as a matching process with missing data so that spectral regions proximal to harmonics are weighted more strongly (de Cheveigne & Kawahara, 1999).

Vowel Short-term Spectrum

Vowels also can be described with respect to their spectra, and some investigators have proposed that a short-term spectrum is better than formant pattern in distinguishing vowels. Of course, the formant pattern is reflected in the spectrum of a vowel, but vowel spectra contain information in addition to formants. A graphical summary of the effects of selected spectral variations on vowel identification is presented in Figure 4–8. Part A shows spectral tilt, in which the spectrum is rotated along a mid-frequency value to change the relative amplitudes of the low- and high-frequency portions. The effects of such spectral changes are usually slight. Part B shows a spectral variation in which the depth of the spectral valleys is altered. This kind of variation also results in relatively little effect on vowel identification. Part C depicts a logarithmic shift in the intensity of the spectrum. Such shifts usually have little perceptual effect, except on loudness. Part D gives an example of shifts in the relative position of spectral peaks. Such modifications frequently have pronounced effects on vowel perception. Finally, part E illustrates a spectral change in which the slope (rate of change in spectrum) is changed in the vicinity of a peak. This spectral alteration also has large effects on vowel identification. A general conclusion to be drawn is that any spectral variation that affects the location of a peak can seriously affect the phonetic interpretation of the vowel spectrum.

In one study that compared formants with spectral-shape features for the automatic classification of vowels, it was concluded that spectral-shape features are a more complete set of acoustic correlates for vowels than are formants (Zahorian & Jagharghi, 1993). This study indicates that a global smoothed spectrum preserves acoustic information more fully than a formant-frequency specification. In fact, the authors noted that, "three formants, even with their bandwidths and amplitudes included, appear to be insufficient to encode all the important properties of natural speech spectra" (Zahorian & Jagharghi, 1993, p. 1975). But they also allowed that no particular set of three global spectral features was better than the three formant frequencies. The superiority of the global spectral-shape features was demonstrated especially when ten or more features were used. It might be concluded that formant information is not the complete acoustic account of vowels, but it is an economic description.

If short-term spectra are averaged over many samples, the result is a long-term average speech spectrum (LTASS). The LTASS is not useful to identify individual speech sounds because their properties are blurred with those of other sounds. However, because vowels provide the dominant energy in speech, they determine in large part the shape of the LTASS. It appears that

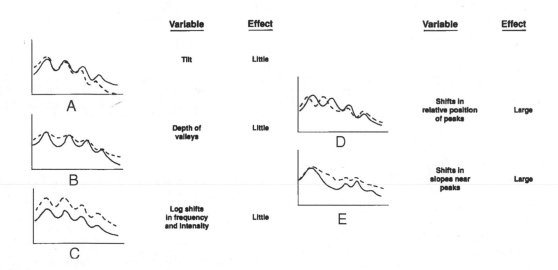

FIGURE 4–8. Effects of various spectral changes on vowel identification. Spectral change variable is illustrated at the left and effect on identification is summarized at the right. Redrawn from J.D. Miller (1984). Auditory processing of the acoustic patterns of speech, *Archives of Otolaryngology, 110,* 154–159. (Reprinted with permission of the Archives of Otolaryngology.) Copyright 1984.

the LTASS is similar across languages (Byrne et al., 1994) but differs between genders (Mendoza, Valencia, Munoz, & Trujillo, 1996). Figure 4–9 illustrates the LTASS for five varieties of English. It can be seen that men have greater energy in the low frequencies, that the strongest energy for men and women is in the range of 125 to 500 Hz, and that energy drops off for frequencies above 500 Hz. The solid line in the different graphs of Figure 4–9 might be taken as an approximation of a universal LTASS, that is, the LTASS across all languages of the world. Gender differences may go beyond those illustrated in Figure 4–9: Mendoza et al. (1996) observed that the LTASS for women differed from that for men in having a greater level of noise in the vicinity of F3 and a lower spectral tilt. These features are considered further in Chapter 6.

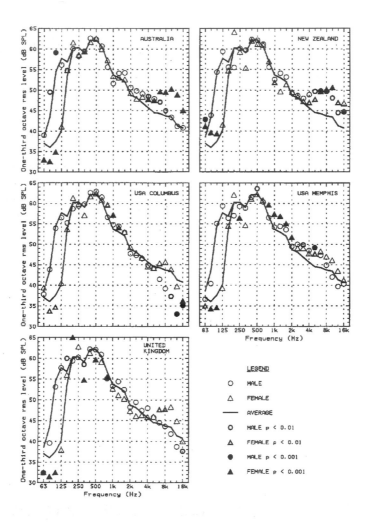

FIGURE 4–9. Male and female long-term average speech spectrum (LTASS) values for five samples of English. Solid line shows LTASS average across 17 speech samples from different languages; males and females separately for frequencies below 160 Hz, combined for higher frequencies. Reprinted from Byrne et al. (1994. Long-term average speech spectra, *Journal of the Acoustical Society of America, 96*, 2113. (Reprinted with permission from the American Institute of Physics.). Copyright 1994.

Vowel Duration

The third parameter, after formant frequencies and spectral shape, is vowel duration. Although duration is neglected in the traditional F1–F2 chart, it is almost always available as a cue in the physical signal of speech, and many languages exploit duration as a vowel feature. Vowels can differ substantially in their durations, as illustrated in Figure 4–10. Among the factors that influence vowel duration are: tense-lax (long-short) feature of the vowel, vowel height, syllable stress, speaking rate, voicing of a preceding or following consonant, place of articulation of a preceding or following consonant, and various syntactic or semantic factors such as utterance position or word familiarity (for a good review, see Klatt, 1976). Some of these are inherent durational attributes (e.g., tenseness or laxness, vowel height), and others are determined by the suprasegmental properties or phonetic context (e.g., stress, speaking rate, consonant environment). Erickson (2000) showed that covariance structure modeling reveals that the effects of various factors on vowel duration may be best understood in terms of a dual population model, with one population being monosyllabic content words and lexically stressed syllables and the other, monosyllabic function words and

lexically unstressed syllables. Both populations show similar effects of intrinsic duration and phrase-final position (so that these two effects may be regarded as vowel general). However, the effects of post-vocalic consonant voicing and position in word were important predictors for vowel duration in content words and stressed syllables, but not in function words or unstressed syllables. Erickson's results indicate that the various influences on vowel duration have somewhat different effects on two major classes of vowels.

Experiments indicate that although duration is not sufficient in itself for identification of any individual vowel, it does help the listener to distinguish spectrally similar vowels, such as /ae/ versus /ɛ/ or to place vowels in categories such as tense vs lax. Hillenbrand, Clark, and Houde (2000) concluded from an experiment using synthesized speech that the effects of vowel duration on vowel recognition are important for the vowel group /ɑ/ /ɔ/-/ʌ/ and the pair /ae/-/ɛ/. Interestingly, some vowel contrasts that are accompanied by consistent differences in duration (e.g., /i/-/ɪ/) were not affected appreciably by the duration cue. Apparently, the presence of a consistent acoustic difference does not necessarily mean that phonetic identification will exploit the difference.

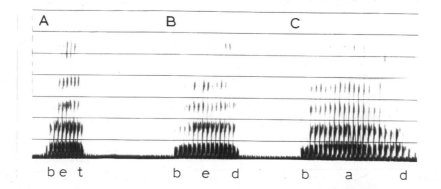

FIGURE 4–10. Spectrographic illustration of variations in vowel duration. Spectrograms are shown for (A) bet [b ɪ t], (B) bed [b d], and (C) bad [baed].

Chapter 3 discussed the measurement of segment durations from various acoustic displays. Vowel duration is one of the most common temporal measures in speech analysis, and it is important to know how accurately this value can be determined. The precision of vowel duration measurements has been estimated in several studies. It appears that measurements are of comparable precision from spectrograms and oscillograms, with a 95% confidence interval of about 10 to 25 ms (Allen, 1978). Similarly, Smith, Hillenbrand, and Ingrisano (1986) concluded that temporal measures from spectrograms and oscillograms are usually within 8 to 10 ms of one another, but measurements from oscillograms tended to yield somewhat longer vowel durations than did measurements from spectrograms. Measurements of duration also can be affected by formant criteria used in spectrography. Blomgren and Robb (1998) measured vowel steady state durations in [Cid] (where C indicates a variable consonant) syllables using a fixed rate-of-change criterion for either the F1 or F2 frequency. Their data from 40 normal speakers indicated that durations were longer for measurements based on F1 than on F2.

Vowel Fundamental Frequency

Vowels also vary among themselves in the fundamental frequency of phonation. These differences often are obscured by the many other factors that govern phonation, such as linguistic stress, speaker emotion, and intonation. However, when these factors are controlled, reliable differences in intrinsic fundamental frequency can be observed. The general rule is that fundamental frequency varies with vowel height, that is, high vowels have a somewhat higher fundamental frequency, on the average, than low vowels. A graphical summary of two classic studies of American English is shown in Figure 4–11.

It is doubtful if these fundamental frequency differences play a major role in

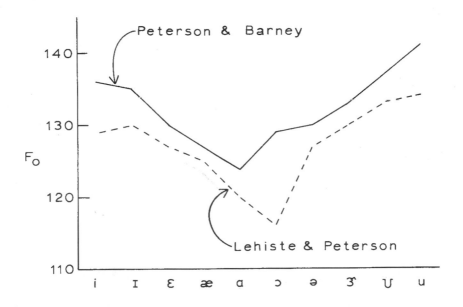

FIGURE 4–11. Mean fundamental frequency for different vowels as reported in two studies (Lehiste & Peterson, 1961; Peterson & Barney, 1952). Note that high vowels are associated with higher fundamental frequencies.

vowel recognition, but they may be secondary cues and possibly can be exaggerated by some speakers to be more salient. As noted in the discussion of formant frequency, vowel f_0 can be combined with formant-frequency measures for the purposes of vowel classification. In Syrdal and Gopal's (1986) analysis, the F1-f_0 Bark difference helped to distinguish the high vowels /i/, /I/, /u/ and /U/ from the lower vowels (Table 4–3). In addition, it was hypothesized by Diehl and Kluender (1989) that intrinsic fundamental frequency is one aspect of enhancement of the speech signal, in which speakers manipulate cues to strengthen phonetic percepts. The perception of vowel height, they argue, would be enhanced by regulating the difference between F1 and f_0. Intrinsic fundamental frequency would achieve the desired effect. However, Whalen and Levitt (1995) questioned the auditory enhancement interpretation and attributed intrinsic fundamental frequency to a universal and inherent aspect of phonation. They reported evidence of intrinsic fundamental frequency in 31 languages representing 11 of the world's 29 major language families. Their cross-language analyses showed a mean intrinsic f_0 effect of 13.9 Hz for males and 15.4 for females. In addition, the general pattern of high f_0 for high vowels and low f_0 for low vowels is consistent across age and gender, at least for American English (Sussman & Sapienza, 1994; Whalen, Levitt, Hsiao, & Smorodinsky, 1995; see also the data compiled in Tables 4–1 and 4–2) but perhaps not for Greek (Fourakis, Botinis, & Katsaiti, 1999).

A number of studies have addressed the origin of these f_0 differences among vowels. The bulk of the evidence agrees with a articulatory-based theory (Honda, 1983), which supposes that elevation of the tongue root for high vowels causes an anterior displacement of the hyoid bone. These effects on extrinsic attachments of the larynx produce increased tension on the larynx, possibly combined with a forward tilt of the thyroid cartilage. This is not to argue that f_0 plays no role in vowel perception, but rather to affirm that the origin of vowel-dependent f_0 differences is found in speech physiology.

A particularly important issue with respect to f_0 is that it, and its harmonics, define the short-term spectrum of a vowel. Peaks in the spectrum (which are often used in inferring formant frequencies) are strongly influenced by harmonic structure. Because many acoustic analyses (and perhaps auditory analysis as well) sample the transfer function at multiples of f_0, estimates of formant structure are based on harmonic properties. This issue becomes especially serious for high f_0 values. For this reason, de Cheveigne and Kawahara (1999) proposed a "missing-data model" in which vowel identification is accomplished with f_0-dependent weighting functions that emphasize spectral regions adjacent to harmonics.

Formant Bandwidth and Amplitude

The conventional F1–F2 chart specifies only the formant frequencies of vowels. But, as discussed in Chapter 2, each formant also can be described by two additional and interactive features, bandwidth and amplitude. In general, any resonance can be described by two numbers, its resonance frequency and bandwidth. Amplitude usually reflects the amount of energy available to the resonator. In describing vowels, it is useful to think of each formant as being described by three numbers: *formant frequency*, *bandwidth*, and *amplitude*. Because the last two typically interact, they need not always be specified individually. However, particularly for some applications in speech synthesis, independent control of bandwidth and amplitude is possible.

Bandwidth is related to *damping*, which is the rate of absorption of sound energy. The greater the damping, the greater the bandwidth of the sound. Sounds that are greatly damped tend to die out quickly, that is, their energy is quickly dissipated.

Sounds that are associated with very little damping tend to be sustained. A practical application of this concept occurs with the acoustic treatment of concert or lecture halls. Frequently, halls that are enclosed with hard, flat walls are not acceptable acoustically. Sounds produced in these halls tend to echo or reverberate. The hard walls reflect the sound energy, so that the energy of a newly produced sound often competes with the reverberant energy of previous sounds, producing a mixture that sounds "muddy." To reduce this unwanted reverberation, acoustic engineers often use draperies or acoustic tiles that absorb sound energy. The greater the absorption of sound, the less the problem with reverberation.

Each formant of the vocal tract during vowel production has a bandwidth. The usual convention in bandwidth measurement is to measure the width of the formant (or any resonance) at a point that is 3 dB below the peak (Figure 4–12). The figure of 3 dB corresponds to the "half-power point," or the point corresponding to half the acoustic power of the sound as determined by the peak. The effect of increasing formant bandwidth is illustrated in Figure 4–12 by the superimposed curves, each of

which represents a resonance with a different bandwidth. If the human vocal tract were a hard-walled tube, like a metal horn, its damping would be considerably less than it is. Because the vocal tract is composed largely of soft tissues, an appreciable amount of the sound produced in speech is absorbed by these tissues.

Formant bandwidths determined by empirical measurement are summarized in Table 4–14. Formant bandwidth generally increases with formant number, so that the higher formants have larger bandwidths than does F1. One exception to this pattern is that the bandwidth for F1 may decrease somewhat as F1 frequency increases from 100 Hz or so to 500 Hz (Hawks and Miller, 1995). For frequencies above 500 Hz, formant bandwidth increases with formant frequency. Hawkes and Miller (1995) suggested that formant bandwidth can be estimated from formant center frequency alone. Their estimates agreed with empirical measurements obtained by Fant (1961) and Fujimura and Lindqvist (1971). The general relation between formant bandwidth (FBW) and formant center frequencies (FF) is as follows:

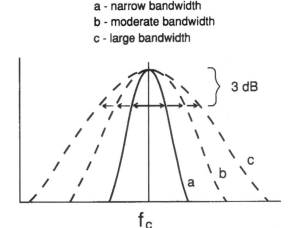

a - narrow bandwidth
b - moderate bandwidth
c - large bandwidth

f_c

FIGURE 4–12. Variations in bandwidth for a fixed center frequency, f_c. Bandwidth is conventionally measured 3 dB down from the energy peak.

1. FBW decreases from about 10 Hz to about 40 Hz over the FF interval of 100 Hz to 500 Hz.

2. FBW is fairly stable at 40—50 Hz over the FF range of about 500 Hz to 1800 Hz.

3. For FF greater than 1800 Hz, FBW increases steeply from about 60 Hz bandwidth at 1800 Hz to over 300 Hz bandwidth at 5000 Hz.

4. The FBW values for women are about 25% larger than the values for men.

Experiments have shown that changing the bandwidth of formants has very little effect on vowel perception. Apparently, the ear is not very sensitive to such changes. Even when the effect of bandwidth reduction is perceptually obvious, as when the bandwith approaches zero, listeners can still identify vowel sounds. It is possible to synthesize a recognizable vowel by generating three simultaneous sinusoids having the frequencies of the first three formants of a vowel (Figure 4–13). The primary perceptual effect of formant bandwidth is on the naturalness of the vowel sound. Vowels that have unusually narrow bandwidths sound artificial even though listeners usually can identify these vowels. One can extend this idea to entire sentences. Remez and colleagues (Remez, Rubin, Pisoni, & Carrell, 1981; Remez, Rubin, & Pisoni, 1983) produced a type of synthetic speech that consisted only of three simultaneous sinusoids, adjusted to vary in frequency according to the formant frequency patterns of human speech. Sentences produced by this "sinusoidal synthesis" were generally intelligible if the listeners were told to expect speech sounds. (Interestingly, if the listeners were told to expect "science-fiction" sounds, they often didn't hear speech at all.) At the other extreme, increasing formant bandwidth eventually can reduce the distinctiveness of vowels because the energy of the different formants begins to overlap. In such an instance, the vowel spectrum loses the sharpness of its peaks and valleys (Figure 4–14). Nasalization of vowels has this effect, and it is interesting that nasalized vowels are less distinctive than their nonnasal counterparts (Lindblom, Lubker, & Pauli, 1977; Lubker, 1979). Therefore, although formant bandwidth is not necessarily a critical factor in vowel perception, there is possibly an optimum bandwidth that facilitates the discrimination and identification of vowels. Perhaps optimum formant bandwidth contributes to the concept of ideal (resonant) voice quality and intelligible speech.

TABLE 4–14
Bandwidths (in Hz) of the first three vowel formants as estimated in eight studies.

	A	B	C	D	E	F	G	H
F1 bandwidth	39	110	130	55	54	40-70	47	30-70
F2 bandwidth	51	190	150	66	65	50-85	48	30-70
F3 bandwidth	80	260	185	89	70	60-100	82	50-135

A - Lewis (1936)
B - Tarnoczy (1948)
C - Bogert (1953)
D - van den Berg (1955)
E - House & Stevens (1958); closed glottis condition
F - House (1960); preferred bandwidths in perceptual judgments
G - Fant (1962); average for 16 vowels
H - Fujimura & Lindqvist (1971); estimated range for closed glottis condition

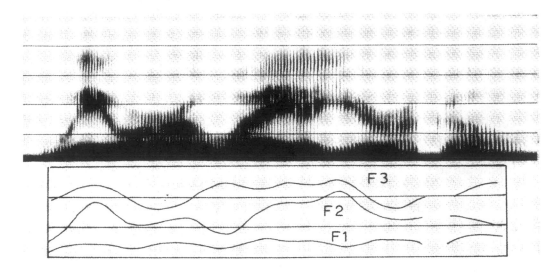

FIGURE 4–13. (Top) Spectrogram of the sentence, *We were away a year ago*, and (bottom) sinusoids that vary in frequency according to the F1, F2, and F3 frequencies in the spectrogram at the top.

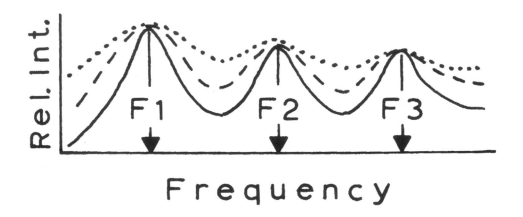

FIGURE 4–14. Effects of increasing formant bandwidth on the spectrum of a vowel sound. Bandwidth increases from the solid to the dashed to the dotted lines.

Formant amplitude is related to formant bandwidth insofar as increases in bandwidth often lead to reductions in overall amplitude. That is, so long as the source energy (that is, the acoustic energy from the larynx) remains constant, increases in formant bandwidth are accompanied by reductions in formant amplitude. The relative amplitudes of the formants in a vowel are determined by the formant frequencies of the formants, the bandwidths of the formants, and the energy available from the source. The last of these probably is quite obvious, given that a resonator cannot create energy but rather depends on the energy from a source such as the vibrating vocal folds. As noted earlier in this paragraph, bandwidth can affect formant amplitude by determining the peak value of the formant. But why does formant frequency pattern affect formant amplitudes? The reason is that in vowel production the formants interact. This interaction can be understood graphically as the algebraic addition of the overlapping formant curves at specific frequencies, as discussed in Chapter 2. When two formants are drawn closely together, they reinforce one another and both their amplitudes increase. When these two formants move apart, their interaction is reduced and both their amplitudes decrease. When F1 moves up in frequency, the higher formants are, in effect, boosted by the high-frequency tail of the F1 curve. When F1 moves down, the higher formants are not as strongly influenced by the high-frequency tail.

Both the amplitudes and frequencies of formants are affected by changes in vocal effort or intensity (see Chapter 7 for additional details). A general finding is that F1 frequency increases with vocal intensity (Huber, Stathopoulos, Curione, Ash, & Johnson, 1999; Lienhard & DiBenedetto, 1999). Lienhard & DiBenedetto also reported that f_0 increases with increasing vocal effort. The frequency changes observed by Lienhard and DiBenedetto were 5Hz/dB for f_0 and 3.5 Hz/dB for F1. They also noted that, as vocal effort increased, the amplitudes in the high frequency range increased more than those in the lower frequencies. With a 10 dB change in overall amplitude, the changes in the formant amplitudes were 11 dB for A1, 12.4 dB for A2, and 13 dB for A3 (where A represents formant amplitude) They attributed this pattern to a change in spectral tilt. That is, with increasing vocal effort, the source spectrum changes so that relatively more energy is available in the higher frequencies. Nawka, Anders, Cebulla, and Zurakowski (1997) reported that male speakers have an increasing envelope peak between 3150 and 3700 Hz. They gave the term **speaker's formant** to this local energy maximum and noted that the spectral slope in this region becomes shallower as sonority or intensity of the voice decreases. They also reported that the energy in this region is about 10 dB higher in professional than nonprofessional voices. Their results point to a possible correlate of sonority.

The amplitude envelope of a vowel waveform determines judgments relating to vowel onset, such as hard (abrupt) or soft (gradual) attack. When the envelope of the vowel waveform reaches its maximum rapidly, listeners are apt to judge the vowel as having a hard attack. But when the envelope reaches its maximum value slowly, listeners tend to judge the vowel as having a soft attack. The perceived abruptness of vowel onset seems to be related to the logarithm of the time over which the amplitude envelope rises from 10% to 90% of its maximum value (Peters, Boves, & van Dielen, 1986). This feature does not necessarily affect vowel identification, but it can determine the likelihood with which listeners will hear a glottal stop at vowel initiation. The faster the rise in the amplitude envelope, the more likely is a judgment of glottal stop occurrence.

Summary of the Acoustic Features of Vowels

A full account of the acoustic cues for vowel perception would seem to require consideration of formant pattern, spectrum, duration, fundamental frequency, formant bandwidth, and formant amplitude (Assman, Nearey & Hogan, 1982; Jenkins, 1987; Miller, 1989; Nearey, 1989). Moreover, particularly when vowels are produced in the context of other speech sounds, it may be necessary to consider various dynamic aspects of the acoustic signal associated with the vowel in its phonetic context. These dynamic aspects involve primarily the formant trajectories of the syllable nucleus but also may include variations in fundamental frequency and formant amplitudes. These contextual changes are discussed in some detail in Chapter 7.

The first two or three formants (F1, F2, F3) are the most important for vowel identification Many English vowels can be satisfactorily distinguished from the first two formants alone. Formant frequencies must be adjusted for speaker age and gender, and it also appears that formant frequencies may vary across languages for the same nominal IPA vowel. The higher formants are not necessarily important for phonetic recognition but they do enhance the naturalness of the vowel, which is why they are typically included in the vowels of synthetic speech (Chapter 8). Vowels are inherently intense sounds and therefore give an overall shape to the LTASS. The first-formant is typically the strongest formant and therefore tends to be highly associated with judgments of loudness and it falls in the most intense region of the LTASS (Figure 4–9). For purposes of vowel classification, the human ear is quite tolerant of changes in formant bandwidths. Under some conditions, the formant bandwidth can be reduced to zero (leaving only a single sinusoid to represent the formant) and speech can still be understood.

Table 4–15 summarizes the relations among various acoustic measures and some phonetic features of vowels. The primary intent of this table is to show that certain phonetic contrasts can be associated with several acoustic differences. For exam-

TABLE 4–15

Differences in acoustic measures for several phonetic contrasts for vowels: low versus high, front versus back, tense versus lax, rounded versus unrounded, and nasal versus nonnasal, soft versus loud.

Measure	Low versus High Vowels		
Mean f_0	Low vowel	<	High vowel
Intensity	"	>	"
Duration	"	>	"
F1 frequency	"	>	"
F1-f_0 difference	"	>	"

Measure	Front versus Back Vowels		
F2 frequency	Back vowel	<	Front vowel
F2-F1 difference	Back vowel	<	Front vowel
F3-F2 difference	Back vowel	>	Front vowel

Measure	Tense versus Lax Vowels		
Duration	Tense vowel	>	Lax vowel
Centralization (Formants)	Tense vowel	<	Lax vowel

Measure	Rounded versus Unrounded Vowel		
F1 + F2 + F3 (Sum of values)	Rounded vowel	<	Unrounded vowel

Measure	Nasal versus Nonnasal Vowel		
Formant bandwidth	Nasal vowel	>	Nonnasal vowel
Intensity	"	<	"
F1 frequency	"	>	"
F2 + F3 frequency	"	<	"

Measure	Soft versus Loud Vowel		
f_0 frequency	Soft vowel	<	Loud vowel
F1 frequency	"	<	"
Formant amplitudes	"	<	"

ple, the phonetic contrast of low versus high is associated with possible differences in five acoustic measures. In the main, the phonetic contrasts of low versus high and of front versus back are best determined as acoustic differences in formant structure. The phonetic difference of lax versus tense can affect formant-frequency pattern but is often readily apparent as a difference in vowel duration. Lip rounding has the effect of lengthening the vocal tract, which causes all formants to assume lower frequencies than for a nonrounded configuration. Therefore, the sum of the first three formants is lower than for a nonrounded vowel. Nasalized vowels, compared to their nonnasal counterparts, tend to have larger formant bandwidths, less intensity, a higher F1 frequency, and lower F2 and F3

frequencies.

Part 2: Diphthongs

Vowels are also called monophthongs, meaning single (*mono-*) voiced sound (*phthong*). The diphthongs are another class of sounds related to vowels. Diphthongs are like vowels in that they are produced with a relatively open vocal tract and a well defined formant structure, and they serve as the nucleus of a syllable. Diphthongs are unlike vowels in that they cannot be characterized by a single vocal tract shape or a single formant pattern. Diphthongs are dynamic sounds in which the articulatory shape (and hence formant pattern) slowly changes during the sound's production.

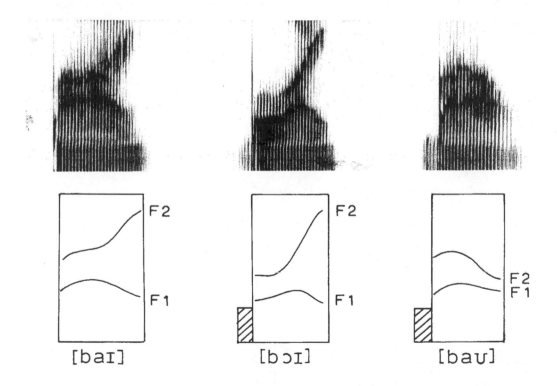

FIGURE 4–15. Spectrograms and extracted F1–F2 patterns for the words *bye, boy,* and *bough.* Note distinctive F1–F2 pattern for each diphthong.

Figure 4–15 shows spectrograms for three English diphthongs in the words *bye*, *boy*, and *bough*.

Most phonetic descriptions specify the starting (or onglide) and final (or offglide) positions of the diphthong. The symbols in the International Phonetic Alphabet reflect this description. For example, the diphthong in the word *eye* is represented by a digraph such as [aI], where the first symbol [a] represents the onglide and the second symbol [I] represents the offglide. A similar approach can be taken to describe the diphthongs acoustically. As shown in Figure 4–16, each diphthong can be represented in the F1–F2 chart by a trajectory that begins with the formant frequencies of the onglide and ends with the formant frequencies of the offglide. Comparisons of the formant frequencies of diphthongs with those of simple vowels have been reported by Holbrook and Fairbanks (1962); Lehiste and Peterson (1961) and Wise (1965.). Limited data have been published for other languages, for example, Chinese (Ren, 1986); Dutch (Collier, Bell-Berti, and Raphael, 1982; Petursson, 1972); Estonian (Piir, 1983); and Spanish (Manrique, 1979).

Particularly when diphthongs are produced in context or at fast speaking rates, considerable variation can occur in both the onglide and offglide formant values. Accordingly, these trajectory descriptions should be regarded more as suggested than as prescribed values. At least for some dialects, the rate of formant frequency change may be a characteristic feature of diphthong production. Gay (1968) reported that the rate of frequency change was essentially invariant despite variations in the onglide and offglide values. Possibly, then, the rate of formant frequency change is a perceptually important feature for the identification of English diphthongs.

Summary

Vowels and diphthongs are associated with relatively well-defined formant patterns, and formant frequencies have been the dominant approach to acoustic characterization of these sounds. This is not to say that formant structure is all that needs to be considered. As noted in this chapter, there are different views of the most accurate and

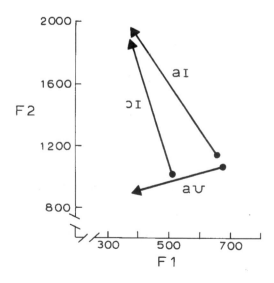

FIGURE 4–16. F1–F2 trajectories for the three diphthongs /aI/, /ɔI/ and /aU/. Arrowhead indicates direction of frequency change.

economical acoustic description of vowels and diphthongs. However, formant pattern clearly has dominated the acoustic study of vocalic sounds, and understanding formant patterns is important with respect to the acoustic theory of speech production (Chapter 2), laboratory measurements, and acoustic descriptions of vowels for different languages. Especially when only a small number of dimensions are used in vowel description, vowel formant frequencies are a reasonable solution.

The Acoustic Characteristics of Consonants

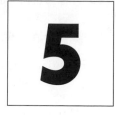

CHAPTER

The acoustic characteristics of consonants are more complicated than those of vowels. All vowels can be described with essentially the same acoustic characteristics, such as duration or formant pattern (or some other spectral information). However, consonants differ significantly among themselves in their acoustic properties, and it is, therefore, difficult to describe all of them with any single set of measures. Some consonants are associated with a significant interval of noise energy (such as the consonants in the word *caustic*) but others have virtually no noise components (such as the consonants in the word *raining*). Some consonants are produced with a period of complete obstruction of the vocal tract but others are produced with only a narrowing of the vocal tract. Some consonants are strictly oral in their sound transmission but others involve a nasal transmission of acoustic energy. Because of these differences, the consonants are discussed in groups that are distinctive in their articulatory and acoustic properties: stops, fricatives, affricates, nasals, glides, and liquids.

The **stops** in English are the phonemes /p b t d k g/ (also known as plosives and stop-plosives). The **fricatives** are /f v θ ð s z ʃ ʒ h/. The **affricates** are / tʃ dʒ /. The stops, fricatives, and affricates comprise the class of *obstruents*. These sounds are produced with a radical constriction (complete closure or narrow opening) of the vocal tract. The **nasal** consonants are /m n ŋ /. The **glides** are /w j/ (also called *semivowels* and *approximants*). The **liquids** are the lateral /l/ and the rhotic /r/. Nasals, glides, and liquids are grouped as the *sonorants* or *nonobstruents*. A great deal of acoustic information has been collected on consonant sounds. Because this background is important to the understanding of consonant acoustics, a selective review of the literature is incorporated in this chapter.

Stop Consonants

The essential articulatory feature of a *stop consonant* is a momentary blockage of the vocal tract. The blockage is formed by an articulatory occlusion, which for English, has one of three sites: bilabial, alveolar or velar (there is also a glottal stop, but this is discussed separately in another section because it is usually considered allophonic in American English). In other languages, stops are produced at a variety of places, including palatal, uvular, and pharyngeal. Stops are abundantly represented in the world's languages and often are among the most frequently occurring consonants in a given language. It also has been argued that stops are the archetypal consonant, involving as they do a radical obstruction of the vocal tract, which makes them a natural opposition to vowels, the sounds made with a maximally open vocal tract. The

terms *stop-plosive* or *plosive* are used by some writers to refer to the consonants /p t k b d g/, but the more general term *stop* is favored in this book. Not all stops involve the pressure release denoted by the word plosive, but all stops necessarily require an articulatory blockage, or stopping

The articulatory and acoustic classification of stop consonants is diagramed in Figure 5–1. The upper part of the diagram applies to word-initial, prevocalic stops, such as those produced in CV syllables. Prevocalic stops have both a closure phase and a release phase (accordingly, they may be called stop-plosives in the strict sense of the term). The articulatory blockage has a variable duration, usually between 50–100 ms and is subsequently released with a burst of air as the air pressure impounded behind the obstruction escapes. Acoustically, the closure phase is associated with a minimum of radiated energy. Because the

STOP CLASSIFICATIONS

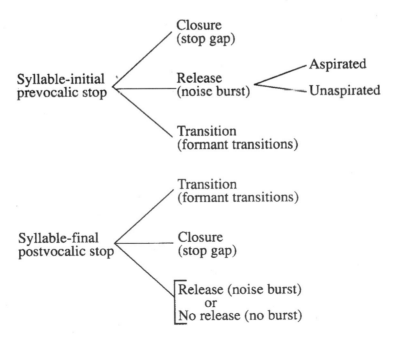

FIGURE 5–1. Diagram of the phonetic classification of the stop consonants.

vocal tract is obstructed, little or no acoustic energy is produced. However, upon the release, a burst of energy is created as the impounded air escapes. This burst is sometimes called a **transient** in recognition of its brevity and fleeting character. However, this terminology is not followed universally. Typically, the burst is no longer than 5 to 40 ms in duration. It is one of the shortest, if not *the* shortest, acoustic events that is commonly analyzed in speech.

Stop releases are classified further as *aspirated* or *unaspirated*. Aspiration is a breathy noise generated as air passes through the partially closed vocal folds and into the pharynx. This noise is essentially that of the glottal fricative [h], as in the word *hat*. Naturally enough, the IPA represents aspiration with a superscript *h*. For example, [tʰ] denotes an aspirated voiceless stop. The aspiration closely follows the release burst and is distinguished from it by the spectrum of noise energy. In English, the voiceless stop plosives have aspirated releases before stressed vowels except when the stops follow /s/. For example, the words *pie*, *too* and *core* are produced with aspirated stops but the words *spy*, *stew* and *score* are produced with unaspirated stops. Both aspirated and unaspirated stops have bursts but only the former have the [h]-like noise following the burst. Figure 5–2 shows spectrograms of aspirated and unaspirated stops. Note that the aspiration appears in a brief interval between the stop burst and the onset of vocal fold vibrations (voicing) for the following vowel. Sometimes the distinction between burst and aspiration is not easily made from a spectrogram. Voiceless stops in prevocalic position are characterized by a delay in voicing relative to the release of the stop. This delay is on the order of 25–100 ms, depending on various factors to be considered later.

The voiced stops in English are normally unaspirated. Because the onset of vocal fold vibration begins close to the burst (with voicing just before, simultaneously with, or just after voicing onset), there is little opportunity for an interval of aspiration. The vocal folds must be adducted for effective voicing, and the generation of turbulence noise requires some degree of glottal opening. Aspiration of stops is phonemic in some languages, but not English. The information given here pertains to English and will not directly apply to all languages.

The information in the next few sections emphasizes syllable-initial prevocalic stop consonants, but some information is given for stops in other contextual positions. The discussion is organized according to the sequence of events in the acoustic pattern, as seen in a spectrogram.

Acoustic Features of Stop Consonants

What we perceive as a stop consonant can correspond to a sequence of acoustic events that are illustrated in the spectrogram of Figure 5–3. This spectrogram represents the word *toss*. The acoustic segments shown from left to right are: a transient (a brief pulse of acoustic energy produced by the initial release of the constriction), a *frication interval* (a period of turbulence noise generated as the constriction is progressively released), and *onset of voicing* (the initiation of vocal fold vibration for the vowel). An interval of aspiration occurs between the frication and the onset of voicing. The **stop gap** that precedes these noise events is the silent interval that appears to the left of the transient. The interval between the transient and the onset of voicing is called the **voice onset time** (**VOT**). VOT has a range of values that are often classified as *voicing lead* or **prevoicing** (voicing begins before the stop is released), *simultaneous voicing* (onset of voicing is simultaneous with the transient), *short lag* (onset of voicing begins shortly after the transient), and *long lag* (onset of voicing begins considerably later than the transient). Finally, **formant transitions** may be seen as the vocal tract configuration changes from the oral constriction

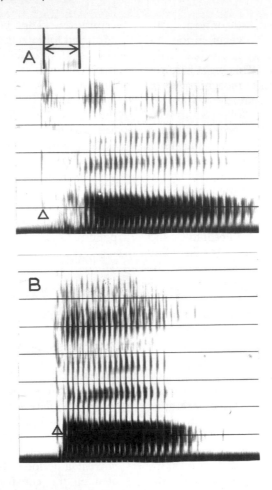

FIGURE 5–2. Spectrograms of (A) aspirated and (B) unaspirated stops. The double arrow in A indicates the interval of aspiration.

for the stop to a relatively open shape for the following vowel. The formant transitions are not always conspicuous for a voiceless stop like that shown in Figure 5–3, but we will see them more clearly in a later section. Klatt (1975a) is a good source for data on the relationships among the temporal measures of VOT, frication, and aspiration in word-initial consonants and consonant clusters. Stevens (1998) gives a detailed theoretical treatment of the various noise events associated with stops. We now consider these acoustic events in more detail, beginning with the stop gap.

The stop gap

Because the stop gap is the acoustic interval corresponding to a complete obstruction of the vocal tract, this interval is an energy minimum in the acoustic signal. That is, little or no sound radiates from the obstructed vocal tract. For voiceless stops, the stop gap is virtually silent because the vocal tract is occluded and the vocal folds are not vibrating (voicing energy is absent). Such silent gaps are illustrated as the spectrogram and waveform in Figure 5–4. This is the first time in this book that we recognize that silence can be a perceptual cue for the identification

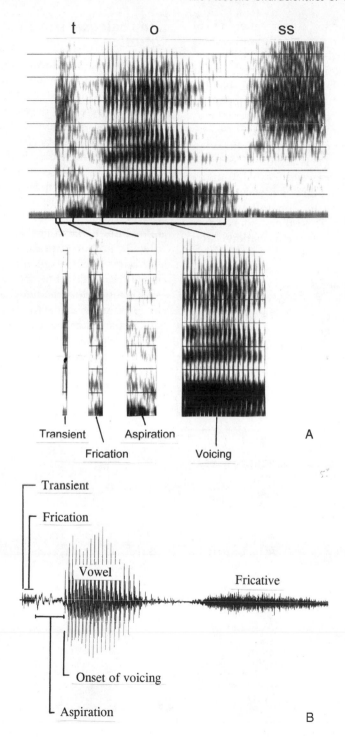

FIGURE 5–3. (A) Spectrogram of the word *toss* showing the acoustic events of transient, frication, aspiration, and voicing. (B) Waveform of the word *toss* labeled to identify the transient, frication, aspiration, onset of voicing, vowel segment, and fricative segment.

of speech sounds. In fact, intervals of silence are very important. For voiced stops in other than word-initial position, the stop gaps usually contain a low-frequency band of energy called the **voice bar**. This band is the energy of the fundamental frequency of phonation. A spectrogram and oscillogram of voiced stop gaps can be seen in Figure 5–5. The primary criteria for identification of stop gaps are: (1) a region of reduced energy, typically between 50 to 150 ms in duration, and (2) other evidence of stop articulation preceding or following (or both) the stop gap. This other evidence may take the form of formant transitions, stop bursts, or aspiration intervals. Of course, not every silent interval in speech is a stop gap. Silent segments also are associated with pauses. Sometimes a silent interval reflects both a pause and a stop gap. For example, if a sentence begins with a stop, the gap for the stop will follow a pre-sentence pause.

Stop release: transient and frication

The lower part of Figure 5–1 shows the classification of stops in word-final, postvocalic position, as the case of VC syllables. These stops can be either released or unreleased. Their only common feature, then, is a period of articulatory closure. When word-final stops are released, the acoustic evidence of the release is a short burst. The optional nature of the stop release is indicated in Figure 5–1. When the stop is not released (that is, when the closure is maintained until well after the utterance is completed), no burst appears. Obviously, then, the burst is not a reliable acoustic cue for word-final stops, but speakers can make a special effort to articulate the stop distinctly by producing a release burst. Particularly when a speaker makes special efforts to be intelligible, as when speaking against a noise background, stop bursts often are

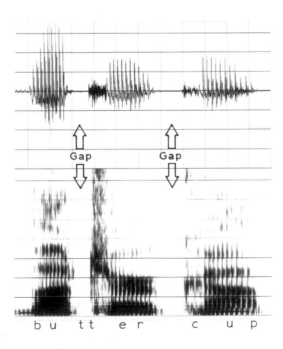

FIGURE 5–4. Waveform and spectrogram of the word *buttercup*. The arrows labeled gap point to the voiceless interval associated with the voiceless stops.

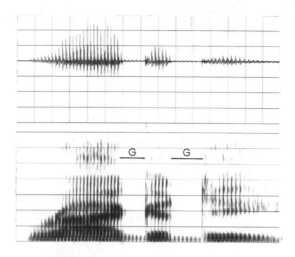

FIGURE 5–5. Waveform and spectrogram of the word *raggedy*. The intervals labeled "G" identify the voiced stop gaps.

accentuated. This and other modifications to promote intelligibility are discussed in a later chapter under the heading of clear speech.

The release burst is a transient produced on release of the occlusion and is rarely more than 20 or 30 ms in duration. As noted earlier, this transient is one of the shortest acoustic events in speech, often no more than 10 ms in duration for voiced stops and somewhat longer for voiceless stops. Accordingly, adequate determination of bursts can be made only if the analysis technique has a suitable temporal resolution. The method of analysis must be able to resolve intervals as brief as 10 ms if stop bursts are to be identified. The burst is a very brief acoustic event that represents the initial release of the impounded air pressure behind the constriction for the stop. The transient is sometimes (but not always) followed by an identifiable segment called frication. The frication phase is noise energy generated at the site of oral constriction. As shown in Figure 5–3, the frication can be identified by spectral properties different from those observed for the burst. Following the burst and frication is still another type of noise that corresponds to aspiration, a noise produced as the vocal

folds begin their adductory (closing) motion. Aspiration is discussed in more detail later. In summary, the release of a stop consonant into a following vowel can be associated with as many as three noise segments: transient, frication, and aspiration.

It has long been recognized that the spectrum of a stop burst varies with the place of articulation. The spectral variation is attributable to the fact that the short noise burst is shaped by the resonance properties defined by a particular articulatory configuration. To a certain degree, the spectral differences are visible even in spectrograms. As Figure 5–6 shows, labials tend to have a low-frequency dominance, alveolars are associated with high-frequency energy, and velars are characterized by a mid-frequency burst. A major research question has been whether these spectral differences are sufficient for phonetic identification.

A classical early experiment on this question was conducted with a pioneering approach to speech synthesis called *pattern playback* (Cooper et al., 1952). With this technique, patterns painted on a belt provide a facsimile of speech. When these patterns are played back through an optical-to-acoustic conversion, identifiable speech

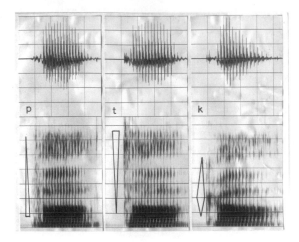

FIGURE 5–6. Waveforms and spectrograms of the syllables [p a], [t a] and [k a]. Line drawings near the onset of each syllable suggest the spectral envelope of each burst—low frequency dominance for [p], high frequency dominance for [t], and mid-frequency dominance for [k].

sounds are produced. Although this technique is crude compared to modern methods of computer speech synthesis, it provided one of the first opportunities to manipulate the acoustic features of speech. This was a landmark development in acoustic phonetics and speech perception.

Liberman, Delattre, and Cooper (1952) used the pattern playback technique to generate the stylized speech stimuli depicted in Figure 5–7. The stop burst is represented acoustically as a short vertical tic or noise pulse with a specified center frequency. The following vowel is represented by two

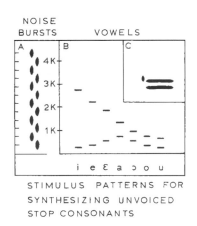

FIGURE 5–7. Representation of synthesized stimuli used in a study of the phonetic classification of various noise bursts. Each noise burst in A was paired with each of the vowel formant patterns in B to yield stimuli such as that shown in C. Redrawn from A. M. Liberman, P. C. Delattre, and F. S. Cooper. (1952). The role of selected stimulus variables in the perception of unvoiced stop consonants, *American Journal of Psychology, 65,* 497–516 (redrawn with permission). Copyright 1952.

static formants. When the synthetic burst and the synthetic vowel are combined as shown in the inset diagram, listeners heard a stop + vowel sequence. The results of the identification experiment are shown in Figure 5–8. A major conclusion is that the phonetic identification of the noise bursts depended on the vowel context. As a general rule, bursts with a center frequency lower than the vowel F2 were identified as [p]; bursts with a center frequency approximating the vowel F2 were heard as [k]; and bursts with a center frequency higher than the vowel F2 were labeled [t]. However, exceptions to this rule are easily seen—for example, some bursts with energy above vowel F2 were heard as [p] when the vowels were [o] and [u]. This experiment established one important result, namely, that stops could be identified solely on the basis of a simplified burst cue. It also raised the possibility that the phonetic interpretation of the burst was influenced by acoustic context, that is, the following vowel.

Some of the earliest spectral data on stop bursts were reported by Halle, Hughes and Radley (1957). Their results indicated that the bilabials [b] and [p] were associated with a primary concentration of energy in the low frequencies, from about 500–1500 Hz. For the alveolars [d] and [t], the spectral pattern either was relatively flat or had a high-frequency concentration of energy (above 4 kHz). The burst spectra for the velars [g] and [k] had strong concentrations of energy in the intermediate frequency regions of about 1.5–4.0 kHz.

Several more recent studies have determined the acoustic properties of bursts. In a series of studies, Stevens and Blumstein (1975, 1978) explored the possibility that a *spectral template* could be associated with each place of stop articulation. The original idea of these templates was as follows: bilabial: a flat or falling spectrum; alveolar: a rising spectrum; and velar: a compact (mid-frequency) spectrum. These templates are illustrated in Figure 5–9. Using these templates to classify naturally produced stops, Blumstein and Stevens (1979) were able to classify stops correctly in 85% of 1,800 stimuli produced by six speakers. A statistical approach to the acoustic classification of word-initial obstruents was taken by Forrest Weismer, Milenkovic, and Dougall (1988). In their analysis, FFTs were treated as random probability distributions for which the first four moments (mean, variance, skewness and kurtosis) were computed. The spectral moments can be

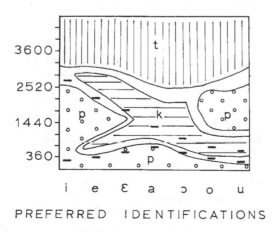

PREFERRED   IDENTIFICATIONS

FIGURE 5–8. Results of identification experiment for the stimuli represented in Figure 5–7. Regions of /p/, /t/ and /k/ responses are shown. Redrawn from A. M. Liberman, P. C. Delattre, and F. S. Cooper. (1952). The role of selected stimulus variables in the perception of unvoiced stop consonants, *American Journal of Psychology, 65,* 497–516 (redrawn with permission). Copyright 1952.

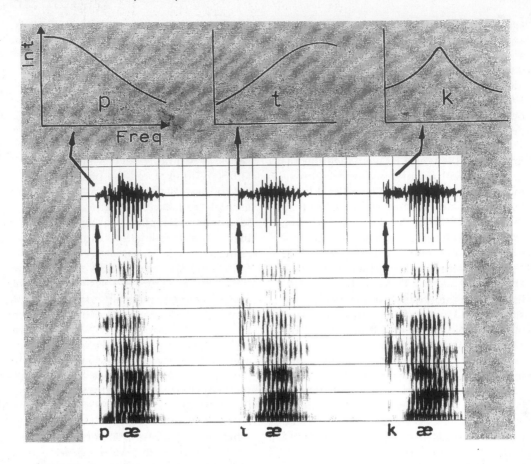

FIGURE 5–9. Spectral patterns of the release burst for bilabial, alveolar, and velar stops. Bilabial: flat falling pattern; alveolar: flat rising pattern; and velar: compact or mid-frequency peak.

interpreted roughly as follows: first moment—mean or center of gravity of the spectrum; second moment—distribution of energy around the mean; third moment—spectral tilt; and fourth moment—degree of peakedness of the spectrum. A dynamic analysis based on moments from the first 40 ms of voiceless stop bursts yielded a correct classification rate of 92%. Moreover, the model constructed from the results for male speakers was able to classify the voiceless stops of female speakers at a rate of about 94%, indicating the generality of the analysis across speaker sex.

Studies of stop recognition from bursts present a mixed pattern of results. The rates of correct stop identification in six studies of American English were: 58% (Winitz, Scheib, & Reeds, 1972), 100% (Cole & Scott, 1974), 97% (Ohde & Sharf, 1977), 0–69% (Dorman, Studdert-Kennedy, & Raphael, 1977), 88% (Kewley-Port, 1983a and b), and 92–94% (Forrest et al., 1988). The large differences in the results of these studies are caused in part by differences in procedures. What may be concluded is that, at least under certain conditions, stops can be identified reliably from bursts alone.

The importance of the burst cue has not been studied extensively in other languages, so it is not possible to make a universal conclusion about the role of the burst in the identification of stop place of articulation. However, studies of French, Spanish, and Dutch support the general conclusion from American English that the burst goes a long way toward identification of stop place of articulation. In a study of stop perception in French, burst information alone was associated with an identification rate for place of 87% (Bonneau, Djezzar, & Laprie, 1996). A near perfect identification of the stops required the presence of all main cues (burst spectrum, burst duration, and onset of vocalic formant transition (which is discussed in a later section). A similar conclusion was reached for Spanish by Feijoo, Fernandez, and Balsa (1999). In a study of stops in Dutch, Smits, ten Bosch, and Collier (1996) found that the identification of stops from burst information alone varied with place, with [k] being highly identifiable but [p] and [t] being rather poorly identified.

Other burst characteristics that have been suggested for stop identification are burst amplitude (Jongman & Blumstein, 1985; Ohde & Stevens, 1983) and relative spectral change from burst onset to voicing onset (Lahiri, Gewirth, & Blumstein, 1984). Jongman and Blumstein determined that burst amplitude could serve as a cue to distinguish alveolar and dental stops, with the former having a larger burst amplitude. Lahiri et al. (1984) tried to classify stops in Malayalam, French and English. They discovered that static spectral features could not distinguish labial and dental stops, both of which have a diffuse-flat spectrum (that is, a spectrum with widely and uniformly distributed energy). However, these stops could be identified with a dynamic cue based on a comparison of the ratio of change in the high frequencies (3500 Hz) to the ratio of change in the low frequencies (1500 Hz) over the time interval from stop release to voice onset. With this criterion, over 90% of the labial and dental stops were correctly classified. Essentially, this dynamic criterion describes a temporal change in spectral tilt. Similarly, Blumstein (1986) used a spectral tilt feature to distinguish palatal and velar stops in Hungarian. Because both these stops have a compact spectrum at burst onset, a static spectral feature is not sufficient for their classification.

Beyond the question of whether the burst cue alone is sufficient to determine place of articulation for stops is the issue of which aspects of the burst are most important. Is a single spectrum of the burst sufficient—as the template approach assumes, or is other information important as well? Kewley-Port's (1983a) study indicated that effective classification of bursts should take temporal factors, and not only spectral shape, into account. Her classification matrix for stops is reproduced in Table 5–1. In this dynamic classification, the burst spectrum is categorized as falling, rising or indeterminate; the onset of voicing is categorized as late, early or indeterminate, and the presence of mid-frequency peaks (1–3 kHz) for at least 15 ms is noted. The bilabial versus alveolar distinction is based almost entirely on spectral tilt (the shape of the spectrum), whereas velars are identified by late voicing onset and the presence of

TABLE 5–1.

Acoustic cues for classification of voiced stop consonants by their noise bursts alone (based on Kewley-Port, 1983a).

Stop	Feature		
	Tilt of burst	Late onset	Mid-frequency peaks
b	falling	no	no
d	rising	?	no
g	?	yes	yes

mid-frequency peaks. More is said about VOT in the next section.

Additional clarification comes from Smits et al. (1996), who determined the importance of various acoustic cues for the perception of the prevocalic Dutch stops [b d p t k]. They concluded that the bursts of voiceless stops were more effective as a cue for place of articulation than were the bursts for voiced stops. As noted earlier, the stop [k] could be recognized nearly all the time from the burst cue alone, but neither [p] or [t] had high rates of identification from their bursts in isolation. For formant transitions, essentially the inverse pattern held: [p] was recognized very well from formant transitions alone, but [k] was very poorly recognized from this cue. The study by Smits et al. demonstrates that the relative value of an acoustic cue for stop identification depends on the voicing and place features of the stop. Moreover, they concluded that the relative perceptual value of burst versus transition depended on the vowel context, with the burst being more important in front-vowel contexts and the formant transitions being more important for back vowels. This research points to an important lesson: the acoustic and perceptual features of consonants can be complex and often are context dependent. The cue of formant transitions is discussed later.

In summary, stops can be identified from their bursts if several features are examined over an interval of about 40 ms extending from the onset of the burst to the onset of voicing. A fairly high rate of correct identification should be possible with the following information: spectrum at burst onset, amplitude of the burst, spectrum at voice onset, and time of voice onset relative to burst onset (VOT). Table 5–2 summarizes the relationship between these acoustic properties and place of consonant articulation.

Voice Onset Time and Other Cues for Voicing

We already have seen that VOT carries information about voicing and place of articulation for a stop. In fact, the voicing feature for syllable-initial stops is specified reasonably well by this single number that gives the interval between the articulatory release of the stop and the onset of vocal fold vibrations. The cross-linguistic application of the measure of VOT was described in a classic article by Lisker and Abramson (1964). This article foreshadowed a large number of studies in which VOT was measured in normal adult speech for several different languages, developing speech in children, and various speech disorders. A basic appeal of VOT is that it is a single acoustic measure that may correlate with the voicing contrasts in all relevant natural languages (Cho & Ladefoged, 1999). The present discussion begins with American English.

For voiced stops in American English, VOTs assume a small range around zero. At VOT = 0, stop release and voicing onset are simultaneous. For example, VOT = 0 for the

TABLE 5–2

Relationship between place of articulation for stops and the acoustic properties of burst onset spectrum, burst amplitude, voice onset spectrum, and VOT.

Place	Feature			
	Burst onset spectrum	Burst amplitude	Voice onset spectrum	VOT
Bilabial	Diffuse flat/falling	Variable	Low frequency dominance	Early
Dental	Diffuse flat/falling	Weak	High frequency dominance	Early
Alveolar	Diffuse rising	Strong	Diffuse rising	– –
Palatal	Compact	Strong	High frequency dominance	?
Velar	Compact	Strong	Low frequency dominance	Late

stop [b] in the word *bye* means that the release of the bilabial closure occurs simultaneously with the onset of voicing for the following diphthong sound. For small negative values of VOT (e.g., VOT= -10 ms), voicing onset briefly precedes the stop release. This situation is also called prevoicing or voicing lead, given that voicing precedes the release. For small positive values of VOT (e.g., VOT = +10 ms), the onset of voicing slightly lags the articulatory release. The term short voicing lag is used to refer to these VOT values. VOTs for voiced stops range from about −20 ms to about +20 ms. Voiceless stops have VOTs that range upward from about 25 ms to as much as 100 ms. The word *range* should be emphasized: There is no single value of VOT that will be used by all speakers or across all phonetic contexts. Generally, voiced and voiceless stops have VOTs in the ranges indicated—the 5-ms gray interval (from 20 to 25 ms) is a kind of boundary region. The VOT ranges for voiced and voiceless stops are illustrated in Figure

5–10. Azou et al. (2000) compiled VOT data from a number of studies of English speakers. The following list shows for each voiced and voiceless stop in English the range of VOT means across 12 published studies: /p/ - 46 to 85 ms; /t/ - 65 to 95 ms; /k/ - 70 to 110 ms; /b/ - 1 to 20 ms; /d/ - 0 to 21 ms; /g/ - 14 to 35 ms. In general, there is at least a 20-ms variation in the means from different studies but a clear distinction between the voiced and voiceless stops. Azou et al. (2000) summarized some of the factors that influence VOT values, including age of speaker, speaking rate, phonetic context, and lung volume at speech initiation (see also Weismer, 1979). One other comment should be made in respect to the paper by Azou et al.: They note that when *double bursts* or *multiple bursts* occurred, they measured VOT from the first burst. Double or multiple bursts are especially likely in speech disorders such as stuttering or dysarthria, but they occasionally occur in normal speech as well.

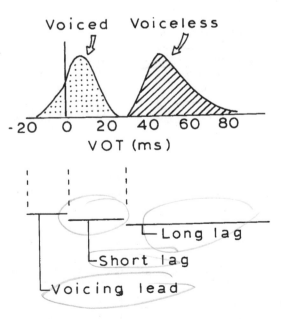

FIGURE 5–10. Distribution of voice onset time (VOT) values for voiced and voiceless stops, showing approximate VOT ranges for voicing lead, short voicing lag, and long voicing lag.

When a number of different languages are considered, the distribution of VOT values is more complicated. A basic question is: How many VOT categories are used across natural languages? In the case of velar stops in 18 different languages, Cho and Ladefoged (1999) suggested that there may be four categories of VOT, with boundaries as follows:

1. About 30 ms for unaspirated stops,

2. About 50 ms for slightly aspirated stops,

3. About 90 ms for aspirated stops, and

4. Over 120 ms for highly aspirated stops.

VOT also interacts with place of consonant articulation, with shorter VOT values occurring for more anterior closures (Azou et al., 2000; Cho & Ladefoged, 1999; Fischer-Jorgensen, 1954; Peterson & Lehiste, 1960). The effect of place of articulation is robust across languages, averaging about 18 ms between coronal and velar stops (Cho & Ladefoged, 1999). As mentioned earlier, the place-dependent nature of VOT values can be a cue to place of articulation of the consonant. The general rule is that bilabials have the shortest VOTs, including frequent prevoicing; alveolars have intermediate VOTs; and velars have the longest VOTs. This apparently is a universal characteristic of VOT and is not unique to American English. Moreover, the VOT cue to place of articulation can be used not only by human listeners, but also by several animal species and by computational learning systems (neural networks) (Damper, Gunn, & Gore, 2000).

VOT often suffices to account for the voicing feature when stops are in syllable-initial position. However, for stops in other positions, we must search for other voicing cues. Here we consider two examples: stops in word-medial position occurring between two vowels (e.g., *rabid* versus *rapid*) and stops occurring postvocalically at the end of a word (e.g., *robe* versus *rope*). For the former, several different cues can apply, including the presence of a voice bar during the stop gap of a voiced stop, a longer stop gap for a voiceless stop, a stronger release burst for a voiceless stop, a longer duration of the prevocalic vowel for a voiced stop, and a higher fundamental frequency for the voiceless stop (Abrahamson, 1977; Lisker, 1978). It should be noted that not all these properties should be expected to occur. One or more of them may suffice for the voicing distinction for a given speaker and a given context.

For postvocalic syllable-final stops, like those in the words *robe* and *rope*, the duration of a preceding vowel tends to be longer before voiced than voiceless consonants (Chen, 1970; House, 1961; House & Fairbanks, 1953; Raphael, 1972). Chen reported that for English, the average ratio of vowel duration for vowels before voiceless as opposed to voiced consonants is 0.61. This is a rather large difference that should be readily perceptible. However, the feature of vowel lengthening does not necessarily constitute the primary cue for a voicing distinction. Perhaps the strongest cue is in the end portion of the vowel (Hogan & Rozsypal, 1980; Revoile, Pickett, Holden, & Talkin 1982; Wardrip-Fruin, 1982; Wolf, 1978). Speakers can signal the voicing contrast in syllable-final position with a variety of cues including presence/absence of voicing during closure, duration of stop gap (with a longer closure for voiceless stops), strength of release burst or presence of aspiration (with a stronger burst or aspiration for voiceless stops), and fundamental frequency (with a lower fundamental frequency for voiced stops, and a lower F1 throughout the preconsonantal vowel) (Castleman & Diehl, 1996; Hogan & Rozsypal, 1980, Summers, 1988; Wolfe, 1978). An example of a pair of words that differ in the voicing feature of a final stop is given in the spectrograms of Figure 5–11. The words are *pod* and *pot*. The former has a conspicuously longer duration of the vowel segment (interval *a*), a lower F1 frequency near the vowel-consonant boundary (the ellipse labeled *b*), and vocal pulsing in the vicinity of the stop gap (the ellipse labeled *c*).

Stevens and Blumstein (1981) hypothe-sized that the voicing distinction is cued by the presence or absence of low-frequency periodic energy in or near the consonant constriction interval. They noted that this low-frequency energy can be analyzed into at least three phonetically distinct proper-ties: (a) voicing during the consonant con-striction interval, (b) a low F1 frequency near the constriction interval, and (c) a low f_0 in this same interval. Castleman and Diehl (1996) grouped these properties in a single hypothesis termed the *low-frequency hypothesis of consonant voicing,* which reflects the idea that the three cues all are associated with low-frequency energy related to f_0 and F1.

The voicing distinction is a good exam-ple of the principle that several different acoustic cues may signal a given phonetic contrast. The listener is able to detect these cues and use them as needed. There may be a hierarchy of acoustic cues for voicing, with timing information used only when other cues are unavailable or ambiguous (Barry, 1979; Hogan & Rozsypal, 1980; Port & Dalby, 1982; Wardrip-Fruin, 1982). Many of these same acoustic cues serve to signal the voicing contrast for other obstruents. Because the voicing cues are especially complicated for stops, the discussion of voicing for these sounds prepares the way to understand voicing for other types of consonants. Despite the multiplicity of

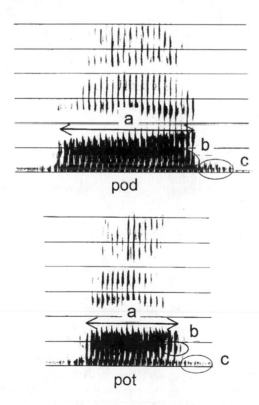

FIGURE 5–11. Spectrogram of the words *pod* and *pot* showing the low-frequency cues associated with the voicing feature. The former has a conspicuously longer duration of the vowel segment (interval *a*), a lower F1 frequency near the vowel-consonant boundary (the ellipse labeled *b*), and vocal pulsing in the vicinity of the stop gap (the ellipse labeled *c*).

acoustic cues for voicing, it is possible that all the cues can be unified in terms of relatively simple concepts. For examples of this attempt, see Lisker and Abrahamson (1971), Slis and Cohen (1969), and Stevens and Blumstein (1981).

Formant transition

For stops in syllable-initial position, the stop release entails a change in vocal tract shape from stop occlusion to vowel configuration. The articulatory transition from stop to vowel is associated with an acoustic transition in the form of shifting formants. These changes in formant frequency reflect changes in the resonating cavities of the vocal tract. The formant shifts in consonant + vowel sequences are called *CV formant transitions*. The formant transitions are a very important acoustic cue for speech perception and have been the focus of numerous research efforts.

When the word-final stop is preceded by a vowel, as in Figure 5–12, an interval of formant transition joins the vowel and consonant segments. The *VC formant transition* can be regarded as the reverse, or mirror image, of the CV formant transition discussed earlier. For CV sequences, the transition is from stop to vowel, whereas for VC sequences, the transition is from vowel to stop. The acoustic transition is largely characterized as formant-frequency shifts; it reflects the underlying articulatory transition between a closed vocal tract and a following vowel, or vice versa. The VC transition carries information regarding place of stop articulation and may also carry information on the voicing feature of the postvocalic stop, as discussed earlier.

In general, changes in vocal tract shape during speech are signaled acoustically by changes in the vocal tract resonances. The acoustic changes have approximately the same duration as the underlying articulatory

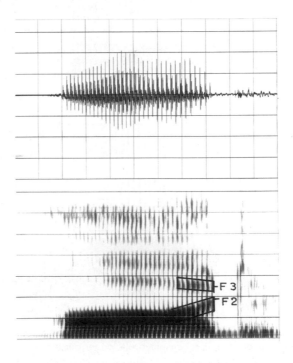

FIGURE 5–12. Spectrogram of the word *odd* showing the vowel-to-consonant (VC) formant transition.

changes. If the articulatory transition from stop occlusion to vowel configuration takes 50 ms, the acoustic transition also has a duration of about 50 ms. One fairly reliable temporal constant of stop articulation is that the transition from stop to vowel or from vowel to stop is about 50 ms in duration. Within this 50-ms interval, all formant frequencies shift from their values for the stop to their values for the vowel. Examples of formant transitions are shown in spectrograms with highlighted formant trajectories in Figure 5–13. This figure illustrates that all visible formants accomplish their frequency shifts within an interval of about 50 ms. This relatively short transition time relates to the fact that stops are made with rapid articulatory movements.

The three syllables shown in Figure 5–13 are a good starting point for a discussion of formant transitions because they represent three different stops produced with the same vowel. In each syllable, the F1 frequency increases from stop to vowel. This change is fairly easily explained from acoustic theory because the F1 frequency during a stop occlusion is theoretically close to zero. Therefore, the F1 frequency will *always increase* during a stop to vowel transition (and will decrease during a vowel to stop transition). A very low F1 frequency usually means that the vocal tract is constricted to some degree for a consonant sound. The ultimate constriction is stop closure and it is for stops that the F1 frequency reaches its minimum, which would theoretically be zero for a hard-walled tube, but since the vocal tract is not really hard-

walled, F1 only approaches zero during stop closure.

The formant frequency changes are not as simple for F2 and F3 as they are for F1. The F2 frequency increases slightly during the transition from [b] to [u], but it decreases slightly for the [g] to [u] transition and decreases markedly for the [d] to [u] transition. This result holds the promise that the F2 transition may be sensitive to place of stop articulation. A similar suggestion is prompted by the results for F3, that is, the F1 transition appears to be a cue to manner of production (degree of constriction), and the F2 and F3 transitions may be cues to place of production. To evaluate this idea, we will revisit a significant part of the history of speech research.

Although formant transitions are evident in natural speech, they can be difficult to measure because of variability in their durations, rate of change, and initial and terminal points. In view of these difficulties in the analysis of natural speech, it was easier to study formant transitions in synthetic speech. Early studies were performed with the pattern playback, which allowed investigators to determine the perceptual qualities of various formant transitions. This work securely demonstrated that variations in the F2 transition between consonant and vowel were sufficient to produce stimuli identified as different stops. The problem that remained was to explain how stop identification related to the form of the transitions. It was immediately clear that a given consonant was associated with a variety of transitions, depending on the vowel

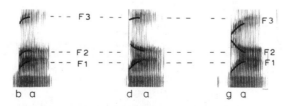

FIGURE 5–13. Spectrograms with highlighted formant transitions for the syllables /ba/, /da/, and /ga/. Note distinctiveness of F2 and F3 transitions, but the uniformity of the F1 transition.

context. Figure 5–14 shows the variety of stylized spectrographic patterns that applied to the three voiced stops [b d g] in seven vowel contexts. Note in particular that [d] could have a rising transition, a flat transition or a falling transition, depending on the vowel that followed it. Obviously, the direction of F2 shift was not in itself a sufficient cue to determine stop identity.

From examination of patterns like those in Figure 5–14, it was recognized that a possible unifying feature of the various F2 transitions was the starting frequency. For example, all the F2 transitions for [b] were consistent with the hypothesis that the F2 starting frequency was very low, somewhere in the region of 600–800 Hz. For [d], the F2 starting frequency appears to be about 1800 Hz. The results are not as simple for [g], but it must be remembered that velar stops are not produced with a single site of contact but rather with a substantial antero-posterior (front-back) range associated with the vowel context. In the case of bilabials and alveolars, for which a definite point of occlusion is maintained across vowel contexts, the evidence for the hypothesized constant starting frequency

of F2 is fairly strong. This starting frequency came to be known as the **locus** (center of gravity or concentration). The F2 locus for bilabials was estimated to be about 800 Hz and the F2 locus for alveolars, about 1800 Hz. At least two F2 loci were needed for [g]—one at about 3000 Hz and one at about 1300 Hz. (These values are for the speech of adult males and must be adjusted for the smaller vocal tracts of women and children.)

These locus values were based on experiments with simplified two-formant stimuli. When F3 is added to the formant pattern, a clearer picture emerges. For one thing, the F2-F3 relationship is important for velars, for which the transitions into a following vowel are characterized by an increasing F3-F2 separation (sometimes described as a "wedge" shape). The results of perceptual experiments should always be interpreted with respect to the acoustic stimuli from which the judgments were obtained.

As a further illustration of the locus concept, Figure 5–15 shows several different F2 transitions for the stop [d] produced with different following vowels. Despite

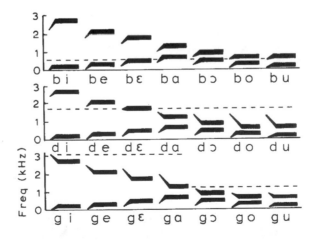

FIGURE 5–14. Stylized spectrograms (F1 and F2 patterns) for CV syllables composed of the stops /b/, /d/, and /g/ and each of seven vowels. The broken line in each CV series is an estimate of the F2 locus for that place of articulation. For example, the locus for the bilabial /b/ is approximately 600 Hz. Adapted from Delattre, Liberman, and Cooper (1955).

the considerable divergence of the patterns, the starting point is essentially the same, that is, the F2 pattern begins approximately at the locus value of 1800 Hz and then moves to the F2 value of the following vowel. Similar ideas can be applied to the F3 transition, and current understanding of formant transitions emphasizes the combined frequency shifts of F1 (a cue for manner of articulation) and F2 and F3 (cues for place of articulation). It also should be emphasized that the formant loci are consistent with the resonance frequencies calculated from acoustic theory for each place of consonant articulation (Stevens & House,

1956), that is, the loci are grounded in acoustic theory.

Confirmation of the perceptual significance of formant transitions has come from contemporary experiments with synthetic speech. When the formant transitions are properly specified, listeners can identify stops even when bursts are omitted from the synthetic stimuli. Spectrographic examples of computer-synthesized stop + vowel syllables are shown in Figure 5–16. As compelling as some of the synthesis experiments have been, analyses of natural speech still do not provide strong support for the locus concept. Kewley-Port (1983b)

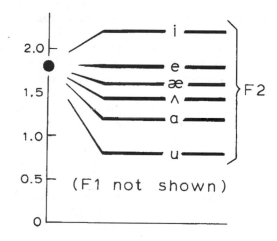

FIGURE 5–15. Composite illustration of the F2 patterns for syllables composed of an alveolar stop /d/ and six different vowels. F2 locus for /d/ is indicated by filled circle on frequency axis.

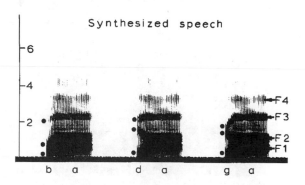

FIGURE 5–16. Spectrograms of synthesized CV syllables. The small filled circles near the onset of each syllable indicate the starting frequencies of F1, F2, and F3.

concluded that none of the individual F1, F2 or F3 transitions were distinctive correlates of place of articulation when they were analyzed with respect to onset frequency and duration. In addition, the formant loci for F2 and F3 were so variable across vowel contexts that determination of a single locus frequency for each stop was tenuous (although the results for [d] did converge on the expected value of 1800 Hz). A summary of Kewley-Port's F2 and F3 loci is given in Table 5–3.

A distinctive property of the F2 and F3 transitions for the velar stop is that both appear to emerge from the mid-frequency noise burst. This pattern is illustrated in Figure 5–17. Notice that F2 and F3 diverge from a common frequency region that is nearly continuous with the burst. The pattern is similar to one that Stevens and Blumstein (1975) described as having a leading edge that is wedge-shaped. The mirror pattern occurs for the VC transition, as shown in the same figure. The F2–F3 divergence or convergence is a useful cue for the velars and is a more reliable crite-

rion than any single locus value. It is questionable if even a 2-valued locus suffices for the velar consonants. In an X-ray microbeam study of 12 speakers of American English, Dembowski (1998) reported that the site of constriction for the velar stops ranged widely over the palate, as though these sounds could be formed quite variably.

Klatt (1979, 1987) suggested a modified-locus approach in which the starting frequency of the F2 transition is plotted against the F2 frequency of the following vowel. The measurement points are shown in Figure 5–18. The frequency coordinates thus determined can be grouped into vowel subsets, such as front vowel, rounded vowel, back vowel and unrounded vowel. Evidence for a locus theory is obtained if the data points fall on a straight line. A linear relationship indicates that the onset frequency of F2 can be predicted from the vowel target frequency. An extension of this idea includes the F3 frequency of the vowel as an additional data point, so that three values are available to establish consonant identity.

TABLE 5–3
F1, F2 and F3 loci for three places of stop articulation (after Kewley-Port, 1983b).

	Locus Estimate		
	F1	F2	F3
Bilabial	near 0	1100–1500	2200–2400
Alveolar	near 0	1800	2500–2700
Velar	near 0	1500–2500	2200–3000

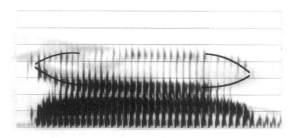

FIGURE 5–17. Spectrograms of the syllable [gæg] with highlighted F2 and F3 transitions. Note wedge-shaped F2–F3 patterns.

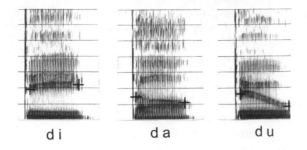

di   da   du

FIGURE 5–18. Illustration of measurement points to determine locus equations corresponding to place of articulation. Measures of F2 frequency are made at F2 onset and at the F2 value for the vowel.

Sussman (1979) examined this possibility for two male speakers and presented locus equations for F2 and F3 of /b/, /d/ and /g/. He reported distinctive slopes for the linear locus equations. For example, for one speaker, the F2 slope value was 0.91 for bilabial place, 0.46 for alveolar place, and 0.67 for velar place. Sussman and colleagues continued this line of investigation by determining locus equations for additional adult speakers of American English (Sussman, McCaffrey, & Matthews, 1991), adult speakers of Thai, Cairene Arabic, and Urdu (Sussman, Hoemeke, & Ahmed, 1993), adult speakers compensating for a bite block (Sussman, Fruchter, & Cable, 1995), and children learning American English (Sussman, Hoemeke, & McCaffrey, 1992). Fruchter and Sussman (1997) showed how the locus equation could accommodate classical data from Liberman et al. (1954) as well as more recent data (Sussman et al., 1991) in the form of identification surfaces for the identification of the stops. Sussman et al. (1998) offered an hypothesis called the orderly output constraint based on the linearity of the locus equations. However, the interpretation and significance of locus equations has been questioned. Brancazio and Fowler (1998) concluded that locus equations failed to account for large proportion of variance in listener judgments of stop consonants, and Lofqvist (1999) argued that locus equations do not appear to be an index of the degree of coarticulation between a consonant and a following vowel. For a more thorough discussion of locus equations, see the article by Sussman et al. (1998) and the associated peer commentary.

Discrimination of pharyngeal and uvular consonants apparently depends largely on F1 characteristics, with the onset F1 frequency being higher for the pharyngeal (Alwan, 1989). Interestingly, the relative value of the F1 onset frequency was related to perception of three places of consonant articulation, with uvular judgments associated with low F1 onsets, pharyngeal judgments with high F1 onsets, and glottal judgments with intermediate onsets. Because Alwan's results were obtained with a single vowel environment, further studies are needed to establish the generality of this acoustic–perceptual relationship.

Although stop bursts and formant transitions have been considered separately, both are often available in speech perception. Therefore, they are complementary cues and their integration probably leads to a stronger phonetic percept than would be formed with either one alone. Furthermore, the relative importance of the burst and formant transition may vary with the voicing and place features of the consonant and even with the vowel context in which the consonant is produced (Smits et al., 1996). One additional important point is that the formant transition cue applies to consonants generally. For instance, it is noted later that the nasal consonants, produced like the stops with bilabial, alveolar and velar articulations, have similar formant transitions. This result is not surprising if we remember that formant transitions are a cue to place of articulation and are not restricted to any given manner of production. An understanding of formant transitions for stops is a foundation for the more general study of formant transitions associated with consonant–vowel or vowel–consonant sequences.

Summary of Correlates of Place of Articulation of Stops

Place of articulation can be cued by different acoustic properties, including burst template (Blumstein & Stevens, 1979; Stevens & Blumstein, 1978), spectral moments (Forrest et al., 1988), formant transitions, and, when available, even the relative VOT value. The following summaries list these different cues for each place of stop articulation assuming a syllable-initial position.

1. Bilabial:

    Template description: diffuse, flat or falling spectrum;

    Spectral moment description: relatively low spectral mean, high skewness, and low kurtosis;

    Formant transition: F2 frequency increases from stop release into following vowel.

    VOT: relatively short; prevoicing likely for voiced bilabial stops.

2. Alveolar:

    Template description: diffuse, rising spectrum;

    Spectral moment description: relatively high spectral mean, low skewness, and low kurtosis;

    Formant transition: F2 frequency decreases from stop release into following vowel except for the high-front vowels.

    VOT: intermediate between bilabials and velars.

3. Velar:

    Template description: compact (mid-frequency emphasis) spectrum;

    Spectral moment description: relatively low spectral mean, high skewness, and high kurtosis, probably reflecting compact spectrum;

    Formant transition: F2 and F3 have a wedge-shaped pattern in which they are initially nearly fused but separate in frequency during the transition.

    VOT: longest values across the 3 places of stop production; long lags likely for voiceless velars.

Fricative Consonants

As discussed in Chapter 2, the essential articulatory feature of a fricative is a narrow constriction maintained somewhere in the vocal tract. When air passes through the constriction at a suitable rate of flow, the condition of turbulence results. Turbulence means that the particle motion in the airstream becomes highly complex, forming small eddies in the region just beyond the constricted segment. The aerodynamic condition of turbulence is associated with the generation of turbulence noise in the acoustic signal. Thus, fricatives are characterized by: (1) the formation of a narrow constriction somewhere in the vocal tract, (2) the development of turbulent airflow, and (3) the generation of turbulence noise. These three characteristics define the essential articulatory, aerodynamic, and acoustic properties of fricatives.

Fricatives are not the only class of sounds involving noise generation. However, compared to stops and affricates, fricatives have relatively long durations of noise, and it is this lengthy interval of aperiodic energy that distinguishes fricatives as a sound class. It is risky to assign a particular duration to fricative noise segments, because the duration is influenced by numerous contextual factors. Klatt (1974, 1976) reported that the duration of fricative [s] can range from 50 ms in consonant clusters to 200 ms in phrase-final position. About all that can be safely said is that when stops, affricates and fricatives are compared in an equivalent context, the fricatives generally have the longest noise segments. In a study of the noise segment durations for stops, affricates, and fricatives in the languages of Mandarin, Czech, and German, Shinn (1984) identified the following durational boundaries: 62 to 78 ms for the stop-affricate boundary, and 132 to 133 ms for the *affricate-fricative boundary*. That is, for his stimuli (isolated meaningful CV syllables), noise segments were likely to be labeled stops if they were less than about 75 ms, affricates if they were in the range of 75 to 130 ms, and fricatives if they were longer than 130 ms. However, these values are only approximate. The boundaries are typically altered for changes in speaking rate and utterance complexity. Energy level may interact with noise duration in determining whether listeners hear an affricate or a fricative. Hedrick (1997) reported that listeners presented with synthetic stimuli heard more palatal affricates than fricatives when (a) presentation level increased, (b) the relative amplitude in the third formant region increased, or (c) frication duration decreased.

Fricatives in English are produced at five places in the vocal tract: labiodental—[f v], linguadental—[θ ð], lingua-alveolar—[s z], linguapalatal—[ʃ ʒ], and glottal—[h]. These fricatives may be classified as **stridents** [s z ʃ ʒ] and **nonstridents** [f v θ ð h]. Some phoneticians use the term *sibilants* (and nonsibilants) rather than stridents (and nonstridents). Stridents have greater noise energy than nonstridents, and the dif-

ference can be important to their perceptual identification (Behrens & Blumstein, 1988a, 1988b; McCasland, 1979; Strevens, 1960)

Fricatives also may be classified with respect to voicing. The voiced fricatives [v ð z ʒ] are produced with two sources of energy, the quasi-periodic energy of vocal fold vibration and the aperiodic energy of turbulence noise. The voiceless fricatives have only the latter source of energy. Voiced fricatives tend to have shorter noise segment durations than voiceless fricatives (Baum & Blumstein, 1987; Crystal & House, 1988). However, there is considerable overlap in the durations of noise segments of voiced and voiceless fricatives when large numbers of these sounds are compared together; that is, the durational differences in noise segments are statistical, rather than categorical. The presence or absence of voicing energy is the dominant cue for the perception of the voicing contrast in fricatives. Furthermore, the presence or absence of voicing energy at the acoustic boundaries of the fricative noise seems to be particularly important (Pirello, Blumstein, & Kurowski, 1997). Pirello et al. used the amplitude of H1 (first harmonic) as an index of voicing during the frication interval.

These classifications of English fricatives are diagramed in Figure 5–19, which serves as the framework for the following discussion of the acoustic properties of these sounds.

Stridents

The strident fricatives possess intense noise energy and are distinguished among themselves with respect to voicing and noise spectrum. The turbulence noise of voiced fricatives is modulated by the laryngeal vibrations. This quasi-periodic modulation is illustrated in Figure 5–20 with both a waveform and a spectrogram for [z] and [ʒ]. The spectrogram reveals how the turbulence noise is pulsed by the voicing source. The voiceless cognates [s ʃ] are shown in Figure 5–21. For these fricatives,

FRICATIVE CLASSIFICATIONS

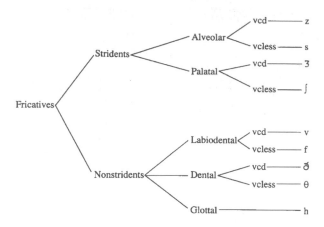

FIGURE 5–19. Phonetic classification of fricative consonants.

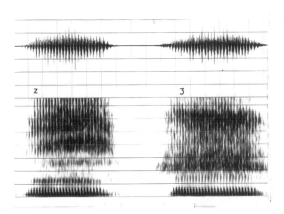

FIGURE 5–20. Waveforms and spectrograms for isolated productions of the fricatives [z] and [ʒ].

continuous noise energy is evident in the waveform and the spectrogram.

It is clear from comparing the spectrograms in Figures 5–20 and 5–21 that the spectra for alveolar fricatives contain relatively higher frequency energy than the spectra for palatals. As a rule of thumb for adult male speakers, the major region of noise energy for the alveolar fricatives lies above 4 kHz. In contrast, the palatal fricatives have significant noise energy extending down to about 3 kHz. These cutoff

values are only approximate and would have to be scaled upward for women and children.

Spectrograms are not ideal for examination of the detailed spectral features of fricatives. For this purpose, it is preferable to use spectra determined by methods such as FFT or LPC. Examples of FFT and LPC spectra for the voiceless stridents are contained in Figure 5–22. As we saw earlier with spectrograms, the alveolar fricative has more energy at higher frequences com-

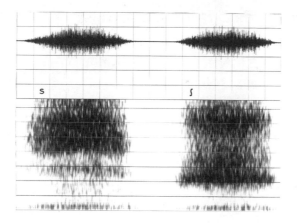

FIGURE 5–21. Waveforms and spectrograms for isolated productions of the fricatives [s] and [ʃ].

pared to the palatal. Both alveolar and palatal fricatives have numerous minor maxima and minima in their spectra (Hughes & Halle, 1956). Apparently, these spectral irregularities are of relatively slight consequence in the perception of these sounds. In a study with synthesized fricatives, Heinz and Stevens (1961) modeled these sounds with a single low-frequency zero (anti-resonance) and a single pole (resonance) applied to a white noise source. Listeners identified the resulting noise as [ʃ] when the center frequency of the pole was below about 3 kHz and as [s] when the center frequency was between about 4–8 kHz. Manrique and Massone (1981) determined the relative importance of different noise regions to fricative identification by filtering the sounds with various low- and high-pass circuits. Identification of [s] appeared to depend on energy peaks at about 5 and 8 kHz whereas identification of [ʃ] was related to a peak at about 2.5 kHz. The results of this filtering study are consistent with the synthesis study of Heinz and Stevens in demonstrating the importance of a low-frequency noise region for [ʃ] and a high-frequency noise region for [s]. Forrest et al. (1988) attempted to classify voiceless fricatives from the first four moments (mean, variance, skewness and kurtosis) computed from FFTs of the frication noise.

Among these statistical measures, skewness was more effective in distinguishing [s] and [ʃ], especially when a Bark transform was applied to the acoustic data. However, the statistical classification did not fare well with the nonstridents [f] and [θ]. Nearly half the [θ] tokens were misclassified as [f].

Another guideline for the spectral distinction between alveolar and palatal fricatives is based on a comparison of the major noise region of the fricative with the formant pattern of a vowel produced by the same speaker. As shown in Figure 5–23, the lower frequency limit of the primary noise energy for [s] in the word *see* is close to the frequency of F4 for the vowel. For the palatal fricative [ʃ] in the word *she* in the same figure, the lower frequency limit of the major noise region is closer to the frequency of F3 for the vowel. As a test of this criterion, you might try to classify each labeled noise segment in Figure 5–24 as either [s] or [ʃ]. Each fricative occurs in a CV syllable, making it convenient to compare the noise region of the fricative with the formant pattern of the vowel.

Several possible cues have been examined for their relevance in distinguishing alveolar and palatal fricatives (especially the unvoiced [s] and [ʃ]) (Jongman, Wayland, & Wong, 2000; Behrens & Blumstein,

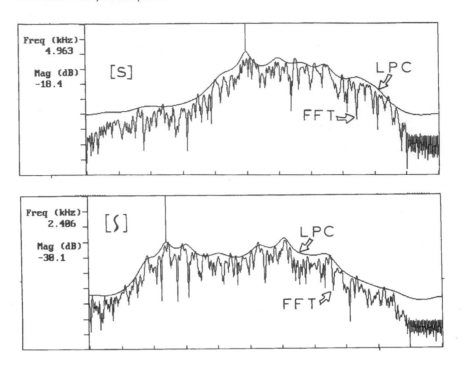

FIGURE 5–22. FFT and LPC spectra for the fricatives [s] and [ʃ]. Values shown at the left pertain to vertical line on spectra.

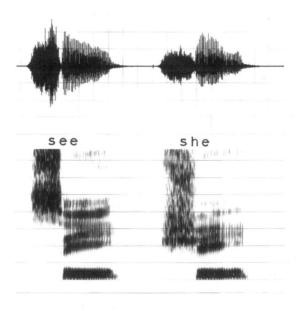

FIGURE 5–23. Waveforms and spectrograms of the syllables *see* and *she*. Notice relationship between the lower-frequency limit of noise energy for the fricative and the formant pattern for the following vowel.

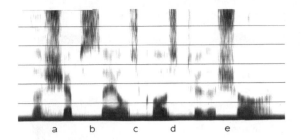

FIGURE 5–24. Spectrogram of the sentence, *"The ship sails close to the shore."* Try to classify the frication intervals (a-e) as either alveolar or palatal.

1988a; Evers, Reetz, & Lahiri, 1998). In general, these studies indicate that amplitude and durational properties do not distinguish these sounds, but spectral features do. The challenge is to select a distinguishing spectral feature that is both reliable and quantifiable. Several candidates can be considered, including spectral moments (Jongman et al., 2000; Forrest et al., 1988), energy in particular spectral regions (Behrens & Blumstein, 1988a), spectral peak (Jongman et al., 2000), and measures of spectral slope (Evers et al., 1998). One of these eventually may emerge as the preferred feature for all languages in which the contrast is relevant. However, for the present, it can be said that [s], compared to [ʃ], tends to have a spectral peak of higher frequency, greater skewness (but not uniformly in all studies), more energy in the 3.5–5.0 kHz frequency range (as opposed to the 2.5–3.5 kHz range), and a shallower slope for the spectral envelope below 2.5 kHz.

As described earlier for stops, consonants are joined to preceding or following vowels by an interval of formant transitions. Fricatives are no exception. The formant transition probably is secondary to the noise spectrum as a cue for the perception of stridents. The spectrum is primary because the noise energy for stridents is intense and phonetically distinctive. Experimental demonstrations of this point were provided by Harris (1958) and La Riviere, Winitz and Herriman (1975). Harris used a splicing technique in which the noise segment of one

fricative was combined with the transition segment of another fricative. The identification of the strident fricatives from their noise segments was unaffected by this procedure, indicating that the noise spectrum was highly distinctive. La Riviere et al. studied fricative identification for edited stimuli in which different cues were available. Their results were like those of Harris in demonstrating that the stridents were well identified from the noise segment alone. However, it also was discovered that the transition interval could aid the identification of the stridents and that the relative value of the noise or transition interval varied with vowel context. For example, the noise segment for [s] was not as effective a cue in the [i] context as it was in the [a] or [u] contexts. It may be concluded that, although stridents can be identified fairly well from their noise segments alone, formant transitions can play a secondary role in improving fricative recognition.

Nonstridents

For these fricatives, we can consider the same major acoustic features discussed for stridents. The voiced nonstridents [v ð] are shown as waveforms and spectrograms in Figure 5–25. The overall noise energy of the nonstridents is obviously less than that for the stridents. Quasi-periodic modulation of the noise by glottal pulses is evident for the voiced nonstridents in Figure 5–26 but is

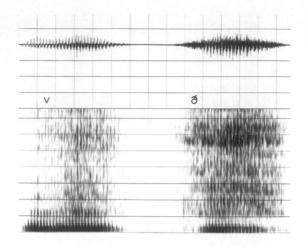

FIGURE 5–25. Waveforms and spectrograms for isolated productions of the fricatives [v] and [ð].

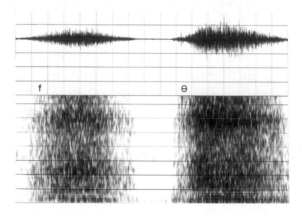

FIGURE 5–26. Waveforms and spectrograms for isolated productions of the fricatives [f] and [θ].

lacking for the voiceless nonstridents shown in Figure 5–26.

As a group, the nonstridents are weak in overall energy and possess fairly flat or diffuse spectra. The spectral flatness is illustrated by FFT and LPC spectra in Figure 5–27. The pronounced difference in energy between stridents and nonstridents makes it unlikely that a strident would be confused with a nonstrident, or vice versa. When confusions occur, they are more likely to be among the stridents or among the nonstridents. The noise energy for nonstridents can extend over an appreciable frequency range, but it is not clear how this energy relates to phonetic identification. Jongman et al. (2000) concluded that the nonstrident fricatives of American English, compared to stridents, had a lower mean amplitude (by about 10 dB), a higher spectral peak, a lower spectral mean (first moment), and a higher spectral variance (second moment). Tabain (1997) concluded that spectral information above 10 kHz for nonstrident fricatives is speaker specific. Therefore, the energy in higher frequencies may not be particularly

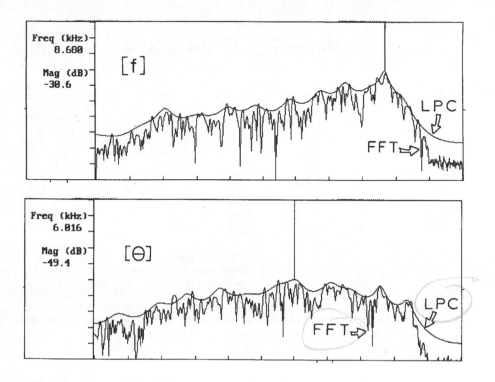

FIGURE 5–27. FFT and LPC spectra for the fricatives [f] and [θ].

important for phonetic identification but could play a role in speaker identification (discussed in Chapter 6).

The experiments by Harris and La Riviere et al. cited earlier indicated that the formant transition is more effective than the noise segment as a cue for perception of the nonstridents. However, in some vowel contexts, the noise segment can aid fricative recognition. The distinctive formant transitions for the labiodentals and the linguadentals arise because the former have a F2 locus of about 1000 Hz compared to a F2 locus of about 1400 Hz for the latter (assuming an adult male speaker). The fricative [h] typically is not associated with formant transitions. Not only is [h] produced at the glottis and pharynx, but it can be almost completely coarticulated with a following vowel's vocal tract shape. For instance, in the word *he* [hi], the vocal tract configuration for the vowel [i] is assumed

during the fricative production. Therefore, formant transitions are virtually absent even though the [h] noise segment often has a fairly marked formant-like structure (as noted by Strevens, 1960). Jongman et al. (2000) found little evidence that formant transitions carried important information relating to place of fricative articulation.

The Problem of Spectrum Characterization

The spectral properties of the noise segments for several voiceless fricatives from different languages are summarized in Table 5–4. Information is given on relative intensity, effective spectrum length and location of prominent spectral peaks. In addition, the rank frequency of occurrence as determined in a sample of 317 languages is noted. Although one should not make too

TABLE 5–4
Spectral properties of voiceless fricatives compiled from several sources. Shown for each fricative is the IPA symbol, place of articulation, rank of frequency of occurrence[a], relative intensity[b], effective spectrum length[c], and spectral peaks[d,e].

IPA	Place	Freq	Intensity	Spectrum	Spectral peaks	Spectral peaks
ø	Bilabial	—	Low	Long	—	—
f	Labiodental	3	Low	Long	1.5, 8.5	(0.5–0.6), 1.0–2.7
θ	Dental	6	Low	Long	—	(0.5–0.6), 1.5–2.3
s	Alveolar	1	High	Short	5.0, 8.0	1.0–2.7. 4.4–9.5
ʃ	Palatoalveolar	2	High	Short	2.5, 5.0	1.0–2.0, 2.3–5.3
ʂ	Palatal	7	High	Short	—	0.9–1.3, 2.7–4.4
x	Velar	4	Medium	Medium	—	1.0–1.7, 3.7–4.4
χ	Uvular	5	Medium	Medium	—	0.9–1.7, 3.1–3.7
h	Glottal	—	Medium	Medium	—	—

Sources: a—rank based on frequencies of occurrence in 317 languages reported by Nartey (1982); b,c—relative intensity and spectral length from Strevens (1960); d—spectral peaks from Manrique and Massone (1981); e—spectral peaks interpreted from tables in Nartey (1982). Values indicate ranges over which prominent peaks occur. Parenthesized values indicate peaks present in some languages or contexts but not others. Sources: Manrique, A.M.B., and Massone, M.I. (1981). Acoustic analysis and perception of Spanish fricative consonants. *Journal of the Acoustical Society of America, 69,* 1145–1153. Nartey, J.N.A. (1982). On fricative phones and phonemes: Measuring the phonetic differences within and between languages. UCLA Working Papers in Phonetics, No. 55, Department of Linguistics, University of California at Los Angeles. Strevens, P. (1960). Spectra of fricative noise in human speech. *Language and Speech, 3,* 32–49.

much of the frequency of occurrence data, it is interesting that the most frequently occurring fricatives among these languages were the stridents [s] and [ʃ]. Perhaps languages tend to select high-energy fricatives with prominent spectral differences. These fricatives should be perceptually salient and discriminable even with unfavorable masking noise.

The acoustic description of fricatives has considerable room for improvement. It has been difficult to identify measures that are economic, valid and reliable. Measures such as effective spectrum length and location of prominent peaks are not always highly repeatable within or across observers. Anyone who intends to make spectral measurements for fricatives is well-advised to read the literature carefully and evaluate the reliability of any measures selected for use. One possibility is the use of spectral moments, either alone, or in combination with other descriptions of spectral shape. Unfortunately, only limited data have been reported on spectral moment

values, and questions remain about technical issues in moment analysis (two of which are the effect of ambient noise and the effect of different values of low-pass filtering). However, two examples of spectral moment description of fricatives should be noted. One is the report on Polish voiceless fricatives from Jassem (1995), for which the spectral moment values are reported in Table 5–5. The other is the detailed study of American English fricatives by Jongman et al. (2000), the major results of which are summarized in Table 5–6.

Affricate Consonants

There are only two affricates in English, [tʃ] and [dʒ]. These are usually described as having a palatal place of articulation and to differ between themselves only in voicing. Some believe that the place of articulation is not truly palatal, at least when compared with the palatal fricatives [ʃ] and [ʒ]. The affricate is a complex sound, involving a

TABLE 5–5

Spectral moments for Polish voiceless fricatives. From W. Jassem (1995), The acoustic parameters of Polish voiceless fricatives: An analysis of variance. *Phonetica, 52,* **251–258. (Reprinted with permission of S. Karger AG, Basel). Copyright 1995.**

Fricative	Mean	Standard deviation	Kurtosis
[f]	3337	0.04982	-1.3006
[s]	6404	0.8425	2.8730
[S]	3870	0.3684	-1.6677
[C]	3874	0.5175	-0.9969
[x]	1792	4.1527	14.5630

TABLE 5–6

Summary of acoustic measures for the fricatives of American English, based on data from Jongman et al. (2000). The measures are mean duration (Dur) in ms, peak amplitude (Amp) in dB, location of spectral peak (Spect pk) in Hz, first moment (M1) in Hz, second moment (M2) in Hz, third moment (M3), and fourth moment (M4). Reprinted from A. Jongman, R. Wayland, and S. Wong (2000), Acoustic characteristics of English fricatives, *Journal of the Acoustical Society of America, 108,* **1252–1263. (Reprinted with permission of the American Institute of Physics.) Copyright 2000.**

Fricative	Dur	Amp	Spect pk	M1	M2	M3	M4
/f/	166	55.7	7733	5108	6.37	0.077	2.11
/v/	80	63.2	7733	5108	6.37	0.077	2.11
/θ/	163	54.7	7470	5137	6.19	0.083	1.27
/ð/	88	62.7	7470	5137	6.19	-0.083	1.27
/s/	178	64.9	6839	6133	2.92	-0.229	2.36
/z/	118	67.7	6839	6133	2.92	-0.229	2.36
/ʃ/	178	66.4	3820	4229	3.38	0.693	0.42
/ʒ/	123	68.2	3820	4229	3.38	0.693	0.42

sequence of stop and fricative articulations. Like stops, the affricates are produced with a period of complete obstruction of the vocal tract. Like fricatives, the affricates are associated with a period of frication. The frication interval for affricates tends to be shorter than that for fricatives. Basically, then, acoustic description of the affricates entails a description of the stop portion and a description of the noise portion.

For the syllable-initial position, the primary acoustic cues that are thought to distinguish affricates from stops are the *rise time* of the noise energy and the duration of frication (Howell & Rosen, 1983). Rise time is a measure of the time over which the amplitude envelope reaches its maximum or near-maximum value. For affricates, the mean rise time measured by Howell and Rosen was 33 ms, contrasted with a mean rise time of 76 ms for the fricatives. Thus, the affricates are characterized by a rapid buildup of acoustic noise energy, though not quite as rapid as that for stop consonants. The difference in rise time between affricates and fricatives is evident in Figure 5–28. Hedrick (1997) observed that perception of the palatal affricate also is influenced by presentation level or by the relative amplitude of energy in the third

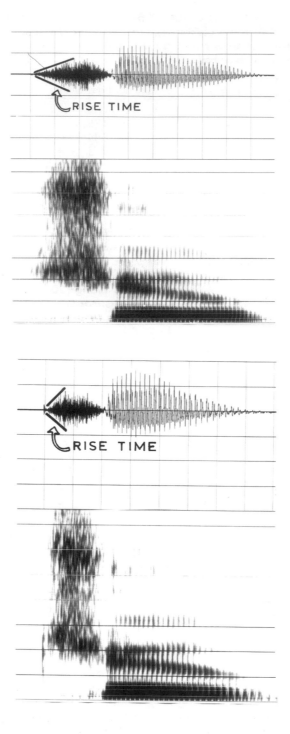

FIGURE 5–28. Waveform and spectrogram for the word *shoe* and the word *chew*. Note gradual rise time of frication energy in the waveform for *shoe* (top) but a rapid rise of frication energy for *chew* (bottom).

formant region. Several factors need to be considered in the acoustic differentiation of affricates and fricatives, and further studies are needed to determine the relative importance of the different cues.

In the postvocalic position, the acoustic cues for the affricate-fricative distinction include the rise time and duration of the noise segment, the presence or absence of a release burst, the duration of the stop gap and the temporal and/or spectral characteristics of the preceding vowel (Dorman, Raphael, & Eisenberg, 1980). These features can be seen in Figure 5–29 which displays the waveform and spectrogram for the word *judge*, which has the voiced affricate in prevocalic and postvocalic positions.

Kluender and Walsh (1992) manipulated frication duration and rise time independently in a study of the perception of voiceless fricatives and affricates. Their results showed that variations in rise time were not a sufficient cue for the affricate/fricative contrast but that variation in frication duration was sufficient. According to this result, speakers may control frication duration as the primary cue for this distinction, with rise time serving only as a secondary or redundant cue.

Nasal Consonants

The nasal consonants, /m n ŋ / in English, are produced with closure of the oral cavity and radiation of the sound through the nasal cavity while the oral obstruction is maintained (Fujimura, 1962; Lindquist & Sundberg, 1972). As explained in Chapter 2, the obstructed oral cavity acts as a shunt or side-branch resonator. That is, even though the oral cavity is closed at some point, it nevertheless contributes to the resonant qualities of the nasal consonants. If it did not, then it would be impossible to distinguish the nasals in sustained, isolated productions. Although the nasal consonants are not always easily distinguished in such productions, they do not sound exactly alike.

The articulatory feature of velopharyngeal opening accompanied by oral cavity obstruction is linked to an acoustic feature of a **nasal murmur**. The murmur is the acoustic segment associated with an exclusively nasal radiation of sound energy. Although nasalization has effects beyond this interval, the murmur is a good place to begin our inquiry into nasal consonants.

As a first look at nasal murmur, Figure 5–30 shows a spectrogram of a sustained production of the nasal consonant [n]. This spectrogram was prepared with an especially wide dynamic range to display the maxima and minima in the sound spectra. Formants are evident as the bands of energy labeled in the illustration. However, notice also the conspicuous band of reduced energy labeled as an antiformant. Another look at the spectral features of the nasal murmurs is given in Figures 5–31, 5–32, and 5–33, which show spectrograms accompanied by FFT spectra for the murmur portion of each nasal. Both the spectrograms and the FFT spectra illustrate that the nasal murmurs are associated with distinct regions of energy, similar to the formant patterns of sustained vowels (monophthongs). However, the figures also show regions of greatly reduced energy. Unlike orally radiated vowels, which theoretically possess only formants in their transfer function, the nasals possess both formants and antiformants. As was discussed earlier, the antiformants can be thought of as interfering with, or preventing, the transmission of energy in the frequency range of the antiformant. Antiformants, like formants, can be described with two numbers, the center frequency and the bandwidth. It is important to recognize that the interaction of formants and antiformants in the spectrum of a nasal sound is not a simple matter of assigning formants to spectral peaks and antiformants to spectral valleys. Although such a result may occur, other spectral consequences may occur as well. For example, if a formant and antiformant have exactly the same center frequency and bandwidth, the

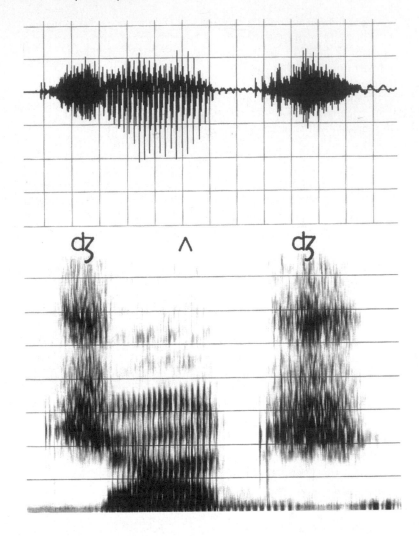

FIGURE 5–29. Waveform and spectrogram for the word *judge* to illustrate a prevocalic and postvocalic voiced affricate.

result of their interaction is a mutual cancellation. In fact, formants and antiformants often occur in pairs. When the members of a pair have the same frequencies and bandwidths, they cancel, but when the formant and antiformant diverge in these values, a particular spectral consequence will be seen.

Figure 5–34 gives a spectral comparison of a nonnasal vowel and a nasal consonant murmur. The murmur is similar to the vowel in having a number of spectral peaks but only one of these, the low frequency **nasal formant**, has an amplitude comparable to that of the vowel formants. The reduced amplitude of the other spectral peaks in the nasal murmur means that the nasal will have less overall energy than the vowel. Indeed, as the spectrogram in Figure 5–35 shows, nasal murmurs usually are easily distinguished from vowels by a comparison of the total energy. We can conclude by stating that the murmur portion of a nasal consonant has a dominant low-frequency

[n]

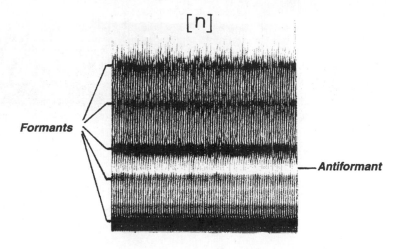

FIGURE 5–30. Spectrogram of a sustained murmur for the nasal consonant [n].

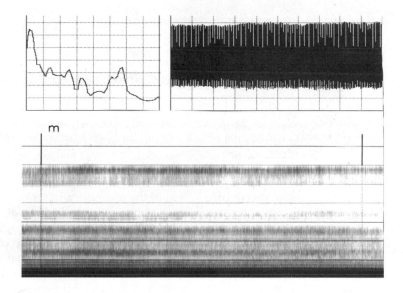

FIGURE 5–31. Three-panel analysis for the nasal consonant [m]. Upper left: long-term spectrum; upper right: waveform; lower half: spectrogram of sustained [m]. Long-term spectrum was calculated for the interval bounded by vertical lines in the spectrogram. This multiple display (and those in the following two figures) was produced with a Kay Elemetrics Corporation Model 5500 Sona-Graph.

resonance, the nasal formant, accompanied by a number of much weaker resonances at higher frequencies. As explained in Chapter 2, the nasal formant is associated with a rather long tube extending from the larynx up through the opening of the nose.

Fujimura (1962) determined that the nasal consonants have three common properties. First, all of them have a first formant of about 300 Hz that is well separated from higher formants. Second, the formants tend to be highly damped (i.e., they have large

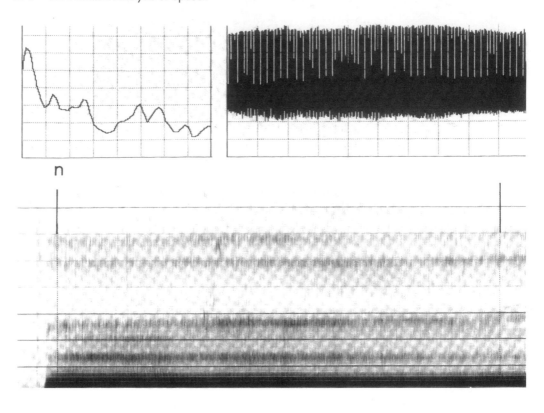

n

FIGURE 5–32. Three-panel analysis for the nasal consonant [n]. Upper left: long-term spectrum; upper right: waveform; lower half: spectrogram of sustained [n]. Long-term spectrum was calculated for the interval bounded by vertical lines in the spectrogram.

bandwidths reflecting a rapid rate of absorption of sound energy). Third, there is a high density of formants and the existence of antiformants.

A close examination of Figure 5–35 reveals that nasal consonants, like other consonants, are associated with formant transitions when they are produced in sequence with other sounds. In fact, the interpretation of the formant transitions associated with nasals is very much like that for their cognate (homorganic) stops. The formant transitions can be interpreted according to place of articulation, so that similar patterns are observed for the stop-nasal pairs, [b]-[m], [d]-[n], and [g]-[ŋ]. This similarity is not surprising given that the F2 transition relates to the place of articulation and that the F1 transition relates to obstruc-

tion of the oral cavity. In many respects, the nasal consonants can be regarded as nasalized stops, that is, they share some fundamental properties with the stop consonants. The major differences between stops and nasals are explained by the effects of nasalization. A stylized representation of a stop-vowel and a nasal-vowel syllable is given in Figure 5–36. Because the stop [d] and nasal [n] are homorganic (having the same place of articulation), they differ only in the articulatory feature of nasality. The acoustic properties of the stop-vowel syllable include the release burst, transition, and the vowel steady state. The properties for the nasal-vowel syllable are the murmur, transition, and vowel steady state. The formant transition segment is highly similar for the two syllables.

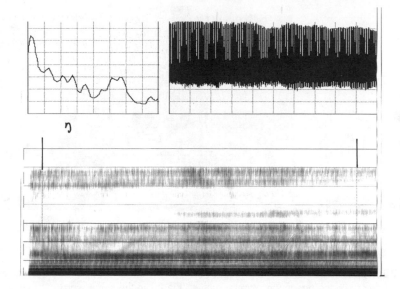

FIGURE 5–33. Three-panel analysis for the nasal consonant [ŋ]. Upper left: long-term spectrum; upper right: waveform; lower half: spectrogram of sustained [ŋ]. Long-term spectrum was calculated for the interval bounded by vertical lines in the spectrogram.

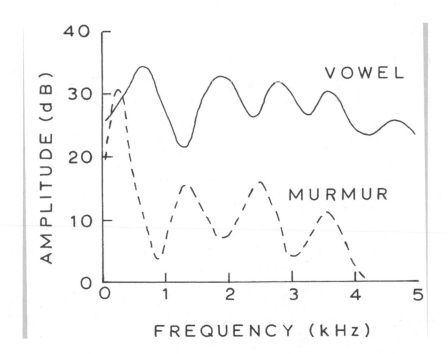

FIGURE 5–34. Idealized spectra of a nonnasal vowel and the murmur portion of a nasal consonant.

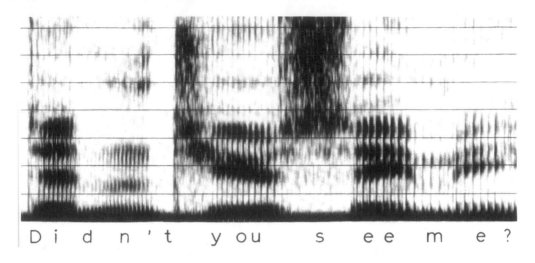

FIGURE 5–35. Spectrogram of the sentence *"Didn't you see me?"* Compare nonnasal vowels, such as the /I/ in *didn't,* with the nasal consonants, such as the [n] in the same word.

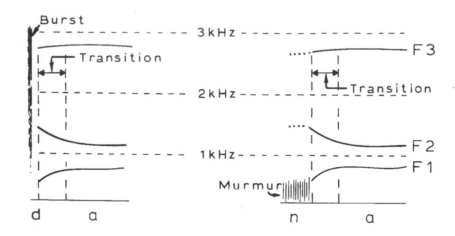

FIGURE 5–36. Stylized representation of stop + vowel and nasal + vowel syllables. Features include the stop burst, formant transitions, and nasal murmur.

Perceptual experiments by Kurowski and Blumstein (1984) demonstrated that the nasal murmur and the transitions are roughly equal in providing information on place of articulation. Their results also indicated that neither the murmur nor the transition is sufficient for consistently accurate perception of place of articulation. When the murmur alone or the transition alone was presented to listeners, the percentage-

correct score for consonant identification was about 80%. Qi and Fox (1992) reported a rate of 86% identification of [m] versus [n] using a fifth-order perceptual linear predictive model. Their results showed that the second transformed pole was significantly lower for [m] than [n]. Apparently, listeners rely on both cues, murmur and transition, and integrate them to form a single phonetic decision. Kurowski and Blumstein's conclusion stands in contrast to earlier work by Liberman et al. (1954) and by Malecot (1956) which indicated that place of articulation for the nasal consonants is cued primarily by the transition segment and not by the murmur. Repp and Svastikula (1988) reported results for nasals in VC syllables that were in substantial agreement with those of Kurowski and Blumstein. Repp and Svastikula concluded that the vocalic formant transitions by themselves conveyed about as much information on place of articulation for [m] and [n] as did the nasal murmurs alone. However, full VC syllables containing [m] or [n] were not identified as well as full CV syllables with the same consonants. A possible reason for the poorer identification of nasals in VC syllables was the "relative absence of a salient spectral change between the vowel and the murmur in VC syllables" (p. 237).

In English, only the nasal consonants /m/ and /n/ occur in word-initial position (/ŋ/ cannot occur syllable- or word-initially), but all three nasals occur word-medially or word-finally. Taken together, the three nasal consonants account for about 10% of the sounds in adult running speech (Mines, Hansen, & Shoup, 1978) and occur at an average rate of about two per second.

The nasalization of the acoustic signal applies not only to the nasal consonants but also to certain surrounding sounds, particularly vowels. In general, vowels preceding or following nasal consonants tend to be nasalized to some degree. Experiments have shown that listeners are sensitive to the vowel nasalization and use this information to make perceptual judgments about the neighboring consonants. In other words, the acoustic cues for nasalization often can be found beyond the nasal consonant segment.

Glide Consonants

The two glides of English are /w/ and /j/. Ladefoged (1975) used the term approximants for these sounds, and the term semi-

vowels also is used. Some writers apply the term semivowels not only to /w/ and /j/ but also to /r/ and /l/ (Espy-Wilson, 1992). All three terms are descriptive: the term glide describes the gradual articulatory motions that characterize these sounds; the term approximant describes the articulatory feature in which the vocal tract is markedly narrowed, but not closed, at some point; and the term semivowel describes the vowel-like nature of these sounds. The glides are necessarily prevocalic (in phonology, a postvocalic variant is sometimes recognized, but we will not do so here). The glide articulation therefore can be understood as a relatively slow movement that proceeds from a vocal tract configuration with a marked narrowing to a vocal tract configuration suitable for the following vowel. For /w/, there are really two regions of narrowing: at the lips and between the lingual dorsum and the palate (or velum). For this reason, /w/ is characterized phonetically as a labio-velar glide, quite similar in vocal tract configuration to the high-back vowel /u/. The labial and lingual movements for this glide are carried out with a close coordination, beginning and ending together. The glide /j/ has a vocal tract narrowing highly similar to that for vowel /i/. The tongue assumes a high-front position, nearly contacting the prepalatal region. The articulatory motion for glides is slow compared to the motion for stops and nasals.

Perceptual experiments have shown that the glides occupy a kind of midway position between stops and vowel-vowel transitions. The glide /w/ stands between the stop /b/ and a transition from vowel /u/ to another sound. Figure 5–37 shows spectrograms for three utterances that differ primarily in the duration of transition: syllable [bi] (as in the word *bee*), syllable [wi] (as in the word *we*), and the vowel + vowel utterance [u: i:] (which might be represented orthographically as something like "oooeee"). The formant patterns for these three utterances are similar in their changes in frequency (e.g., the F2 transition extends over about the same frequency

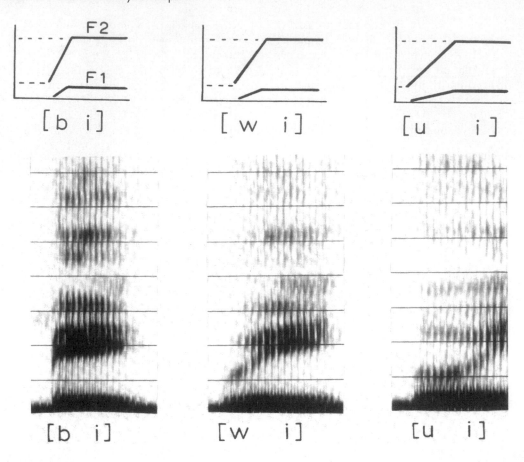

FIGURE 5-37. Stylized F1 and F2 patterns and spectrograms for the utterances [bi], [wi], and [u:i:]. The frequency extent of transition is constant across the utterances but the duration of transition varies.

range), but they differ in the duration of transition. The transition duration is briefest for the stop [b], somewhat longer for the glide [w] and longest for the vowel + vowel utterance.

The glide /j/ stands midway between the alveolar stop /d/ and a transition from vowel /i/ to another vowel. Stylized spectrograms illustrating this relationship are presented in Figure 5-38. The sample utterances are the syllable [du] (as in the word *do*), the syllable [ju] (as in the word *you*), and the vowel + vowel sequence [i: u:] ("eeeooo" as it might be rendered in a comic strip). The formant patterns for the three utterances are similar in their fre-

quency extent but different in the time taken to accomplish the shift in frequency. The transition is briefest for the stop [d], longer for the glide [j], and longer yet for the vowel + vowel utterance.

The perceptual experiments conducted by Liberman et al. (1956) showed that the duration of transition accounted for listener responses to phonetic contrasts like those depicted in Figs. 5-37 and 5-38. When the transition duration was shorter than about 40–60 ms, listeners tended to hear a stop consonant. When the transition duration was greater than 40–60 ms but less than 100–150 ms, the listeners usually judged the sound to be a glide. Finally, when the tran-

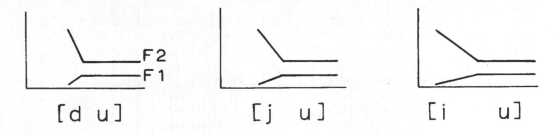

FIGURE 5–38. Stylized F1 and F2 patterns for the utterances [du], [ju], and [i:u:]. The frequency extent of transition is constant across the utterances but the duration of transition varies.

sition duration exceeded about 100 ms, the listeners heard a vowel of changing color, that is, a vowel + vowel sequence. However, a qualification should be added: the phonetic interpretation of transition durations is affected by speaking rate (Miller & Liberman, 1979; Miller & Baer, 1983). This effect can be studied by changing the duration of the test syllable. Shorter syllable durations are heard as being produced with a faster rate. When syllable duration is changed, a given transition duration sometimes is judged differently by a listener. For example, a transition duration that is heard as a stop at a slow rate (long syllable duration) is heard as a glide at a fast rate (short syllable duration). It appears that listeners use rate information to make segmental decisions from acoustic patterns. Therefore, segmental (phonetic) decisions are not entirely independent of speaking rate (an issue discussed in Chapter 6).

It also has been suggested that amplitude rise time can distinguish stops and glides. Shinn and Blumstein (1984) reported that subjects in their study categorized sounds as either /b/ or /w/ depending on the amplitude envelope of the syllable, and apparently ignored temporal information on the formant transitions. However, conflicting results were reported by Nittrouer and Studdert-Kennedy (1986) and Walsh and Diehl (1991), who found that rise time was a far less effective cue than duration of transition. Although the reasons for these conflicting results are not clear, it seems

prudent to accept the general conclusion that rise time is not a particularly salient cue for manner distinctions (Diehl & Walsh, 1986; Kluender & Walsh, 1992). Rise time may serve as a redundant cue or a cue that is speaker-dependent.

Liquid Consonants

The liquids /r/ and /l/ have some consonantal properties similar to stops and other properties similar to the glides. The similarity to stops is dynamic in nature: at least in some phonetic contexts, the articulatory movements for /r/ and /l/ are quite rapid. The similarity to glides is mainly in a shared sonorant (resonant) quality: both liquids and glides have a well-defined formant structure associated with a degree of vocal tract constriction that is less severe than that for the obstruents (stops, fricatives and affricates) but arguably more severe than that for vowels. Waveform and spectrograms are shown for productions of the words *rye* and *lie* in Figure 5–39. Note that there is an overall similarity in the pattern but that they differ in F3 and certain dynamic features.

Both [r] and [l] have a potentially sustainable characteristic articulation, although a steady state often may not be evident for occurrences of these sounds in connected speech. That is, a speaker can, upon request, sustain a sound with the essential quality of either [r] or [l]. Information about

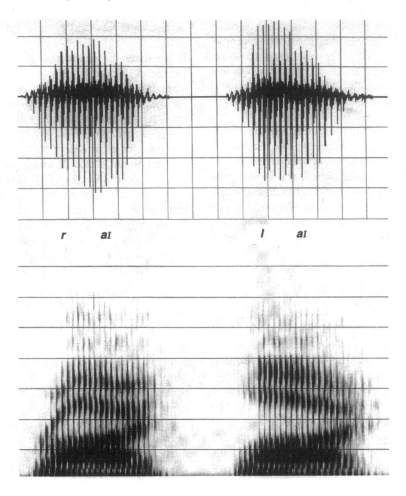

FIGURE 5–39. Waveform (top) and spectrogram (bottom) for the words *rye* and *lie*. Notice in particular the difference in the pattern of F3, which has a low onset frequency for [r] and a high onset frequency for [l].

these sounds can be obtained from the steady state production and from the transitional segment in connected speech.

When comparisons are made in minimal-pair words, F1 frequency distinguishes the glides /w/ and /j/ (which have a low F1) from the liquids /l/ and /r/ (which have a higher F1) (Lisker, 1957; O'Connor et al., 1957; Espy-Wilson, 1992). The two liquids are distinguished especially by F3 frequency. Indeed, the most distinctive property of /r/ is a lowered F3 which is narrowly separated from F2 (Lehiste, 1964;

Espy-Wilson, 1992). Among English sounds, /r/ has the lowest F3 frequency, and this feature alone (or a small F3–F2 separation) often can be used to identify the occurrence of this liquid. This feature stands out clearly in Figure 5–40. As discussed in Chapter 4, a low F3 frequency also is a distinguishing feature for the rhotacized vowel /ɝ/. Generally, for English, /r/-coloring is associated with a low F3 that is close to F2. Nolan (1983) reported the following mean formant frequencies for /r/ produced in a list of words by fifteen

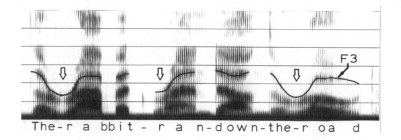

The-r a bb i t - r a n-d o w n-t h e-r oa d

FIGURE 5–40. Spectrogram of the sentence, "*The rabbit ran down the road,*" with the F3 trajectory highlighted. Arrows point to /r/ segments.

17-year-old males: F1—320 Hz; F2—1090 Hz, F3—1670 Hz. An examination of data from Hagiwara (1995) shows that for adult male speakers, F3 has a modal value of about 1500 Hz (range of about 1300 to 1800 Hz). However, for adult female speakers, Hagiwara's results show a bimodal distribution, with some women having a relatively low F3 mean of about 1700–1800 Hz and others having a relatively high F3 mean of 2200 Hz or above. Hagiwara suggested that the extent of F3 lowering is best determined in relation to a neutral value of F3, rather than in relation to some speaker-independent critical frequency value.

The /l/ is described phonetically as a lateral because the tongue tip makes a midline closure at or near the alveolar ridge, so that sound energy is radiated on either side (laterally) of the occlusion. For at least some variants of /r/, there is a marked narrowing, without closure, of the vocal tract in the palatal region. Recall from Chapter 2 that a bifurcation of the vocal tract produces antiformants, and the lateral channels for /l/ constitute such a bifurcation. Antiformants arise during the time in which the lateral articulation is in effect. Thus, /l/ shares with the nasal consonants a steady state segment for which the transfer function contains both formants and antiformants. Both the lateral and nasal consonants also have most of their energy in the low frequency region below 5 kHz. Not surprisingly, then, the lateral and the nasals can be somewhat similar in their

acoustic appearance and are subject to perceptual confusions for one another. A spectrogram of syllable-initial [l] with a prolonged onset is shown in Figure 5–41. Mean formant frequencies for [l] in three different studies were as follows: Nolan (1983): F1—360 Hz, F2—1350 Hz, F3—3050 Hz; Lehiste (1964): F1—295 Hz, F2—980 Hz, F3—2600 Hz; Al-Bamerni (1975): F1—365 Hz, F2—1305 Hz, F3—2780 Hz. The F1 and F2 values for [l] are similar to those for [r], but the F3 value for [l] is about 1 kHz higher than that for [r].

Figure 5–42 depicts the differences in formant pattern between [r] and [l]. This figure shows a schematic spectrographic representation in which three acoustic cues are manipulated to produce stimuli that vary from *rock* to *lock*. One is a temporal cue in which the steady state and transition durations of F1 are varied from an [r] pattern (short steady state and long transition) to an [l] pattern (long steady state and short transition). Another cue is the relative onset frequency for F2, which varies from a relatively low value for [r] to a relatively higher value for [l]. The third cue is the relative onset frequency for F3, varying from a relatively low F3 for [r] to a relatively high F3 for [l].

Phonetics books frequently comment on the allophonic complexity of the liquids. For example, /l/ has both light and dark variants and its formant pattern varies with the vowel context (Tarnoczy, 1948; Lehiste, 1964; Nolan, 1983). Various writers describe

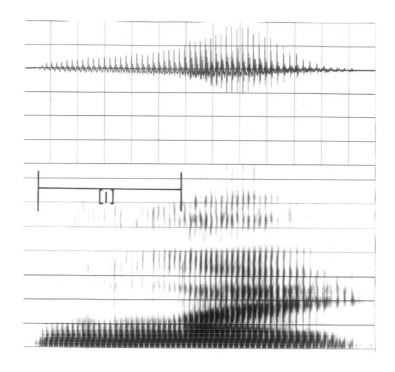

FIGURE 5–41. Waveform and spectrogram of the word *law* produced with a prolongation of the /l/ steady state (labeled on spectrogram).

for /r/ syllabic and nonsyllabic variants, initial and final variants, as well as articulatory variants such as retroflex and bunched (Lehiste, 1964; Shriberg & Kent, 1982). These variants complicate the description of the articulatory or acoustic properties of the liquids, and this limitation should be kept in mind whenever generalizations are proposed. It seems necessary to recognize at least two major variants of each liquid: prevocalic and postvocalic. Justification for such a classification comes from Lehiste (1964) for /r/ and from Giles (1971), Lehman and Swartz (2000), and Narayanan, Alwan, and Haker (1997) for /l/. These studies indicate that prevocalic liquids differ from postvocalic liquids, and that these two categories may predominate over other allophonic distinctions. Lehman and Swartz (2000) reported that prevocalic [l] had a lower F1 and higher F2 frequency than postvocalic [l]. Another difference was

that F2 and F3 were frequently weak or absent for prevocalic but not postvocalic [l].

A further complication is that many phoneticians classify postvocalic [r] as a vowel. We will not attempt to resolve these issues here; it is sufficient it to say that [l] and [r] can be acoustically described in terms of formant pattern.

Note on Sonorants: Nasals, Glides, and Liquids

The nasals, glides, and liquids are classified together as *sonorants*. These sounds derive essentially all their energy from vocal fold vibration, and because the vocal tract is not radically constricted at any point, this energy excites all the formants (though some may be weak in amplitude relative to others). The sonorants can be characterized as sounds with a substantial amount of

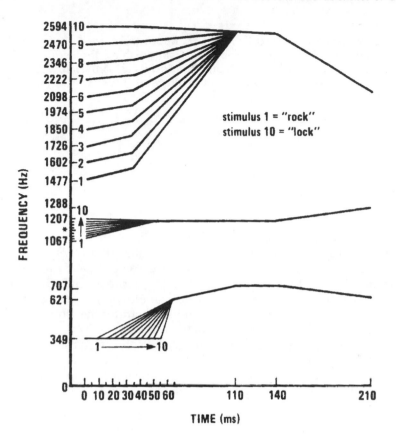

stimulus 1 = "rock"
stimulus 10 = "lock"

FIGURE 5–42. F1, F2, and F3 patterns used in synthesizing a range of stimuli between *rock* and *lock*. Reprinted from L. Polka and W. Strange, (1985). Perceptual evidence of acoustic cues that differentiate /r/ and /l/. *Journal of the Acoustical Society of America, 78,* 1187–1206. (Reprinted with permission of the American Institute of Physics.) Copyright 1985.

low-frequency energy. Espy-Wilson (1992) defined an acoustic correlate of the sonorant feature as the band-limited energy over the frequency range of 100 to 400 Hz. For sonorants, the energy in this limited bandwidth is nearly equal to the overall energy of the sound (i.e., the energy computed for the total bandwidth of analysis). In contrast, the nonsonorants (obstruents) have relatively little energy in the low frequencies compared to the high frequencies. Espy-Wilson (1992) also compared prevocalic /w j l r/ with respect to their bark-difference values (Table 5–7). It appears that bark-difference values hold potential to distinguish among these sounds.

The Allophones [ɾ] and [ʔ]

Several allophones (nonphonemic variants) have been mentioned in the preceding sections. For example, the released and unreleased allophones of the stop consonants were discussed as a part of the general section on stops. But because they have special properties, the two allophones [ɾ] and [ʔ] are given a separate section in this chapter. [ɾ] is described phonetically as a lingual flap (or, alternatively, as a one-tap trill). This sound is made as a very rapid tongue movement from one vocal tract configuration, typically for a vowel, to a brief contact

TABLE 5–7
Bark-difference values for prevocalic /w ȷ l r/. Reprinted from C. Y. Espy-Wilson (1992), Acoustic measures for linguistic features distinguishing the semivowels / w ȷ r l/ in American English, *Journal of the Acoustical Society of America, 92*, 736–757. (Reprinted with permission of the American Institute of Physics.) Copyright 1992.

	B1–B0	B2–B1	B3–B2	B4–B3
/w/	2.4	3.6	6.4	2.5
/ȷ/	1.7	10.2	1.7	1.6
/l/	2.6	4.9	5.5	2.3
/r/	2.8	6.0	2.1	3.9

with the alveolar ridge or the postdental region. The contact is followed by a rapid movement away from the constriction. The flap is an allophone of both [t] and [d] in words like *latter* versus *ladder*, and *writer* versus *rider*. In its spectrographic appearance, the flap is remarkable primarily for its brevity. Compared to distinctive productions of [t] and [d], the flap has a short overall duration and a very brief closure period. These features are illustrated in Figure

5–43.

The glottal stop [ʔ] is used allophonically for the stops [t] and [d], and occasionally for other phonemes, depending on dialect and idiolect. It is hard to identify a good keyword for the glottal stop, because of the variability in its use among speakers and dialects. Some British speakers use [ʔ] in the word *bottle*. In addition, the glottal stop serves a junctural role. Abutting words that end and begin with vowels often are

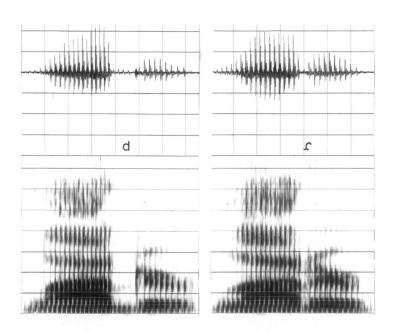

FIGURE 5–43. Waveforms and spectrograms for the word *ladder* produced with an intervocalic stop [d] (left) and an intervocalic flap [ɾ] (right).

produced with a glottal stop between the vowel elements. Thus, the name *Anna Adams* might be realized phonetically as

[ae n ə ʔ ae d ə m z]

to distinguish it from the similar sound pattern in *Ann Adams*. The glottal stop also is used by many speakers to make the distinction *Lee owes* versus *Leo owes*.

This use of the glottal stop can be quite frequent for some speakers. A likely acoustic correlate for glottal stops in prevocalic position is the rate of increase in the amplitude envelope of the vowel waveform (Peters et al., 1986). In medial positions, the glottal stop is an interruption of voicing accomplished by a momentary adduction of the vocal folds. The interruption can be observed on acoustic displays as a gap or period of reduced acoustic energy that may be accompanied by an abrupt onset of vocal fold vibration (Figure 5–44). Because the articulation is carried out at the level of the larynx, the effects on formant pattern are subtle. In particular, the glottal stop usually is not associated with marked formant transitions typical of the oral stops because the formation of a glottal stop does not affect the shape of the cavities above the larynx, which determine resonances. However, it appears that a genuine stop articulation at the glottis is not required for perception of

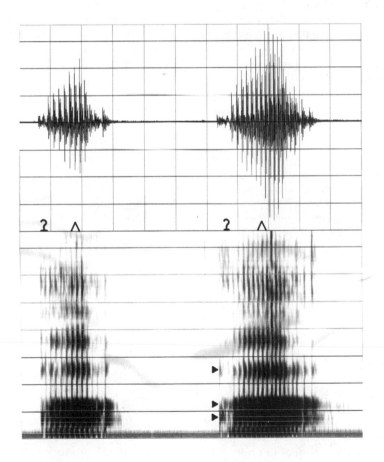

FIGURE 5–44. Waveform and spectrogram for the utterance [ʔ ʌ ʔ ʌ]. Note glottal stops in initial and medial positions. Small arrows point to F1, F2, and F3 frequencies, which are essentially continuous from glottal stop release into the following vowel.

a glottal stop. Hillenbrand and Houde (1996) noted that it is sufficient for the speaker to produce a dip in the f_0 contour or a dip in the amplitude contour. A glottal stop in word-initial position often is acoustically evident through the rapid rise of energy for the voiced sound. This short rise time resembles "hard glottal attack," or a forceful and abrupt onset of voicing energy. Upon release of the glottal stop in word-initial position, a brief burst of energy often can be seen in oscillograms or spectrograms. Usually, the spectral composition of the burst is continuous with that for the following vowel, as would be expected if the acoustic energy produced at the level of the vocal folds activated the formants appropriate for the following vowel sound. A glottal stop is one manifestation of the more general phenomenon of glottalization, which can serve a variety of purposes in speech (Dilley, Shattuck-Hufnagel, & Ostendorf, 1996). This topic is revisited in Chapter 7.

Although some phonetics books describe the glottal stop as voiceless, this classification should not be taken too literally. Given that the glottal stop is produced with a sustained closure of the vocal folds, the laryngeal dynamics of the sound are rather like those for voiced stops. The stop is made with a gesture of glottal adduction. Any similarity with the laryngeal dynamics of voiceless sounds occurs only with an abductory gesture.

Other Consonant Characteristics

Secondary Articulations

The discussion to this point has assumed that a single, primary place of articulation describes consonant production. However, consonants often have *secondary articulations* and these are essential to understanding the acoustic-phonetic features of consonants in many languages. A given consonant may be labialized, palatalized, pharyngealized, glottalized, and so forth. The secondary articulation accompanies the primary articulation; for example, a labialized [t] has an alveolar (primary) articulation and a labial (secondary) articulation. In general, the acoustic effects of the secondary articulations can be understood in reference to the corresponding primary articulation. For instance, the effect of palatalization as a secondary articulation can be understood by considering how palatalization as a single process affects the acoustic structure of a sound. This is not to say that secondary articulations do not deserve study in their own right.

For present purposes, we consider as an example of secondary articulation the *emphatic sounds* in Classical Arabic. These sounds are produced with a coronal articulation as primary and a pharyngeal articulation as secondary. Emphatic sounds differ from their non-emphatic cognates in having an oropharyngeal constriction (Ali & Daniloff, 1972, Laufer & Baer, 1988) and an altered formant pattern of increased F1 and decreased F2 (El-Halees, 1985). Notice that these formant frequency changes are consistent with principles explained in Chapters 2 and 4. A constriction in the pharyngeal region generally has the noted effects on the first two formants. Another example of secondary articulation is the palatalization of consonants in Russian and other Slavic languages. It is also possible for two secondary articulations to co-occur. Ladefoged (1993) gives the example of Twi and other Akan languages spoken in Ghana in which labialization co-occurs with palatalization.

Consonant Reduction

The information given so far assumes that the consonants are precisely and carefully produced. However, when consonants (and vowels) are produced in casual conversational speech, the acoustic cues can be changed. These changes are called *reductions* and they usually take the form of attenuated or less distinctive acoustic properties (van Son & Pols, 1999). This issue is taken up in a later chapter, especially in connection with the topic of speaking style.

Speaker Differences

The information in this chapter has simplified the account of consonant acoustics by neglecting such speaker variables as sex, age, and dialect. Ultimately, these factors must be considered to account for particular acoustic patterns. These are considered in Chapter 6.

The "Speech Banana"

Figure 5–45 shows the *"speech banana,"* a graph that depicts some of the primary acoustic components of the speech signal. Frequency is scaled on the abscissa, and sensation level (or hearing loss) is represented on the ordinate. Essentially, this graph shows the relative energy for selected acoustic components of speech. Fundamental frequency, f_0, typically ranges from about 60 to 250 Hz. Vowel formants (F1, F2, F3, F4) occupy the frequency range of about 0.25 to 4.0 kHz (assuming adult male speech) and they are shown as relatively intense components (i.e., high sensation levels). The main consonant area corresponds to the frequency region of the lowest three vowel formants. Formant transitions for consonants are located in about this range. The high consonant area represents the turbulence energy for sibilant fricatives.

Nonspeech Noises

The acoustic techniques discussed in this chapter and other chapters can be applied to a variety of sounds, including human nonspeech noises. As an example, consider

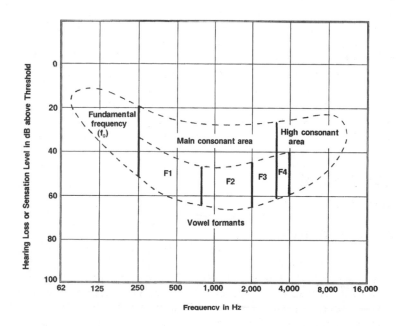

FIGURE 5–45. The "speech banana" that graphically summarizes some of the major acoustic energy regions for speech. The banana-like shape encloses the labeled energy regions.

the sounds of snoring. It is important clinically to determine the site of airway obstruction related to the snore. Miyazaki et al. (1998) used acoustic analysis to determine the obstruction site. Their data for 75 adults with sleep-related respiratory disorders showed that the fundamental frequency of the snore distinguished the following obstruction sites: soft palate type, tonsil/tongue base type, combined type, and larynx type.

Summary

Consonant sounds involve a variety of acoustic characteristics and, therefore, a variety of possible measures by which they can be characterized. A good way to retain the information is to think of the conso-

nants in major sound classes, as presented in this chapter. The most effective acoustic analysis is determined with respect to the properties of the sound to be analyzed. Whereas formant pattern often suffices as a general-purpose acoustic description of vowels, there is no single acoustic portrait that is suitable for the different types of consonants. It is useful to distinguish noise consonants (fricatives and affricates) from those that do not have prolonged noise intervals. It is also useful to distinguish sonorants (those having well-defined formant patterns) from those that do not. Despite the complexities, the traditional place–manner description of articulatory phonetics remains a helpful framework for the classification and description of acoustic features.

The Acoustic Correlates of Speaker Characteristics

Speech carries several kinds of information, including information about the person who produced it. Usually, we can infer several characteristics about a speaker even from hearing just a few words of conversation. We can often make fairly accurate guesses about gender, age, emotional state, language background, and even physical health. This chapter examines the acoustic correlates for various characteristics of speakers, beginning with age and gender.

Gender and Age

To a large extent, the early work in acoustic phonetics focused on the adult male speaker. There were a number of reasons for this focus, including social and technical factors. Only rather recently has the study of acoustic phonetics been broadened to encompass significant research on populations other than men. This is not to say that children and women were neglected altogether in the early history of acoustic speech research. Peterson and Barney's (1952) classic study included acoustic data on vowels for men, women and children, making it clear that acoustic values vary markedly with age and gender characteristics of speakers (see Chapter 4).

The problem is that the research effort given to the speech of women and children has been on a smaller scale than that given to the speech of men. Consequently, there is a continuing need to gather acoustic data for diverse populations. The concentration on male speakers had several consequences, not all of which facilitated research on the speech of women and children. One consequence was the choice of an analyzing bandwidth (300 Hz for the "wide-band" analysis) on early spectrographs that worked well enough for most adult male voices but was deficient for many women and children. The unsuitability of the analyzing bandwidth probably discouraged acoustic analyses of women's and children's speech.

The implications of the male emphasis may have reached even to theory; Titze (1989) commented, "One wonders, for example, if the source-filter theory of speech production would have taken the same course of development if female voices had been the primary model early on." (p. 1699) Klatt and Klatt (1990) remarked on the same point: "informal observations hint at the possibility that vowel spectra obtained from women's voices do not conform as well to an all-pole [i.e., all formant] model, due perhaps to tracheal coupling and source/tract interactions." (p. 820) The acoustic theory for vowels discussed in Chapter 2 assumed that the vocal tract transfer function is satisfactorily represented by formants (poles) and that antiformants (zeros) are required only for modifications such as nasalization. It is advisable to bear in mind that this theory is predicated largely on the characteristics of adult male speech and that it may have to be altered to account for the characteristics of both children and women. Some of these theoretical modifications are noted in this chapter.

One might think that acoustic data for women and children could be extrapolated quite easily from data collected for men's speech. After all, the acoustic theory outlined in Chapter 2 tells us that the length of the vocal tract is one determinant of formant frequencies. Given that resonance frequencies change systematically as the length of a pipe is changed, one might expect that scaling factors could be determined to permit the derivation of acoustic data for women and children from the data for men. Such scaling factors have been

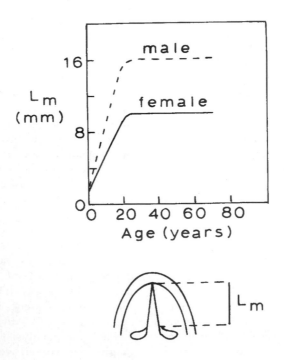

FIGURE 6–1. Variation in length of the vocal fold with age in males and females. Redrawn from I. Titze, (1989). Physiologic and acoustic differences between male and female voices, *Journal of the Acoustical Society of America, 85,* 1699–1707. (Reproduced with permission from the American Institute of Physics.) Copyright 1989.

proposed but they are calculated with difficulty and have limited accuracy. Even if accurate factors could be determined, the speech of women and children present some special problems that must be taken into account in both theory and analysis. The following sections review some of these problems.

Women's Speech

Simply listening to the voices of various speakers tells us that women generally have higher-pitched voices than men. Indeed, women's voices are on the average about one octave, or about 1.7 times, higher than men's. This difference in fundamental frequency relates primarily to the membranous length of the vocal folds (Titze, 1989). Figure 6–1 illustrates the scaling of the glottis in terms of three variables that account for differences between men's and women's voices. A scaling factor (computed by Titze to be about 1.6) based on the membranous length L accounts almost entirely for differences in mean fundamental frequency, mean airflow and aerodynamic power. An additional scaling factor of about 1.2 based on vibrational amplitude A accounts for the power differences between men and women's voices.

But women's voices may differ from men's in many ways. In particular, it has been suggested that women's voices have the following attributes (relative to men's):

- breathy
- weak
- more glottal leakage (air escaping through the glottis even during its "closed" phase
- less abrupt flow termination
- larger open quotient (meaning that the vocal folds are open longer during each glottal cycle)
- more symmetric vocal pulses (about the same time given to the opening and closing portions
- shorter pulses

- higher fundamental frequency
- different range of fundamental frequency
- lower Sound Pressure Level
- more dominant fundamental frequency (first harmonic)
- steeper spectrum slope (i.e., a faster roll-off of harmonic energy with frequency)
- more noise fill in interformant regions
- higher formant frequencies
- larger formant bandwidths
- different coupling, or interaction, between subglottal and supraglottal cavities
- greater interaction between source and filter

These various items are not necessarily independent of one another; for example, breathy voice, glottal leakage, more dominant first harmonic, and noise fill may all be related. The list is simply a compilation of characteristics that may have to be taken into consideration for a full understanding of women's voice. For additional discussion, see Hanson (1997), Hanson and Chuang (1999) and Klatt and Klatt (1990).

It was recognized early on in attempts to produce women's speech from speech synthesis that a woman's voice is not simply a man's voice produced with higher fundamental and formant frequencies. Attempts to use this simple alteration met with limited success. The voice simply did not sound feminine. More recent work (Hanson, 1997; Klatt & Klatt, 1990) shows that synthesis of women's voices should include provision for: (a) a voicing source model that offers flexible control of open quotient, spectral tilt, aspiration noise associated with breathiness, flutter timed to glottal pulses, and diplophonic double pulsing; (b) an extra pole-zero pair to simulate a tracheal resonance, and (c) pitch-synchronous adjustment of the first-formant bandwidth to simulate one component of source/tract interaction. Price (1989) noted that the glottal waveforms for female voices tended to have shorter closed quotients and less sharp excitation than the waveforms for male voices. Hanson (1997) emphasized that the more open glottal configuration typical of women's voices results in (a) a glottal volume–velocity waveform that has greater low-frequency and weaker high-frequency components, (b) a stronger source of aspiration noise, and (c) larger bandwidths of the formants, particularly F1. In addition, the amplitude of the first harmonic (H1) relative to that of the third formant (F3) is almost 10 dB lower for males than females (Hanson & Chuang, 1999). This amplitude difference reflects a difference in spectral tilt, that is, females tend to have more spectral energy in the higher frequencies.

The higher fundamental frequency of women's voices can present occasional difficulties in acoustic analysis. As fundamental frequency increases, there is a corresponding increase in the interval between harmonics of the laryngeal source spectrum (Figure 6–2). At some harmonic spacings, it becomes difficult to discern the location of formants in the spectrum. The problem is essentially one of sampling: widely spaced harmonics do not reveal much detail about the spectral envelope from which formant estimates are typically made. Early spectrographs were particularly limited in the analysis of high-pitched women's speech because they were equipped with a standard 300-Hz analyzing filter for wide-band analysis. This filter worked satisfactorily for most men's voices because it typically embraced at least two harmonics and therefore resolved formants rather than harmonics. But for many women's voices, this filter bandwidth corresponded to a harmonic interval. As a result, spectrograms had harmonic-formant interaction, as illustrated in Figure 6–3. This

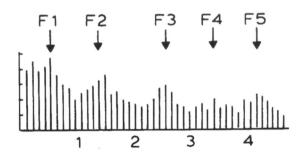

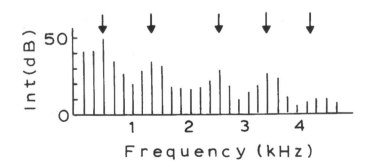

FIGURE 6–2. Effect of change in fundamental frequency on vowel spectrum. Top: spectrum for vowel produced with low fundamental frequency; bottom: spectrum for same vowel produced with high fundamental frequency. Approximate formant frequencies are shown by arrows.

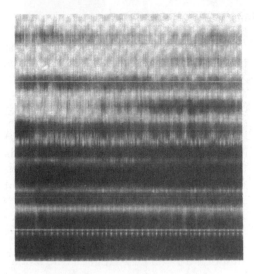 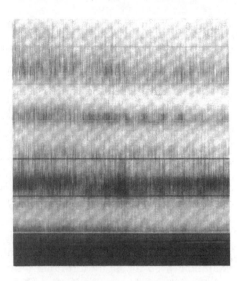

FIGURE 6–3. Spectrograms to illustrate formant–harmonic interaction. The sound on the left was produced with a high fundamental frequency, so that the analyzing bandwidth resolves individual harmonics of the voice. The spectrogram at the right is the same vowel spoken by that same woman but with a lower fundamental frequency, so that the analyzing bandwidth resolves formants.

occurrence made it difficult or impossible to tell when a band of energy on the spectrogram represented a formant or a harmonic. There is a practical lesson here: if the formants of a vowel produced by a woman or child are obscure with the standard or default analyzing bandwidth of acoustic analysis, it often is helpful to increase the bandwidth (decrease the number of points in a FFT) and repeat the analysis.

As a rule, the bandwidth of the analyzing filter should be 2 to 3 times as large as the speaker's fundamental frequency if the object is to identify formants. For example, the analyzing bandwidth for a woman who has a fundamental frequency of 300 Hz should be at least 600 Hz. There are upper limits to the size of the analyzing filter because making the bandwidth too large defeats the purpose of acoustic analysis. For instance, a filter as wide as 1000 Hz would likely embrace not only harmonics but closely spaced formants as well. One approach taken to analyze women's and children's speech with the fixed-bandwidth analyzing filters on older spectrographs

was to play back the speech signal at a slower speed than the speed used for recording. When the slowed signal was fed to the spectrograph, the effective result was a change in analyzing filter bandwidth proportional to the difference in recording/playback speed. Fortunately, modern systems for acoustic analysis typically offer a range of analyzing bandwidths. The task is to select the bandwidth that is optimal for a particular speaker.

A number of studies point to the conclusion that women's voices differ from men's on dimensions other than fundamental frequency. These dimensions are pertinent to the optimal analysis of women's speech. A frequently reported characteristic of women's voices is that they are breathier than men's. Several acoustic correlates have been identified in the study of breathiness and related features in women's voices. Henton and Bladon (1985) determined that for speakers of RP (Received Pronunciation) British, the amplitude of the first harmonic, relative to the amplitude of the second harmonic, was about 6 dB stronger for women than for men. Klatt and Klatt (1990) reported a similar difference for male and female speakers of American English but noted that there was considerable variation within their male and female groups. Bless, Biever, and Shaikh (1986) concluded from stroboscopic observations of the larynx that women were four times as likely as men to have a posterior glottal chink during the closed period of the cycle. Using inverse-filtered, glottal-flow waveforms, Holmberg. Hillman, and Perkell (1988) found greater acoustic evidence of breathiness for women than for men. Similarly, Klatt and Klatt (1990) discovered a tendency for female voices to have a greater excitation of F3 by aspiration noise ("noise in F3") than male voices. Klatt and Klatt also concluded that the partial glottal opening in breathy voices causes an increase in the bandwidth of the first formant, "sometimes obliterating the spectral peak at F1 entirely" (p. 835). They commented that this effect, combined with the appearance of extra pole-zero pairs associated with tracheal coupling, can create problems for models that expect a formant-like representation of sounds across speakers who differ in age and sex.

Another issue in the acoustic analysis of women's speech is the overall frequency range of analysis. Typically, the frequency value for a particular acoustic feature will be on the order of 20% higher for a woman than for a man. Because women's vocal tracts are generally shorter than men's, women have higher values for formant frequencies, as shown in Figure 6–4 (see also Tables 4–1 and 4–2 for a comparison of data on formant frequencies of vowels produced by men and women). It has been suggested that the greater dispersion of vowels in the F1-F2 plane is behavioral as well as anatomic in origin (Diehl et al., 1996). According to Diehl et al., the greater dispersion for women's vowels helps to overcome the problem of harmonic sampling in vowel recognition. That is, because women have a higher f_0, their spectral harmonics are more widely spaced and this wide spac-

ing makes it more difficult to determine formant locations.

Women's shorter vocal tracts affect the frequency characteristics of other sounds as well. Fricatives produced by women generally have higher regions of spectral energy compared to fricatives produced by men (Whiteside, 1998). This upward shift of frequency values in women's speech should be taken into account especially for sounds with high frequency components. Unfortunately, the data on women's frication and burst spectra are not abundant. As discussed in Chapter 5, the most extensive data have been published on adult male speakers. One general principle is clear: although a frequency range of 8 kHz may be quite satisfactory for the analysis of fricative energy for men, this range may not be adequate to represent the fricative energy for women. Therefore, when it is planned to study fricatives produced by women, it is a good idea to extend the frequency range of spectral analysis beyond that which suffices for male speakers.

Wu and Childers (1991) showed that digital signal processing and pattern recognition techniques can be used with great accuracy in the automatic recognition of speaker gender. They concluded that gender information in speech is time invariant, phoneme independent, and speaker independent for a given gender. In a companion article, Childers and Wu (1991) examined the fine details of gender differences in vowel production. They determined that there was redundant information on gender in the formant and fundamental frequency features of vowels but that the single feature that best discriminated male and female speakers was the F2 frequency. In general, female vowels were associated with a higher f_0, higher formant frequencies, lower formant amplitudes, wider bandwidths, and a steeper spectral slope.

In summary, there is much to consider in analyzing women's speech. The points mentioned above should be weighed in the choice of analysis tools and parameters. For example, the all-pole model assumed in

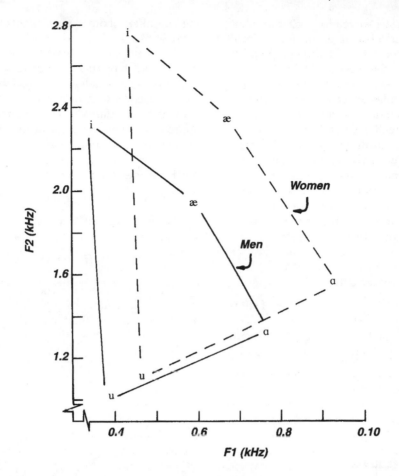

FIGURE 6–4.   F1–F2 chart for the vowels of American English produced by men and women. From *The speech sciences. A volume in the speech sciences* (1st ed.), by Kent, copyright 1998. Reprinted with permission of Delmar, a division of Thomson Learning.

many LPC analysis routines may not be well-suited to breathy women's voices, which may be characterized by tracheal pole-zero pairs, enlarged F1 bandwidth and significant noise excitation of the F3 frequency region. Moreover, consideration should be given to bandwidth values—both the overall bandwidth of speech energy and the analyzing bandwidth for spectral computations. These considerations in acoustic analysis have a parallel in matters of theory and data interpretation. In general, the best measures are those based on a sound theoretical framework.

Children's speech

Because children have shorter vocal tracts and shorter vocal folds than adults, it is expected that children will have relatively higher fundamental and formant frequencies than adult speakers. This statement is generally true, but it should be recognized that children are a diverse population having a range of speech characteristics. Grouping all children together risks a heterogeneity that may preclude any useful generalizations. To a first approximation, we may say that the speech of prepubescent children is characterized by higher formant and fundamental frequencies than those observed for adult speech. After puberty, the situation changes markedly, particularly for males. The well-known "voice change" in adolescent males brings about a sizeable reduction in vocal fundamental frequency, which typically drops by about an octave. In addition, male vocal tracts lengthen appreciably during adolescence, which leads to a lowering of formant frequencies. The following sections consider the major ways in which developmental processes affect the acoustic characteristics of speech, beginning with infancy.

Infant Vocalizations.

Although a relatively small number of studies have been published on infant vocalizations, the available reports give a general picture of these early sounds. Compared with speakers of other ages, infants have the shortest vocal folds and the shortest vocal tracts (Figure 6–5), and it is expected that they would have the highest fundamental and formant frequencies. Acoustic research summarized by Kent and Murray (1982) has shown that infants have the following approximate means for the acoustic characteristics of a mid-central vowel:

Fundamental frequency—400 Hz,

First formant frequency—1000 Hz,

Second formant frequency—3000 Hz, and

Third formant frequency—5000 Hz.

The fundamental frequency of an infant is 3 to 4 times as high as that for an adult male (recall that the laryngeal harmonics are integer multiples of the fundamental frequency, so that the harmonics of

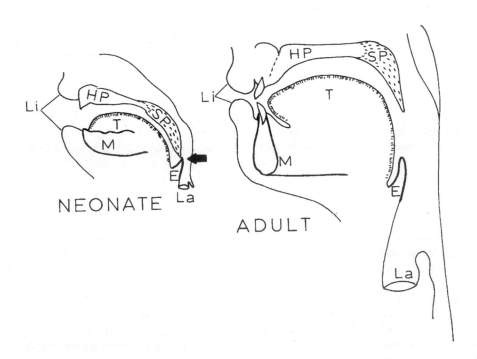

FIGURE 6–5. Drawing of the vocal tracts of an infant and adult. Key: Li = lip, J = jaw, T = tongue, HP = hard palate, SP = soft palate, E = epiglottis, La = larynx. The filled arrow points to the approximation of velum and epiglottis in the infant; note that this anatomic feature is not seen in the adult.

an infant's voice will be about 400 Hz apart). The formant frequencies of an infant's neutral vowel are spaced at intervals of about 2000 Hz, compared to about 1000 Hz for adult males (for whom the first three formant frequencies of the mid-central vowel are about 500, 1500 and 2500 Hz). Using the formulas given in Chapter 2, we can calculate the length of the infant's vocal tract given these acoustic measures of formant frequency. The estimated length of about 8 cm agrees quite well with actual measurements made of an infant's vocal tract length.

The mean value of fundamental frequency of 400 Hz should not be taken too strictly. Infants have large ranges of fundamental frequency, with minimum values reaching down to the adult male range and maximum values extending to 1000 Hz or higher. This large range can make the measurement of fundamental frequencies of infants rather challenging, especially for analysis instruments that have a limited range of measurement. However, range is not the only obstacle, as discussed later in this chapter.

Several other characteristics of infant vocalizations have been noted in acoustic studies. One of these is the relative frequency of occurrence of intonation contours. Kent and Bauer (1985) and Robb, Saxman, and Grant (1989) reported that Rise–Fall, Flat and Fall contours were the most frequently occurring. For example, Kent and Bauer's data showed that Fall and Rise–Fall together accounted for about 77% of the intonation contours produced by five one-year-olds. In the Robb et al. study, the three contours Rise–Fall, Flat and Fall accounted for 67% of the contours in comfort-state vocalizations. The age of 4 months appears to be important in the emergence of intonation types. Hsu, Fogel, and Cooper (2000) reported that before this age, vocalic sounds typically were accompanied by simple melodic contours, but after 4 month there was a greater likelihood that syllabic sounds were associated with complex melodic contours.

Infants also tend to produce a large variety of phonation types. Observations have been made of harmonic doubling (the abrupt appearance and often equally abrupt disappearance of a harmonic series at one-half the original fundamental frequency), fundamental frequency shift, biphonation (a double series of fundamental frequencies), vocal tremor (a periodic variation of fundamental frequency and/or voice amplitude), and noise components (Kent & Murray, 1982; Kent & Bauer, 1985; Michelsson & Michelsson, 1999; Robb & Saxman, 1988). Robb and Saxman (1988) determined that 6% of 1200 noncry vocalizations from 14 infants had instances of harmonic doubling, fundamental frequency shift or biphonation. These variant phonation types can present problems for vocal analysis, especially for unwary investigators. Figure 6–6 shows a narrow-band spectrogram of an infant vocalization in which several phonation types appear. Such rapid and extreme variations in phonatory characteristics are not uncommon.

The overall frequency range of analysis is an important consideration in the analysis of infants' vocalizations. The fundamental frequencies of infants and young children may exceed the nominal range of some analysis systems. Also, the frequency values for some acoustic properties may be considerably higher for children than for adults. Bauer and Kent (1987) reported that the primary energy ranges for fricatives produced by infants sometimes fell above 8 kHz, the upper frequency limit of conventional spectrography. Examples of frication spectra obtained from infants are shown in Figure 6–7. Notice that for these samples, significant regions of noise energy extend to 12 kHz. It is always wise to determine carefully the upper limits required for an analysis before setting analysis parameters, for example, sampling rate for A/D conversion.

Consideration of the acoustic properties summarized so far suggests that the analysis of infant vocalizations can be challenging even for such relatively simple objectives as formant-frequency measure-

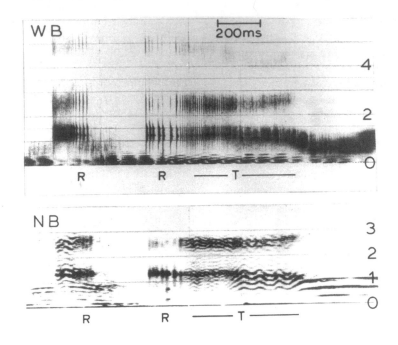

FIGURE 6–6. Wide-band (WB) and narrow-band (NB) spectrograms of an infant's vocalization. Note variation in phonatory pattern, including vocal roll or fry (R) and tremor (T).

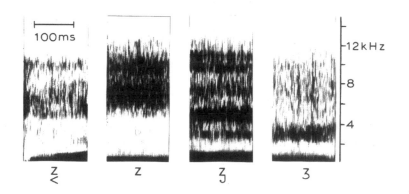

FIGURE 6–7. Spectrograms of fricatives produced by infants younger than one year. Phonetic symbols are shown at the bottom of each sample.

ment. Harmonic–formant interaction is a particular problem, but it is by no means the only one. Frequently, infant vocalizations involve nasalization (which increases formant bandwidths and introduces additional formants and antiformants), variable voice quality, and other features that make formant estimation difficult. Nonetheless, if analysis parameters are chosen carefully even parametric procedures such as linear prediction have been reported to perform fairly well in formant analyses of infant cry and other vocalizations (Fort et al., 1996). This is not to say, however, that there is complete agreement on the preferred methods of analysis. In a study of infant cry, Robb and Cacace (1995) observed large differences in the estimation of F2 and F3 using the methods of sound spectrography, LPC, and power spectrum analysis. The three methods yielded comparable estimates of the F1 frequency, but the mean values of F2 and F3 differed by as much as 500 to 1000 Hz. Robb and Cacace concluded that "serious questions arise whether formant estimates of cry are accurate or appropriate for use as a metric of infant vocal tract resonance" (p. 57). With this caveat in mind, we can use published data on infant cry (Colton & Steinschneider, 1980; Robb & Cacace, 1995) to develop the following tentative characterization of cry in the typically developing infant: mean f_0 of about 500 Hz, mean F1 frequency in the range of 1100 to 1600 Hz, mean F2 frequency in the range of 2200 to 3200 Hz, mean F3 frequency in the range of 3700 to 5300 Hz, and a mean duration in the range of 1 to 2 s. As a point of comparison, Kuhl and Meltzoff (1996) determined the formant frequencies for /i/-like, /a/-like, and /u/-like vowels produced by infants aged 12, 16, and 20 weeks. The F1 frequencies for these three vowel categories in the data for the 12-week-olds were 782, 934, and 732 Hz, respectively. The F2 frequencies were 3121, 2606, and 2199 Hz, respectively. There is a good general fit of the formant-frequency data between the cry and vowel data, which gives confidence in these estimates of formant structure in early infant vocalizations.

Acoustic methods also have been applied to the study of infant babble, the multisyllabic sequences that emerge in the second half of the first year of life. Oller (1986) described the acoustic properties of what he called the *canonical syllable*, which is intended to represent the great majority of syllables in the world's languages. Presumably, the emergence of this syllable is a major accomplishment in vocal development. Oller offered the following acoustic properties for the canonical syllable:

1. The power envelope has peaks and valleys that differ by at least 10 dB.

2. The peak-to-peak duration of the syllable is in the range of 100–500 ms.

3. The nucleus of the syllable is associated with a periodic source (i.e., voicing energy) and a relatively open vocal tract that affords full resonance (i.e., has a well-defined formant pattern).

4. The syllable possesses at least one margin of low resonance and relatively obstructed vocal tract. This margin has properties like those of obstruent consonants.

5. Smooth formant transitions occur between the margin(s) and nucleus, with a transition duration in the range of 25–120 ms.

6. The intensity range should be greater than about 30 dB.

7. The range of fundamental frequency should not exceed about one octave (doubling).

The canonical syllable may be an important unit for the integration of the perception and production of speech. It may well be a precursor of early words and has attracted much attention in the study of typically and atypically developing children. The values given above should be regarded as hypothetical and subject to revision by research. For a more recent definition of canonical babble, see Oller (2000). A good sign of progress in the acoustic characterization of babble is the development of a computer program for automatic babble recognition (Fell et al., 1999). Following canonical babbling (babbling formed largely of canonical syllables), the infant usually begins to produce early words. The ages of these accomplishments vary considerably among children, but canonical babbling typically appears between 7 to 10 months of age, and the child's first words generally occur between 10–15 months. It seems reasonable to expect that experience in syllable babbling assists the child with the production of early words.

Formant-frequency Changes with Development

As children grow, their vocal tracts lengthen and their formant frequencies are expected to decrease accordingly. Data on F1 and F2 frequencies are compiled for various age groups in Table 6–1 and 6–2, respectively. Although these data do not always show a uniform change across increments in age, the overall trend is a decrease in formant frequencies with age. In fact, formant frequencies probably continue to decrease across the age span for most people, because the facial structures grow gradually larger even into old age (Kent & Burkhard, 1981). There is therefore a kind of acoustic "lifeline" in which the formant frequencies for a particular sound gradually decrease over an individual's lifetime (Figure 6–8). However, the most striking period of change is in puberty and adolescence, especially for males (Lee, Potamianos, & Narayanan, 1999).

TABLE 6–1

First formant (F1) frequencies of the vowels /i/, /ae/, /a/, and /u/ for various age groups of children from infancy to young adulthood. Data sources are: H (Hodge, 1989), EH (Eguchi & Hirsh, 1969), B (Bennett, 1981), PG (Penz & Gilbert, 1983), BP (Busby & Plant, 1995); AK (Assmann & Katz, 2000), and LPN (Lee, Potamianos, & Narayanan, 1999). Notes: Bennett's data are for 7- and 8-year-olds but are listed in the 8-year-old group; B-M = Bennett's data for males; B-F = Bennett's data for females; BP-M = Busby and Plant data for males; BP-F = Busby and Plant data for females; data from Busby and Plant were estimated from graphs; LPN-M = Lee et al. data for males; LPN-F = Lee et al. data for females.

Age group	Vowel /i/	/ae/	/a/	/u/
7.7 to 9.5 mos.				
H	655	1401	—	558
1 year				
H	589	1169	1072	594
3 years				
H	512	1248	1072	530
AK	427	1256	1060	502
5 years				
H	440	1141	1010	478
BP-M	540	990	1190	540
BP-F	515	1170	1250	530
AK	472	1161	1066	471
LPN-M	467	1010	1166	477
LPN-F	466	1055	1224	501
7 years				
EH	411	736	950	481
PG	510	1032	827	543
BP-M	460	950	1000	470
BP-F	495	1000	1125	525
AK	358	1074	954	491
LPN-M	425	882	984	449
LPN-F	467	1023	1067	506

(continued)

| | Vowel | | | |
Age group	/i/	/ae/	/a/	/u/
8 years				
PG	531	1166	918	573
EH	397	685	921	450
B-M	470	878	—	—
B-F	482	1020	—	—
LPN-M	414	873	969	458
LPN-F	428	1021	1108	426
9 years				
H	401	1010	919	453
PG	544	1034	847	544
EH	403	647	921	469
BP-M	490	875	950	450
BP-F	520	1050	1100	460
LPN-M	382	872	1011	471
LPN-F	455	948	1063	505
10 years				
LPN-M	424	904	970	482
LPN-F	472	970	1037	496
11 years				
BP-M	455	850	945	460
BP-F	445	950	1025	475
12 years				
LPN-M	358	818	891	424
LPN-F	439	836	939	452
14 years				
LPN-M	350	767	844	401
LPN-F	415	824	893	433
16 years				
LPN-M	296	684	741	348
LPN-F	423	835	851	447
18 years				
LPN-M	283	686	737	337
LPN-F	418	914	932	480

Developmental studies of speech acoustics must account for several influences, including body size (given that length of the vocal tract is correlated with body size), developmental changes in vocal tract anatomy, sex of the speaker, individual articulatory patterns, and dialectal/idiolectal factors. In addition, the relative importance of these factors probably varies with age of the speakers. Published data for vowels produced by infants are limited, which prevents confident statements about developmental patterns between birth and 2 or 3 years of age. Robb, Chen, and Gilbert (1997) concluded from a cross-sectional study of 20 children that average F1 and F2 frequencies changed little over the period from 4 to 25 months of age. However, they did report a significant decrease in the average bandwidths for both F1 and F2. In a study of four children over the developmental period of 15 to 36 months of age, Gilbert, Robb, and Chen (1997) noted essentially constant F1 and F2 frequencies before 24 months but significant decreases in both frequencies between 24 and 36 months.

TABLE 6–2

Second formant (F2) frequencies of the vowels /i/, /ae/, /a/, and /u/ for various age groups of children from infancy to young adulthood. Data sources are: H (Hodge, 1989), EH (Eguchi & Hirsh, 1969), B (Bennett, 1981), PG (Penz & Gilbert, 1983), BP (Busby & Plant, 1995); AK (Assmann & Katz, 2000), and LPN (Lee, Potamianos, & Narayanan, 1999). Notes: Bennett's data are for 7- and 8-year-olds but are listed in the 8-year-old group; B-M = Bennett's data for males; B-F = Bennett's data for females; BP-M = Busby and Plant data for males; BP-F = Busby and Plant data for females; data from Busby and Plant were estimated from graphs; LPN-M = Lee et al. data for males; LPN-F = Lee et al. data for females.

Age group	Vowel /i/	/ae/	/a/	/u/
7.7 to 9.5 mos.				
H	3542	2710	—	1052
1 year				
H	3545	2600	1594	1423
3 years				
H	3474	2502	1594	1179
AK	3437	2503	1656	1891
5 years				
H	3380	2419	1490	1391
BP-M	3000	2625	1900	2425
BP-F	3250	2775	2050	2800
AK	3535	2505	1602	1711
LPN-M	3071	2534	1750	1508
LPN-F	3019	2613	1842	1709
7 years				
AK	3402	2324	1565	1838
EH	3204	2299	1652	1525
PG	3165	2167	1224	1492
BP-M	2625	2250	1700	2425
BP-F	2925	2600	1950	2750
LPN-M	3002	2441	1536	1700
LPN-F	3026	2433	1647	1840
8 years				
PG	3164	2117	1306	1342
EH	3104	2222	1729	1437
B-M	3067	2149	—	—
B-F	3296	2355	—	—
LPN-M	3031	2370	1522	1577
LPN-F	2997	2419	1660	1539
9 years				
H	3134	2110	1383	1203
PG	3178	1980	1394	1515
EH	3106	2295	1785	1392
BP-M	2450	2200	1675	2200
BP-F	2725	2325	1775	2375
LPN-M	2979	2319	1601	1603
LPN-F	3061	2415	1676	1764

(continued)

Age group	Vowel /i/	/ae/	/a/	/u/
10 years				
LPN-M	2959	2269	1558	1656
LPN-F	2969	2318	1663	1747
11 years				
BP-M	2500	2290	1570	2300
BP-F	2750	2300	1800	2400
12 years				
LPN-M	2755	2090	1432	1576
LPN-F	2884	2215	1612	1661
14 years				
LPN-M	2671	1982	1379	1537
LPN-F	2693	2010	1556	1693
16 years				
LPN-M	2334	1762	1261	1368
LPN-F	2776	2050	1412	1691
18 years				
LPN-M	2289	1759	1269	1144
LPN-F	2801	1955	1473	1771

Taken together, the studies by Robb et al. (1997) and Gilbert et al. (1997) indicate a stability of formant frequencies (and, therefore, little change in vocal tract length) from about 4 to 25 months, but a decrease in formant frequencies (and presumably a lengthening of the vocal tract) between 25 and 36 months. The reduction in formant bandwidth observed by Robb et al. (1997) could be the result of less nasalization and/or a change in the biomechanical properties of the tissues of the vocal tract. See Robb et al. (1997) for discussion of this point.

At some point in development, boys and girls have vocal tracts that differ in length (and possibly shape as well) and, therefore, have different formant frequencies. Tables 6–1 and 6–2 show that sexual dimorphism of the vocal tract emerges by the age of at least 7 or 8 years (Bennett, 1981; Busby & Plant, 1995; Lee et al., 1999; Whiteside & Hodgson, 2000). Considering the data for 7- and 8-year-old boys and girls from Tables 6–1 and 6–2, it can be seen that boys have consistently lower formant frequencies across all vowels. The size of the difference varies from as little as about 4% for F2 of vowel /i/ to as much as 13.5% for F1 of vowel /æ/. The largest sex differences occur for F1 for the low vowels /ae/ and / [ɑ] / and for F2 of vowel /ɑ/. These differences in vowel formant frequencies may reflect some articulatory differences between boys and girls in addition to presumed differences in vocal tract length. For example, the large difference in F1 frequencies for the low vowels might mean that boys produce these vowels with a relatively more open jaw position.

The pattern of formant-frequency change as a function of age is not necessarily simple because the growth of the vocal tract is not just a matter of overall lengthening. Particularly in males, the vocal tract has disproportionate growth in the pharyngeal region compared to the oral region. A classic paper on normalization of formant-frequencies for speakers of different ages and both genders is Fant (1975). It is not entirely clear if a uniform scaling factor suffices to normalize vowel formant frequencies for both boys and girls (Kent, 1976; Lee et al., 1999; Whiteside & Hodgson, 2000).

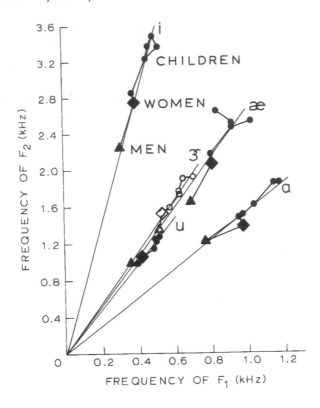

FIGURE 6–8. Variation in F1 and F2 values for five American English vowels, as produced by groups of children, women, and men. The filled circles represent data for different age groups of children. The data are plotted to show "isovowel lines" or lines that connect the mean F1–F2 data for the various age–sex groups.

Lee et al. (1999) observed a linear change in formant frequencies for males between the ages of 11 to 15 years and concluded that their data are consistent with a hypothesis of uniform axial growth. However, White (1999) concluded that vowel dependent differences between boys and girls indicated non-uniform differences in the dimensions of male and female vocal tracts. White also noted that these sex differences were not consistent with data for adult vowels. White's data for 29 11-year-old children showed that formant frequencies were higher for speech than for singing and also were higher for girls than for boys.

Assuming that dialectal, speaking style, and articulatory variations are controlled, differences in formant frequencies are associated with structural differences in the vocal tract, particularly differences in overall length. That is, formant frequencies are an index of anatomic growth of the vocal tract. But speech development also reflects phonetic mastery and maturation of speech motor skills, which are addressed in the following sections.

Temporal Patterns

Speech development is much more than changes in vocal tract size and geometry. It also involves increasing precision of control and the reliable production of phonetic and phonologic cues. Compared to adults, children tend to have longer segment durations (slower speaking rates) and greater variability in repeated productions of an utterance (Kent & Forner, 1980). Figure 6–9 gives a spectrographic comparison of an adult's and child's production of the phrase *took a spoon*. The slow rate of production for the child is evident both in the overall duration of the phrase and in the greater durations of most, but not all, segments. These effects are consistent with motor development generally. As children acquire a motor skill, their performance typically becomes faster and more reliable. Studies of temporal patterns in children's speech are helping to shape the understanding of speech development (Allen & Hawkins, 1980; Nittrouer, 1993, 1995; Nittrouer & Studdert-Kennedy, 1986; Nittrouer, Studdert-Kennedy, & McGowen, 1989; Whiteside & Hodgson, 2000).

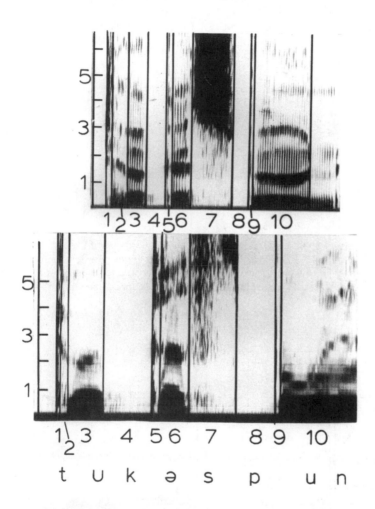

FIGURE 6–9. Spectrograms of the phrase *"took a spoon"* produced by an adult male (top) and a young child (bottom). The numbers identify the following acoustic segments: 1—release burst of [t], 2—aspiration interval, 3—vowel [ʊ], 4—stop gap for [k], 5—release burst for [k], 6—vowel [ə], 7—frication for [s], 8—stop gap for [p], 9—burst for [p], and 10—vowel [u]. Note generally longer segment durations and higher frequency energy for the child's production. Reprinted from R. D. Kent, (1981). Sensorimotor aspects of speech development, In R.N. Aslin, J.R. Alberts, and M.R. Peterson (Eds.) *Development of perception* (Vol. 1). (Reproduced with permission of Academic Press, New York). Copyright 1981.

Acoustic methods are useful in studying phonetic and phonologic variations in children's speech. Consider the child who deletes the [s] fricative in words like *spoon*. Recall that voiceless stops following [s] are unaspirated. If a child deletes the [s], is a following stop aspirated or unaspirated? The former would be predicted if the deleted fricative is not represented in the child's phonologic representation, that is, the representation is something like [p u n]. But the unaspirated allophone would be predicted if the phonologic representation includes the "missing" [s], in which case the representation would be similar to the adult [s p u n]. Figure 6–10 shows two wide-band spectrograms of the phrase *took a spoon* recorded from the same child within the same session. Note that the fricative [s] is deleted in both productions of the phrase. The top pattern shows an aspirated stop [p] but the bottom pattern shows an unaspirated stop [p]. Apparently, the child was uncertain about which stop allophone to use. The spectrograms give clear evidence of the child's uncertainty.

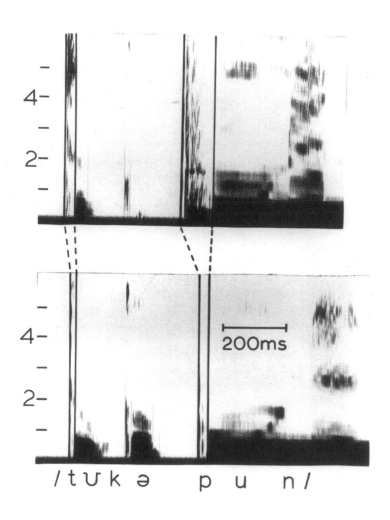

FIGURE 6–10. Spectrograms of the phrase *"took a spoon"* produced by a young child. The [s] in *spoon* is deleted and the following [p] is produced as an aspirated allophone at the top and as an unaspirated allophone at the bottom.

Children's Voices

Children's voices may present some of the same complications reviewed earlier in this chapter for women's voices. A particular problem is that the relatively high f_0 of most children makes it difficult to select an analyzing bandwidth that resolves formants but not harmonics. It sometimes can be helpful if the phonation has noise components, because the aperiodic energy can make it easier to identify formants. Changes in f_0 also can be helpful because they can change the formant–harmonic relationship. Of course, there is no guarantee that either noise or f_0 variation will occur in a natural speech production. White (1999) used a deliberate f_0 sweeping production to study vowel formants in 11-year-old children who were experienced choir singers.

In addition to having a high f_0, children often can be highly variable in their speech and voice characteristics, for example, producing an utterance with widely ranging values of fundamental frequency, intervals of breathiness or laryngealization, and unexpected nasalization. In view of these possible complications, it is prudent to preview speech samples before performing detailed analyses that might be affected by characteristics such as those noted. A real-time spectrographic display is very useful in previewing speech samples. Above all, it should not be assumed that the default values of analysis parameters (usually determined from the speech of adult males) will be optimum for the analysis of children's speech. Generally, analysis parameter values for women's speech will be more suitable than values for men's speech when analyzing the speech patterns of children.

Lee et al. (1999) observed that f_0 differences between male and female children were statistically significant beginning with the age of 12 years. As noted earlier in this chapter, sex differences in formant frequencies appear to emerge by the age of 7 or 8 years. The change in mean f_0 is pronounced for males between the ages of about 12 and 15 years. For example, Lee et al. (1999) reported a 78% decrease in f_0 for males between these ages. No significant change was observed after the age of 15 years, which indicates that the voice change is effectively complete by that age (cf. Busby & Plant, 1995; Hollien et al., 1994; Kent, 1995).

Effects of Aging on Speech

Especially with advanced age, speech may undergo various changes that can be readily perceptible to listeners. Therefore, we often can be fairly accurate in judging a speaker's age just from the sound of his or her voice. Studies have shown that aging can affect the voice (Linville, 1996, 2000; Linville & Fisher, 1985), formant frequencies (Endres, Bambach, & Flosser, 1971; Rastatter & Jacques, 1990), and aspects of the motor control of speech production (Weismer & Liss, 1991). To be sure, speech is a robust function that serves most of us throughout life. However, the changes that occur with aging can be significant in some individuals, leading to reduced intelligibility and altered voice quality.

Speaker Verification, Identification, and Elimination

A day rarely goes by that we do not recognize people from the sounds of their voices. We often can recognize a friend over the telephone even from the merest greeting, and we can identify famous people (actors, singers, athletes, politicians) from recordings of the voices. For all this, however, the human ability to identify others from their voices is not impressively accurate. The shortcomings have been studied in *earwitness* research. In applications to criminal proceedings, earwitness is testimony based on recall of auditory events, such as spoken messages at the scene of a crime. Studies have shown that the accuracy of earwitness is rather low (Olsson, Juslin, & Winman, 1998). Is it possible to use acoustic analysis for such purposes? This question raises the issues of *talker verification, identification* and *elimination*.

Talker verification tests a claim of identity. The typical procedure is to determine if a speech sample from a given individual who claims to be person A matches a stored reference sample previously obtained from Person A. One application of talker verification is as a security measure to allow access of approved individuals to restricted areas or sources of information. If a person wants to gain access, then his or her speech must match a prerecorded sample. Talker identification is a decision process in which a speech sample from an unknown talker is attributed to an individual in a known population, such as employees in a high-security facility, or suspects in a criminal investigation. Talker elimination is the inverse process of identification and involves a decision that a speech sample from an unknown talker cannot be attributed to individuals in a known population. Most forensic applications (criminal investigations) involve speaker identification or elimination.

The application of acoustic analysis to these problems assumes that individual speakers can be distinguished from the acoustic properties of their speech. It seems likely that acoustic differences would emerge in the comparison of certain large subgroups of talkers, such as age-gender subgroups (men vs. women, adults vs. children) and some dialect subgroups (Southerners vs. Easterners). Is it also possible that an individual talker can be distinguished from any other talker? In other words, is it possible to make *voiceprints* that identify individuals as accurately as fingerprints?

Characteristics that might be used for talker identification can be conceptualized according to the source–filter model described in Chapter 2. Voice source features include:

1. Average f_0,

2. Time-frequency pattern of f_0 (f_0 contour),

3. f_0 fluctuations, and

4. Glottal wave shape.

Vocal tract resonance features include:

1. Shape of spectral envelope and tilt,

2. Absolute values of formant frequencies,

3. Time-frequency pattern of formant frequencies,

4. Long-term average spectrum (LTAS), and

5. Formant bandwidths.

Although it is over 25 years old, the largest and most comprehensive study of talker identification by spectrograms is the investigation reported by Tosi et al. (1972). This study was based on 250 men drawn from what was considered to be a "homogeneous population" of 25,000 men speaking general American English (male students at Michigan State University). The examiners were 29 individuals who had received a month's training in spectrographic identification. A total of nearly 35,000 identification trials were conducted, with each trial based on subsets of 10 or 40 speakers drawn from total sample of 250 talkers. The experiment included several aspects, including: comparison of open versus closed tests, use of noncontemporaneous reference and test samples, and context variation. Of these conditions, the one that compares most closely with the kind of test conducted by a forensic specialist is the open test with noncontemporaneous samples extracted from continuous speech. Forensic tests frequently must use conversational speech samples (continuous speech) obtained at different times (noncontemporaneous samples) from a suspect who may or may not be in the reference sample (open test). An example is a person who makes a threatening telephone call which is recorded by the person receiving the threat. A suspect is later taken to the police station and is asked to produce a speech sample that can be compared with the recorded telephone message. For this condition, Tosi et al. reported error rates of 6.4% for false identification (identification of a subject who was not the actual speaker) and 12.7% for false elimination (rejecting from the candidates the actual speaker). The examiners also rated the certainty or confidence of their judgments, with 60% of the incorrect judgments being associated with an "uncertain" rating. The authors suggested if the examiners had been allowed to use a "no opinion" category of decision when they were not certain, then the error rates would have been 2.4% for false identification and 4.8% for false elimination.

The status of talker identification by spectrograms was assessed in a highly important paper authored by a select panel of scientists (Bolt et al., 1970). They concluded that talker identification by this method is subject to a high error rate and that the "available results are inadequate to establish the reliability of voice identification by spectrograms." A quarter century has passed since the Bolt et al. report appeared, but no research papers have appeared to provide a definitive answer to the question of the reliability of spectrographic talker identification (Kent & Chial, 1997).

Recognition of the sex of a talker can be accomplished even from short vowel segments using information on f_0 and vocal tract length cues (formant frequencies) (Bachorowski & Owren, 1999). When both types of information were used together, classification of talker sex was virtually perfect. It is expected that these two information sources reflect the difference in size between the vocal structures of men and women. The question arises if these information sources can be used to predict body size within a sex group. The answer appears to be "no." Vandommelen and Moxness (1995) reported that listener estimates of talker height and weight were generally inaccurate. Furthermore, they found no correlations between several acoustic measures (f_0, formant frequencies, and energy below 1 kHz) and actually measured talker height and weight.

Sociolinguistic Issues: Studies of Dialect and Foreign Accent

Acoustic methods also have been applied to the study of dialect and foreign accent. Only a brief coverage of this topic is included here, primarily to show the ways in which acoustic analysis or speech synthesis can be informative. One of the major questions is: What acoustic properties are must useful in characterizing dialect or foreign accent? The answer may well depend on the languages or dialects involved, but recent research points to some potentially general results.

Arsland and Hansen (1997) studied foreign accent by analyzing temporal features, intonation patterns, and frequency characteristics for native-produced versus Mandarin-, German-, and Turkish-accented English utterances. The temporal features included voice onset time and word-final stop closure duration. The latter feature was particularly important in distinguishing Mandarin-accented versus native English. A detailed frequency analysis of foreign accented speech revealed that the mid-frequency range of 1500 to 2500 Hz is especially sensitive for detecting non-native speaker pronunciation variations. Wayland (1997), in a study of the production of Thai vowels, consonants, and tones by native speakers of Thai or English also concluded that the spectral properties of f_0 and formant frequencies distinguished the speaker groups more effectively than the temporal properties of VOT and vowel duration. Wayland reported that the rating scores for the non-native speakers were lower for level than contour tones, which may indicate different degrees of difficulty for different tones.

The voicing contrast for postvocalic English consonants was examined in speakers of Japanese and Mandarin Chinese (Crowther & Mann, 1992) and Arabic (Crowther & Mann, 1994). The productions were analyzed to determine the use of two major voicing cues, preceding vocalic duration and F1 offset frequency. The results varied with language background of the speakers, with the English speakers being highly sensitive to vocalic duration, the Mandarin and Arabic speakers being relatively insensitive to this cue, and the Japanese speakers being in between these two groups. All three non-English groups appeared to be more sensitive to F1 offset frequency than to vocalic duration.

Several studies point to the general conclusion that the age of learning a second language is critical (Flege, MacKay, & Meador, 1999; Flege, Yeni-Komshian, & Liu, 1999; Munro, Flege, & MacKay, 1996). The younger, the better. However, it also appears that even with early and/or extensive exposure to a second language, the mastery of that language may be limited in regard to certain aspects of phonetic perception (Bosch, Costa, & Sebastian-Galles, 2000; Takagi & Mann, 1995).

Speech Disorders

Speech disorders often present additional challenges to acoustic analysis. Some speech-disordered persons have highly variable phonatory and articulatory function, so that analysis parameters are not equally suitable over a stretch of speech. For example, a speaker may have rapid and marked changes in fundamental frequency during a speech sample of interest, or there may be alternations between a fairly smooth phonation and a very breathy or rough phonation. Therefore, analysis parameters that work well for one portion of the signal may not be appropriate for another portion. Rapid variations in phonatory and articulatory characteristics of speech can occur particularly in speakers who are deaf or dysarthric.

A comprehensive account of the acoustic analysis of speech disorders would require several volumes. However, certain issues are encountered frequently enough that some preparation can be given in a few pages. What follows, then, is a highly selective description of the application of acoustic analysis to speech disorders. Effective acoustic analysis of disorders of voice, speech, and language builds on information presented in earlier chapters. Certain caveats and modifications should be kept in mind in the analysis of atypical or abnormal patterns.

Voice Disorders

A large number of papers have been published on the acoustic correlates of voice quality and voice disorders, but there is continuing uncertainty on which acoustic measures are optimal for analysis of voice. One reason for the uncertainty is that different measures may be preferable for particular types of voice quality or types of voice disorder. In addition, some measures that work well for mild voice disorders may not be useful for more severe disorders. Another difficulty is that studies of the correlations between perceptual ratings of voice and acoustic measures of voice often have produced discrepant results.

A recent book on the subject (Kent & Ball, 2000) describes various approaches to the measurement of voice quality, including selected acoustic methods. The number of possible acoustic measures is huge, and they can be computed with a variety of algorithms (see Buder, 2000, for an extensive listing). Some of the more commonly used measures include jitter (cycle-to-cycle variations in the fundamental period), shimmer (cycle-to-cycle variations in glottal amplitude), harmonics-to-noise ratio (the ratio of periodic to aperiodic energy in a voiced waveform), spectral tilt, and f_0 statistics. Commercially marketed systems offer the capability for multidimensional analyses of voice samples. These analyses generally permit a rapid calculation of the values and convenient displays of the data. An example of one such display is shown in Figure 6–11.

Velopharyngeal Incompetence (Hypernasality)

A particularly troublesome feature of many speech disorders is unexpected nasalization, arising from *velopharyngeal incompetence*, or inadequacies in adjustments of velopharyngeal opening and closure. Nasalization can severely compromise the acoustic analysis of a speech signal. In speakers with severe velopharyngeal incompetence, the entire signal can be influenced by a high degree of damping (resulting in reduced signal energy and increased formant bandwidths) and by antiformants (which can further reduce overall energy of the signal and can complicate the identification of formants). A severely nasalized speech signal usually has a greatly reduced acoustic contrast among its segmental components. An example of such reduction is given in Figure 6–12, which shows spectrograms for a normal speaker's produc-

tion of *Mama made apple jam*, and a recitation of the same sentence by a speaker with severe velopharyngeal incompetence. When dealing with nasalized speech, it should be remembered that the acoustic correlates of nasalization are numerous and complex in their potential effects on the acoustic signal. Interpretation of acoustic records can therefore be difficult. For example, the following correlates of nasalization may appear in spectrograms of nasalized vowels (Kent, Liss, & Philips, 1989):

1. Increase in formant bandwidth, so that formant energy appears broader;

2. Decrease in the overall energy of the vowel (compared to non-nasalized vowels);

3. Introduction of a low-frequency nasal formant with a center frequency of about 250–500 Hz for adult males;

4. A slight increase of the F1 frequency and a slight lowering of the F2 and F3 frequencies; and

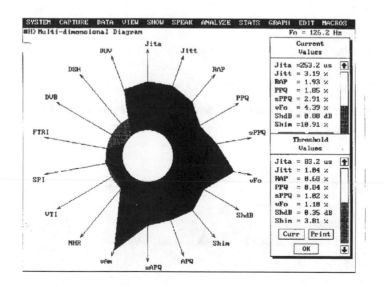

FIGURE 6–11. Example of analysis of a vowel phonation with the MDVP™ from Kay Elemetrics. The graph shows the results of a multidimensional analysis that includes parameters such as jitter, shimmer, tremor, frequency variation, and amplitude variation.

5. The presence of one or more antiformants.

Because nasalization is associated with a complex set of acoustic features, it is not always immediately evident from a given analysis, such as a spectrogram, if the pattern is influenced by nasalization. However, it appears that certain spectral regions are particularly useful in making this determination. Some examples are summarized next.

Analyses of one-third-octave power spectra showed that hypernasal vowels tend to have increased power level in the region between F1 and F2 and reduced power level in the F2 and F2 regions (Kataoka et al., 1996). In a study of nasalization in English and French, Chen (1997) defined nasalization indexes based on two amplitude difference values derived from the following measures: P0, the amplitude of an extra peak in the low frequencies; P1, the amplitude of an extra peak located between the first two formants; and A1, the amplitude of the first formant. Difference values were determined for A1-P1 and A1-P0. The A1-P1 difference averaged more than 10 dB between oral and nasalized vowels produced by speakers of American English. Plante, Berger-Vachon, and Kauffman (1993) reported that particular LPC coefficients were sensitive to the presence of nasalization in vowels produced by children. A distinction between nasalized and nonnasalized speech also has been demonstrated with an analysis based on the Teager energy operator under certain filtering conditions (Cairns, Hansen, & Riski, 1996). Although nasalization poses challenges to acoustic analysis, a clearer understanding of the acoustic correlates of nasal speech is emerging.

Speech of the Deaf or Profoundly Hearing Impaired

A general difficulty in acoustic analysis of speech disorders is that individuals with the same disorder may vary greatly from

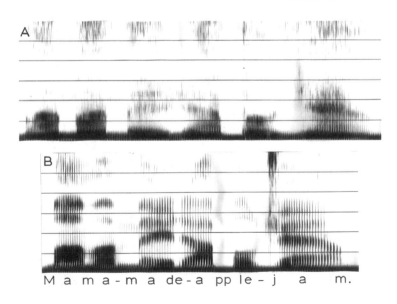

M a m a - m a de - a pp le - j a m.

FIGURE 6–12. Spectrograms for the sentence *"Mama made apple jam"* produced by a speaker with velopharyngeal incompetence (hypernasality) at the top (A) and by a speaker with normal nasality at the bottom (B). The pattern in A has a general loss of acoustic contrast among its component segments.

one another in their acoustic speech characteristics. Speakers with profound hearing loss are notable for such inter-individual variability. Some examples are shown in Figure 6–13 and 6–14. Figure 6–13 contains several spectrograms of a portion of the simple phrase *took a spoon* produced by six deaf adolescents. These spectrograms focus on the production of the fricative [s] in the word *spoon*. The following patterns can be seen: (a) This speaker produced a fairly normal fricative, as evidenced by the conspicuous noise energy at higher frequencies; (b) Here the speaker interrupts the frication segment so that its midsection is nearly silent, somewhat resembling a stop gap; (c) This attempt begins with a fairly good fricative but it is cut short and followed by a noticeable silent gap; (d) The production is characterized by a burst of diffuse noise energy closely preceding the onset of the vowel [u]; (e) The speaker represented here tended to laryngealize consonant segments, as indicated in this spectrogram by the continuation of voicing through the marked interval and the appearance of pronounced

glottal pulses; and (f) In this case, there is no frication energy, but the location of the [s] is marked by a silent interval of approximately the expected duration of the [s] energy in normal speech.

Figure 6–14 gives examples of phonatory, resonance and prosodic variations in the speech of the deaf. All the patterns shown are for the first three words of the sentence, *Buy Bobby a puppy*. Spectrogram *a* shows the result for a speaker with a continuously breathy voice. Note that there is little evidence of periodic voicing energy (absent or weak vertical striations) and that the formants are excited by noise. The interformant regions tend to be filled with noise. In spectrogram *b*, the speaker tends to laryngealize consonants and word boundaries, and to produce speech with little variation in f_0 or F2. The f_0 contour is superimposed as the broken line averaging a little less than 125 Hz, and the F2 frequency is drawn as a solid line on the spectrogram. This is a pattern of continuous voicing (i.e., voicing that continues through intervals that should be voiceless) with a

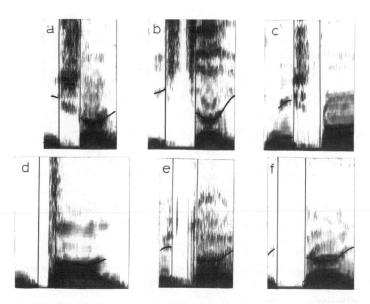

FIGURE 6–13. Spectrograms of the phrase *"a spoon"* (extracted from the sentence *"I took a spoon and a dish"*) produced by speakers with profound hearing loss or deafness. The individual patterns a–f are described in the text.

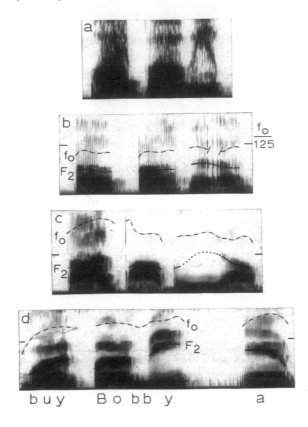

FIGURE 6–14. Spectrograms of the first three words of the sentence *"Buy Bobby a puppy"* produced by individuals with profound hearing loss or deafness. The fundamental frequency (f_0) contour is superimposed on the spectrograms in b, c, and d. See discussion in text.

reduction of f_0 to mark consonants and word boundaries. Note the *glottal roll* (or vocal fry) near the end of the pattern. Spectrogram *c* is the result for a speaker with a highly variable f_0 (see the superimposed broken line representing the f_0 contour) and a strong tendency toward nasalization. The latter results in a virtual disappearance of F2 energy (see dotted line). Finally, spectrogram *d* shows the pattern for a speaker who produced nearly equally stressed, widely separated syllables in a kind of sing-song cadence. This speaker's speech is slow (compare the duration of *c* with that of the other three patterns) and deliberate (note the distinct formant patterns).

The variability among deaf speakers is further illustrated in Figure 6–15, which shows the F1–F2 trajectories for the diphthong in *buy* produced by 23 deaf adolescent speakers. The trajectories are drawn as straight lines connecting the apparent onglide of the diphthong with its apparent offglide. The trajectories differ in onglide frequency, offglide frequency and, to a lesser extent, even the direction of movement in the F1–F2 plane (e.g., some speakers have a downward rather than the expected upward frequency shift for F2).

Dysarthria — *parkinson*

Acoustic contrast among speech segments is reduced in a number of speech disorders. One in particular is the dysarthria (neurologic speech disorder) associated with Parkinson's disease. Some speakers with

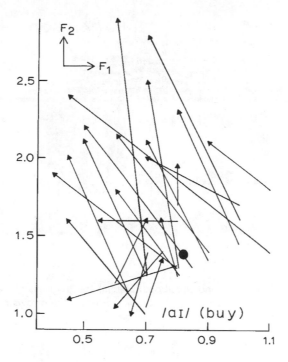

FIGURE 6-15. Productions of the diphthong /aɪ/ by a large number of individuals with profound hearing loss or deafness. The result for an individual speaker is represented in the F1–F2 plane as a line running from the onglide to the offglide (arrowhead). The mean F1 and F2 values for the onglide are indicated by the filled circle.

this disease have a dysarthria in which words are uttered in short rushes or accelerated patterns. Figure 6–16 shows narrow-band (top) and wide-band (bottom) spectrograms for a short-rush production of the words *something beyond his reach*. The pattern is continuously voiced (as evident by the continuous voicing bar and the uninterrupted glottal-pulse vertical striations) and poorly articulated (note the incomplete stop gap and weak fricatives). The speaker may accomplish the rapid speaking rate by neglecting many phonatory and articulatory adjustments to give a "blurred" effect to the overall pattern. A comparison between a neurologically normal speaker and a speaker with Parkinson's disease is shown in Figure 6–17 for the phrase *strikes raindrops*. Even a casual inspection of the two spectrograms reveals the diminished acoustic contrasts for the individual with Parkinson's disease. Spirantization of stop

gaps is readily observed: note the presence of noise energy in the expected stop gaps for the labeled stops. Spirantization results from incomplete articulatory closure, which permits the generation of turbulence noise at the constriction.

Acoustic analyses can be helpful in the study of speech disorders that disturb timing and sequencing. One such disorder is *verbal apraxia* (or *apraxia of speech*), which is a disorder of the sequencing or programming of speech movements. In this disorder, speech tends to be slow, intermittent and variable. Figure 6–18 shows spectrograms for productions of the word *please* by (*a*) a neurologically normal speaker and (*b*) and (*c*) two individuals with apraxia of speech. Differences in word duration are immediately evident, with the productions in *b* and *c* being more than twice the duration of that for the normal control. The second formant (labeled in each spectrogram)

apraxia
verbal
SP
programm

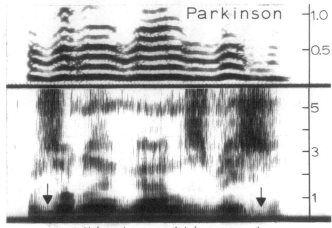

FIGURE 6–16. Narrow-band (top) and wide-band (bottom) spectrograms of the phrase *"something beyond his reach* produced by a speaker with Parkinson's disease. The arrows point to intervals of continuous voicing (voicing of segments that should be unvoiced).

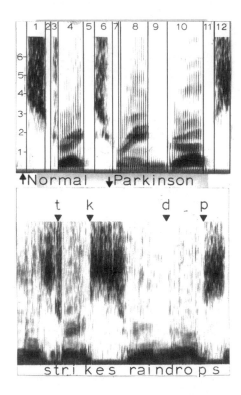

FIGURE 6–17. Spectrograms of the phrase *"strikes raindrop"s* produced (top) by a person with normal speech, and (bottom) and individual with Parkinson's disease and dysarthria. The arrowheads in the result for the speaker with Parkinson's disease indicate spirantized stop gaps (that is, stop gaps containing frication energy).

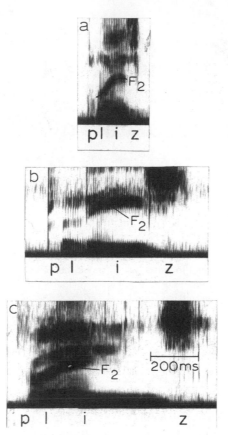

FIGURE 6–18. Spectrograms of the word *please* produced by (a) a person with normal speech, and (b and c) persons with apraxia of speech. The apractic productions are greatly lengthened compared to the normal pattern. Reprinted from R. D. Kent and J. C. Rosenbek, Acoustic patterns of apraxia of speech, *Journal of Speech and Hearing Research, 26,* 231–249. (Reproduced with permission from the American Speech-Language-Hearing Association, Rockville, MD.) Copyright 1987.

has a much slower trajectory for the speakers with apraxia. This analysis shows that the dyspraxic productions are longer, and, moreover, have slower rates of acoustic (and, by inference, articulatory) change.

A general question about dyspraxic speech is whether the errors are phonemic (substitutions of one phoneme for another) or involve phonetic distortions (such as might result from incoordination). Figure 6–19 illustrates the use of a spectrogram to evaluate a particular error in dyspraxic speech. The word analyzed is the monosyllable *shush* in which the vowel is preceded and followed by a voiceless consonant. The

illustration shows both wide-band (top) and narrow-band (bottom) spectrograms. The word was produced disfluently with a false start, as indicated by the initial frication segment followed by a pause and then production of the whole word. Note that the initial fricative production of *shush* is not entirely voiceless: evidence that vocal fold vibrations begin during the fricative interval appears in both the wide-band spectrogram (note circled voice bar) and narrow-band spectrogram (note circled harmonic pattern). Apparently, this speaker commits errors in the coordination of voicing with oral articulatory function, such

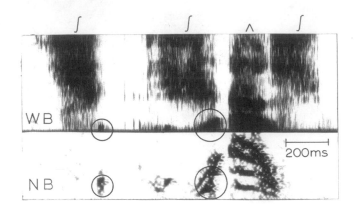

FIGURE 6–19. Wide-band (top) and narrow-band (bottom) spectrograms of a dysfluent production of the word *shush* by a person with apraxia of speech. The circled segments indicate brief voiced intervals during the production of the initial fricative (which should be voiceless). Reprinted from R. D. Kent and J. C. Rosenbeck, Acoustic patterns of apraxia of speech, *Journal of Speech and Hearing Research*, 26, 231–246. (Reproduced with permission from the American Speech-Language-Hearing Association, Rockville, MD.) Copyright 1987.

that the resulting pattern is not a phonemic error but a phonetic or motoric lapse.

Variations in VOT for the prevocalic stop [d] in *dad* are illustrated in Figure 6–20. Results are shown for four speakers with apraxia, arranged in order of increasing duration of prevoicing. The VOT interval is highlighted with a vertical bar and attached arrow. The speaker represented in (d) has a particularly long interval of prevoicing. Azou et al. (2000) describe a number of abnormalities in VOT that are useful in the study of apraxia of speech, dysarthria, and aphasia.

A related speech disorder in children is often given the label of *developmental verbal apraxia*. Children with this disorder have considerable difficulty in producing speech with normal rate and phonetic accuracy. Figure 6–21 contains three spectrograms showing a normal speaker saying the word *spaghetti* (top) and two attempts by a child with apraxia to say the same word. The characteristics of slowness, intermittency, and variability are represented acoustically by long overall duration and long segment durations (slow speaking rate); long and

variable pauses (intermittent, broken speech); and inconsistency between the two productions (variability). Similar characteristics have been observed in adult (or acquired) apraxia of speech (Kent & Rosenbek, 1983).

Children's Phonologic Disorders

These disorders occur with considerable frequency and often require speech therapy. One fairly common pattern is final consonant deletion, in which the child omits the final consonant of a word or syllable (e.g., [k ae t] is produced as [k ae]). A particular consequence of final consonant deletion is that the child cannot distinguish singular and plural forms of words that add /s/ or /z/ as a plural marker. For example, the child presumably cannot distinguish the singular *toe* from the plural *toes*, both being produced as [toU]. But these children may be marking the plural form with other means. Tyler and McOmber (1999) used acoustic analysis to show that four children

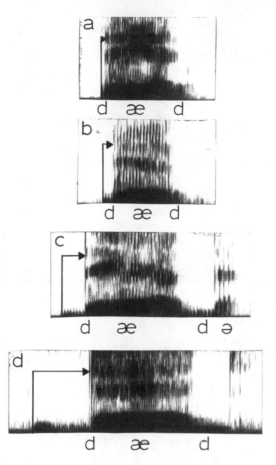

FIGURE 6–20. Spectrograms of the word *dad* produced by (a) a person with normal speech, and (b–d) persons with apraxia of speech. The interval marked by an arrow is the voice onset time (VOT) for the initial [d].

who had the error of final consonant deletion produced plural forms that were, in fact, different from singular forms. They relied on one or more suprasegmental parameters to make the distinction.

Documenting Changes in Speech

A promising role of acoustic methods in speech pathology is to monitor changes in speech production that may occur as the result of management or as the result of disease progression. Acoustic analysis permits a quantification of selected features of speech production. One example is the use of acoustics to study the change in speech in an individual with amyotrophic lateral sclerosis, a degenerative and fatal neurologic disease. Sample spectrograms of the word *sigh* by a woman with amyotrophic lateral sclerosis (Lou Gehrig's disease) are shown in Figure 6–22 for two different times: shortly after the initial diagnosis (top) and several months after diagnosis. This individual is capable of at least a weak [s] in the early sample but generates little or no [s] frication in the later sample. Acoustic methods can be used to detect subtler

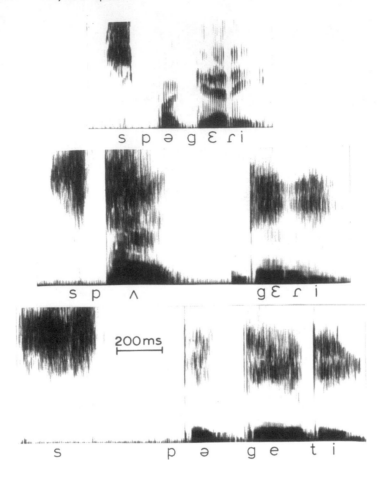

FIGURE 6–21. Spectrograms of the word *spaghetti* produced by a normal adult speaker (top) and (middle and bottom) a child with developmental apraxia of speech. The child's productions are characterized by lengthened segments and a highly variable pattern.

changes as well, possibly changes that cannot be reliably detected by the ear alone.

The spectrograph made possible an objective examination of speech disorders. However, one problem with the spectrograph is that it often leaves the user with a considerable analysis task. The spectrogram in itself is rarely sufficient; the user has to derive measures, often by a rather tedious process. Much faster analyses, resulting in quantitative measures, are being used today. For example, LPC formant tracking identifies formant patterns automatically, thus saving the effort and time that otherwise

would be given to manual formant tracing from spectrograms. A sample of automatic quantitative analysis is given in Figure 6–23. The analysis pertains to a dysarthric speaker's production of the sentence "*The potato stew is in the pot.*" The multi-parameter analysis of Figure 6–23 shows, in the top four panels, the four spectral moments (kurtosis, skewness, standard deviation, mean); the panel third from the bottom, LPC formant tracks for the first three formants; and, in the bottom two panels, the fundamental frequency contour and rms envelope. This multi-parameter analysis yields a great deal

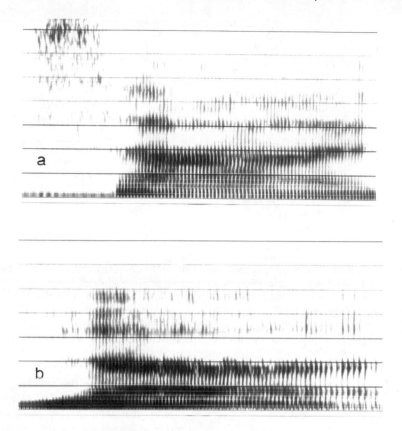

FIGURE 6–22. Spectrograms of the word *sigh* produced by a woman with amyotrophic lateral sclerosis (Lou Gehrig's disease). The result in (a) was recorded at an early point in the disease and the result in (b) was recorded at a later point when the disease was highly advanced.

of information about the speech pattern, all of it obtained semi-automatically on a personal computer.

For more detailed discussions of the acoustic characteristics of disordered speech, the reader is referred to an article on acoustic characteristics of dysarthria by Weismer (1984), a more recent article also on the topic of dysarthria (Kent et al., 1999), and a collection of articles on spectrographic analysis edited by Baken and Daniloff (1990).

Psychiatric Disorders

Some psychiatric disorders are associated with fairly distinctive patterns of spoken language, including some features that can be studied acoustically. Only two examples of this effort are considered here. In a study of 20 male offenders (ten psychopaths and ten nonpsychopaths), it was determined that the psychopaths spoke more quietly and did not differentiate neutral and affective words (Louth et al., 1998). The authors interpreted these results to mean that psychopaths are insensitive to the emotional connotations of language. Acoustical properties of speech may be useful in identifying individuals with depression, and, furthermore, it is possible that acoustic analyses may discriminate between depressed and suicidal speech. France et al., (2000) reported acoustic analyses of the speech of individuals with dysthymia, depression, or high risk for suicide.

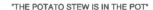

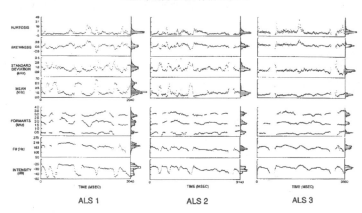

FIGURE 6–23. Multiparameter acoustic analysis of the sentence "*The potato stew is in the pot*" produced at three different times by a speaker with a neurodegenerative disease (amyotrophic lateral sclerosis). Data are shown for the four spectral moments (kurtosis, skewness, standard deviation, mean), the first three formants derived from LPC formant tracking, f_0, and rms contour. Note the diminishing acoustic contrast across the four different recording sessions, which reflects the increasing severity of the disease. The histograms on the sides of each panel represent the cumulative data for each parameter.

Expanding the Acoustic Phonetic Data Base

The preceding comments indicate that the data base of acoustic phonetics is expanding to include a much broader range of speakers than has been studied in the past. Data are being collected on infants, children, women, speakers of various dialects and individuals with various speech and voice disorders. This broader research effort is important to make the acoustic analysis of speech, automatic speech recognition, and speech synthesis and other speech technologies applicable to diverse populations of speakers. Much work remains to be done, but, fortunately, current methods of acoustic analysis are much more adaptable to different speaker characteristics than was the spectrograph of the 1950s and 1960s. The spectrograph was a powerful tool in its day, but modern computer systems for speech analysis go far beyond the spectrograph in speed, flexibility and ease of use.

For many applications, including the evaluation of speech recognition systems, it is useful to have a database of speech samples. Several such databases have been established and among the most frequently used are the TIMIT database (Garofolo et al., 1993), the WSJ database (Paul & Baker, 1992), and BREF (Gauvain et al., 1990). TIMIT consists of a set of constructed sentences read by a variety of American English speakers. WSJ consists of extracts read from the *Wall Street Journal*. BREF contains extracts from the French newspaper *La Monde*.

Suprasegmental Properties of Speech

7

CHAPTER

Most of what has been said so far oversimplifies the problem of speech analysis in various applications. The simplification arises largely from the fact that important sources of variability, as well as sources of information, have been neglected. Some of the sources of variability have been mentioned, but it is the task of this chapter to consider them in more detail and to relate them to additional sources of information in speech. In particular, this chapter will consider phonetic context and suprasegmentals. Phonetic context refers to the phonetic environment in which a sound occurs, including neighboring sounds and prosodic characteristics of the utterance. It is only rarely that a speech sound occurs in isolation from other sounds. More generally, a given target sound is produced in a sequence of sounds and these neighboring sounds influence the production of the target sound. Suprasegmentals are the prosodic features and various other modifications whose effects transcend the boundaries of individual phonetic elements. The suprasegmentals are superimposed on phonetic sequences, giving these sequences a coherence and unity that obscures the ostensible discreteness of their phonetic constituents. Although it is somewhat of a simplification, it can be said that speech is a series of phonetic elements (the segments) produced in a framework of intonation, stress, rhythm, loudness, and rate (the suprasegmentals). Extracting the individual phonetic elements from this framework is highly challenging, which is why it is difficult to instruct machines to accomplish speech recognition.

Coarticulation

The descriptions of speech sounds in the earlier chapters have largely ignored the effects of context, that is, the production of sounds in combinations to form syllables, words and phrases. It is, in fact, rather artificial to describe a sound in terms of its isolated, discrete production. Speech usually

223

involves strings of sounds uttered in rapid succession. In such strings, the individual sounds can lose some of their distinctiveness and even take on some of the properties of surrounding sounds. Frequently, the boundaries between sounds are blurred. To take one example, consider the simple word *am* [ae m]. In the typical production of this word, the vowel [ae] is nasalized, that is, produced with some degree of nasal resonance owing to the fact that the velopharyngeal opening for the nasal consonant [m] is anticipated during the vowel. In effect, an articulatory (and acoustic) feature of the consonant is produced *in advance* during the preceding vowel. As another example, most speakers produce the word *stew* [stu] with lip rounding that begins during the [s]. The lip rounding is actually required for the rounded vowel [u] but begins well before the vowel itself is articulated. No such lip rounding is observed for the [s] in a word like *stay*, which does not involve a rounded vowel.

From these examples, we can see that the segments of speech interact, such that some of their features are intermingled. The term **coarticulation** (or **coproduction**) refers to events in speech in which the vocal tract shows at any one instant adjustments that are appropriate for two or more sounds. The direction of a coarticulatory effect can be described as forward (anticipatory) or backward (retentive). In **forward coarticulation**, an articulatory feature for a phonetic segment is apparent during the production of an earlier segment. Consider the examples in the preceding paragraph. For the word *am*, the property of nasalization (open velopharyngeal port) occurs during the vowel that precedes the nasal consonant. Thus, this word shows evidence of the forward coarticulation of nasalization. In the second example, forward coarticulation of lip rounding is evident for the [s] in the word *stew*. In **backward coarticulation**, an articulatory feature for a phonetic segment is carried over to a later segment. For example, in the word *no* ([noU]), the nasalization for the nasal consonant [n] is

carried over to the vocalic element. Some degree of backward coarticulation is inevitable because the articulators are not capable of infinite speed. It takes time to make articulatory adjustments, and backward coarticulation reflects the physical inertia of the articulators.

Coarticulation is reviewed in depth by Sharf and Ohde (1981) and Farnetani (1997), who consider physiologic, acoustic and perceptual aspects of this speech phenomenon. They also review models of speech production that attempt to account for the coarticulatory patterns of speech. A more recent review of speech production models also is available in Kent, Adams and Turner (1996). For the purposes of this text, coarticulation is mainly of interest in understanding the modifications of a given sound by the context in which it appears. The discussions of vowel and diphthong production in Chapter 4 and consonant production in Chapter 5 should be tempered with the knowledge that sounds in context often are mutually influenced. Some investigators of coarticulation described the process as one of "feature spreading" insofar as a feature of one sound is anticipated during an earlier sound in the string or retained by a later sound. Whether or not this characterization is theoretically correct, it does convey the idea of the coarticulatory effects that can be observed in the acoustic signal.

Recall that in the word [ae m], the vowel [ae] is nasalized because of the influence of the following nasal consonant [m]. The nasalization is present as a modification of the vowel [ae] produced nonnasally. Specifically, antiformants may be present, along with the appearance of a low-frequency nasal formant and a broadening of formant bandwidths. These acoustic features of nasalization are in effect "spread over" to influence the production of the vowel segment.

Figure 7–1 shows several examples of coarticulation. Notice that in each case illustrated, there is a *spreading*, *shingling*, or *blending* of articulatory features across neighboring speech sounds. All three of these words—spreading, shingling, and blending—are used here because they have somewhat different connotations and because all three have been used to describe coarticulation. Spreading suggests an expanding or stretching; shingling describes an overlapping; and blending denotes a fusing or intimate mingling. Spreading might be preferred over the other terms if coarticulation can be likened to a process in which a feature is stretched, rubberlike, to exceed its typical boundaries. For example, if lip rounding for a round vowel is anticipated during earlier segments, one might say that the rounding feature is expanded or stretched. Shingling is a good term to refer to modifications in which a particular feature or property is shifted in time relative to other features. Such a time shift does not reform a sound segment so much as it allows it to be penetrated by a particular feature. For example, some accounts of nasalization propose that a nasality feature is shingled from a nasal phone to its preceding or succeeding phone. Blending is the preferred term if a sound segment is reshaped to accommodate its phonetic neighbors. That is, the segment undergoes a significant revision that takes into account its overall nature vis-a-vis the nature of the sounds that surround it. Blending can be more drastic than either spreading or blending. These concepts recur in the following discussion.

The preceding paragraph discussed concepts that are largely temporal in nature. These concepts are relevant to determining the temporal domain of coarticulation. However, coarticulation can be considered also from the point of view of the range of spatial values assumed by an individual articulator. Keating (1990) described a window model of coarticulation based on the idea that, for a particular physical dimension (e.g., jaw position, velopharyngeal opening), each feature value of a segment is associated with a range of possible spatial values. This range of values is called a window and comprises

"an undifferentiated range representing the contextual variability of a feature value" (Keating, 1990, p. 455). This proposal helps to account for spatial variations in the production of a given sound in different phonetic contexts.

To a certain extent, coarticulation can be described in an abstract way that does not involve physical time. For instance, if individual sounds can be defined by a cluster of co-occurring features, then re-specification of features produces an abstract pattern of coarticulation. Ultimately, however, coarticulation is played out in time, and it is the temporal complexity of the process that confronts the laboratory scientist. The discussion here pertains mostly to physical time, and rather less to an abstract phonologic time. Some features are particularly likely to have a large temporal range. Among these features are lip rounding and nasalization, which are sometimes described as relatively sluggish. Other features tend to affect only the immediately adjacent segments. The preceding statement may be a simplification in that coarticulatory effects may extend over longer intervals than has sometimes been supposed. Magan (1997) observed coarticulatory effects between vowels in nonadjacent syllables, a finding that is not predicted by some contemporary models of speech articulation.

When sounds are produced in context, a number of temporal adjustments usually occur. Generally, a sound produced in context is shorter than the "same" sound produced in isolation. In addition, the duration of a segment tends to become shorter as more elements are added to the sound string. For example, when elements are added to a given consonant to produce two- and three-element consonant clusters (such as /p/, /sp/ and /spr/), the duration of the consonant decreases (Haggard, 1973; Schwartz, 1970; Umeda, 1977). A similar effect occurs for syllables. The duration of a monosyllabic base, such as *stick*, becomes progressively shorter in syllable-suffixing sequences like *stick, sticky,*

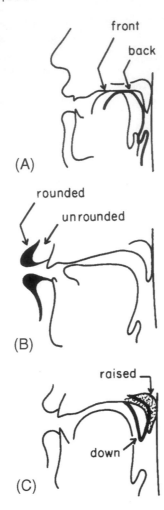

FIGURE 7-1. Examples of coarticulation: (A) variation in place of articulation of velar consonant, depending on vowel context; (B) variation in lip rounding for /s/, depending on following vowel; and (C) variation in velopharyngeal articulation during vowel, depending on following consonant.

stickiness (Lehiste, 1972). These durational effects occur even as the speaker tries to produce speech at a constant rate. This is an essentially automatic and nearly obligatory adjustment that the competent speaker makes. If a word like *stickiness* is produced without such temporal compression, it can sound stilted and unnatural.

As a final note to this section on coarticulation and context effects, it has been suggested that the acoustic cues to phonetic identity are weak and dispersed, rather than

being strongly tied to discrete segments (Nearey, 1992; van Son & Pols, 1999). By this reasoning, it is not expected that the acoustic cues for speech perception are always tightly associated with the traditional notion of a phonemic segment. According to van Son and Pols (1999), "human listeners extract an important fraction of the information needed to identify phonemes from outside the conventional segment boundaries" (p. 1). The authors termed this information *"perisegmental speech."*

Suprasegmentals

A major consequence of coarticulation is that the articulatory and acoustic characteristics of phonetic elements are affected by the surrounding elements. Therefore, allowances should always be made for contextual effects. The acoustic descriptions offered in this chapter do not take account of all the coarticulatory variations in speech, which are too numerous to summarize briefly. The acoustic properties for any given element will depend on a number of factors, including those associated with phonetic context, speaker, speaking style (e.g., casual versus formal), speaking rate, dialect and situation. A speaker can adjust speech patterns in a number of ways and for a number of purposes. Few systematic investigations have been conducted to show the nature of these variations. Some very brief comments will be given here on some selected factors and their acoustic effects. The comments are arranged under the headings of clear speech, prosody (intonation) and speaking rate. These are suprasegmental properties of speech in the sense that they typically have effects that are expressed beyond segmental boundaries. Frequently, suprasegmental features are described in terms of units larger than segments, for example, syllables, phrases or breath groups. This is not to say that suprasegmental properties are without effects at the segmental level.

Clear Speech

One factor is the difference between **clear speech** (speech produced in an effort to be highly intelligible) and *conversational speech* (in which clarity may be compromised). Figure 7–2 gives a spectrographic comparison of clear and conversational speech. Compared to conversational speech, clear speech is (1) slower (by virtue of longer pauses between words and lengthening of some speech sounds), (2) more apt to avoid modified or reduced forms of consonant and vowel segments, and (3) characterized by a greater RMS intensity of obstruent sounds, particularly stop consonants (Picheny, Durlach, & Braida, 1985, 1986, 1989). When speakers make an effort to be easily understood, they modify their articulation to make speech slower and more acoustically distinctive. In conversational speech, vowels often are modified or reduced, thus losing some of their acoustic distinctiveness. Similarly, stops occurring in word-final position in conversation frequently are not released, so that the burst cue is not available to listeners. However, in clear speech, vowels are not likely to be modified or reduced, and stop consonants (and consonants in general) tend to be released.

The question arises: Do the acoustic differences between clear and conversational speech hold implications for understanding the intelligibility differences among individual speakers? Recent research indicates an affirmative answer. Bond and Moore (1994) studied the acoustic–phonetic differences between a speaker with relatively high intelligibility and two speakers with relatively low intelligibility. The high intelligibility speaker had many acoustic-phonetic properties that had been previously described for "clear" speech. Bradlow, Torretta, and Pisoni (1996) studied both global and fine-grained differences among speakers as these differences correlated with interspeaker differences in intelligibility. They concluded that global characteristics did not correlate strongly with intelligibility, but the fine-grained characteristics did. The profile of a highly intelligible speaker was one who produced sentences with a relatively wide range of f_0, a relatively expanded vowel space that includes a substantial F1 variation, precise articulation of the point vowels, and a high precision of inter-segmental timing. It appears, then, that there is an important linkage between two general approaches to the study of intelligibility differences. Those acoustic differences that account for intelligibility differences between clear and conversational

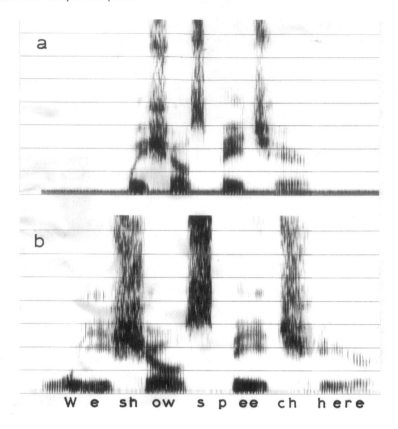

FIGURE 7–2. Spectrographic comparison of conversational speech (A) and clear speech (B). Both spectrograms are for the sentence, *"We show speech here."*

speech are largely congruent with the differences between speakers who have inherent differences in intelligibility.

Lindblom (1990) proposed that speakers vary their speech output along a continuum from *hypospeech* to *hyperspeech* (the *H&H hypothesis*). This hypothesis is based on the idea that speakers adapt to the various circumstances of communication, in effect tuning their production patterns to communicative and situational factors. Lindblom cites evidence that "clear speech" (hyperspeech in the H&H hypothesis) is not simply loud speech; it involves an articulatory reorganization (Moon & Lindblom, 1989). Adams (1990), however, concluded from an X-ray microbeam study of speech movements that changes in speech clarity did not reflect a reorganization of speech

motor control. The changes that Adams did observe, such as increases in maximum displacement and peak velocity of articulatory movements, occurred so as to maintain a fixed velocity/displacement ratio.

Prosody

Imagine how many ways a speaker can produce the simple sentence, "I'll give it to you." It could be a declarative (a factual statement), a question ("I'll give it to you?"), or a checked form in which the speaker requests more information, as in, "I'll give it to you-—PAUSE (on Monday? Tuesday?)." It could convey a wide range of emotion, from a graceful offering to a reassuring agreement to a grudging or even bitter concession, for instance. The sentence can be produced with different stress patterns, by placing the emphasis on the capitalized words in the following versions: "I'LL give it to you." "I'll GIVE it to you." 'I'll give it to YOU." It also could be produced with different internal pausing, such as a pause after *it*, or a pause after *to*. All these modifications fall in the category of *prosody*. For the purposes of this book, prosody will be defined as the suprasegmental features of speech that are conveyed by the parameters of fundamental frequency (perceived primarily as vocal pitch), intensity (perceived primarily as loudness), and duration (perceived primarily as length). The term suprasegmental indicates that the phenomena of interest are not confined to phonetic segments. In fact, they often are observed over much larger intervals—syllables, words, phrases, sentences, and even discourses.

The term prosody is not easily defined in a way that agrees with all that has been written about it. Definitions disagree in some respects, so the reader should be wary in applying any one definition to different writings on the subject. One major disagreement is with the pair of terms, prosody and *intonation*. Some writers regard them as synonyms, while others mark an important distinction between them. We follow Johns-Lewis (1986) in considering intonation to be a part of prosody. Intonation is similar to prosody in that its parameters are vocal frequency, intensity, and duration, but intonation refers to a narrower range of phenomena, generally the patterns of pitch rises and falls and the patterns of stress in a given language. Prosody includes these effects but also embraces *tempo* (pause and lengthening), vocal effort, loudness, and other phenomena. Some writers include speaking rate as a part of tempo, and therefore as a part of prosody. Because these terms are defined differently by different authors, care should be taken in comparing differing sources of information.

The purpose here is not to provide a rigorous and comprehensive definition of prosody and related concepts. This is a mat-

ter of intense debate about linguistic theory and goes beyond the modest scope of this chapter. Rather, the purpose is simply to summarize the acoustic correlates of basic prosodic phenomena: vocal fundamental frequency, intensity, and duration. The measurement of all three parameters was discussed in Chapter 3. The ways in which these parameters are regulated will determine how the sentence, "I'll give it to you" takes acoustic form and is perceived. These parameters influence each other in complicated ways; we will sketch a few basic prosodic effects without attempting to describe their interactions in detail.

It may be helpful to picture prosody in broad relief and then proceed to a discussion of some of its detailed features. Prosody has been described with respect to three general types of phenomena in language: *phrasal stress*, *boundary cues*, and *meter* (Gerken & McGregor, 1998). These classes of prosody are used here to introduce the general issues of prosodic description and analysis.

Phrasal stress is the phenomenon of word prominence in a phrase, that is, one word in a group of words is considered to be more prominent, more salient, or more accentuated. If we consider any particular grouping of words, a speaker usually will place more prominence on one word compared to others. You might try a simple experiment in which speakers are asked to read a short phrase or sentence printed on a card (e.g., the phrase, "I put the fork and spoon on the plate"). Listen to the various productions. Can you tell which word (or words) was given prominence by a particular speaker? With respect to lexical stress, many authors distinguish stress from *accent*. Stress is considered to be an abstract feature at the level of the lexicon, whereas accent is a phonetic feature with correlates in production, acoustics, and perception.

Boundary cues are pauses, changes in duration, or adjustments of pitch that mark the ends of language units. Speakers can use boundary cues to mark major linguistic structures and to give form to a conversation or a reading sample. An important example is *phrase-final lengthening*, in which a word or syllable that precedes the end of a major syntactic unit is lengthened. Lengthening is common for the final word of a sentence, but it also can occur for the final word of a phrase within a larger sentence. For example, the slashes in the following sentence indicate major syntactic breaks (one slash for a phrase boundary and two slashes for a sentence boundary) and the words printed in bold would typically be lengthened: I saw the **sign**/ that was on the **wall**//. A variety of other boundary cues are discussed later in this chapter.

Meter (or rhythm) is the pattern of stressed and unstressed syllables for words and phrases. It is assumed that in American English, syllables usually have a strong-weak (SW) alternation, and this alternation gives a particular rhythm to the language. The SW pattern is a general tendency and should not be expected to occur without violation. It is linked to a stress unit called the *foot*, which is a SW syllable pair. .

These are interrelated phenomena, but we might say that meter defines the rhythmic flow of an utterance, lacing its syllables together in an alternating strong–weak sequence. This sequence is interrupted or modulated by boundary cues (edge effects) at the ends of linguistic units, especially phrases or sentences. Within any given phrase, the speaker may choose one word to receive special prominence and therefore assigns a phrasal stress pattern. Imagine the different patterns of phrasal stress that could be given to the following sequence.

> CV CVC CV CV CVC CV
> CV CVC
>
> my dog saw the cat at the
> door

Syllables

Before proceeding to a more detailed discussion of prosody, we should take a moment to discuss the syllable because this unit figures prominently in many theoretical and analytical accounts of prosody. In the foregoing discussion, and in much of what follows, the syllable is assumed as a unit relevant to the understanding of prosody. What exactly is a syllable? Handel (1989) offers two definitions. First, a syllable can be defined physically as a sonority or loudness peak surrounded by segments with progressively decreasing sonority values (Selkirk, 1984). With this definition, it should be possible to determine syllables quite readily from an analysis of sound energy (such as the RMS amplitude envelope); however, the procedure is not always straightforward. Second, a syllable can be defined phonologically as a phoneme combination with a vowel center bounded by a permitted consonant or consonant combination (O'Connor & Trim, 1953). Of course, sometimes there are no consonants. Another problem is that some consonants seem ambisyllabic, that is, belonging to syllables on either side of the consonant.

In another approach to defining the syllable, Hayes (1984), writing on metrics and phonologic theory, states that "syllables correspond one-to-one with terminal nodes of the metrical pattern." This idea is illustrated in Figure 7–3. With this definition, syllables are a metrical concept and are therefore fundamental to the prosodic description of language.

Phrasal stress

One way to study prosody is to consider its shape on several levels of linguistic or communication structure. At the level of the discourse, for instance, *new*, as opposed to *given*, *information* is highlighted prosodically. Behne (1989) showed that in a mini-discourse like:

"Someone painted the fence."

"Who painted the fence?"

"Pete painted the fence."

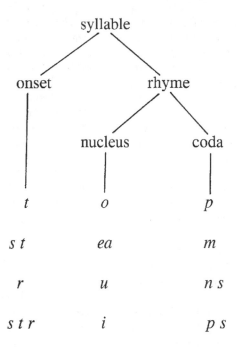

FIGURE 7–3. One model of syllable structure. The syllable divides into an onset and rhyme, with the latter dividing further into a nucleus and coda. Several examples of individual syllables are shown orthographically at the bottom of the figure. Either the onset or coda can be null, as in the words *on* and *no*.

The new information ("Pete" in the above exchange) is made longer and higher in fundamental frequency. She also showed that the same cues are deployed somewhat differently in French. Prosodic cues vary across languages, just as segmental ones do. The major point for present purposes is that speakers and listeners know the means by which new information can be distinguished from given (previous) information.

Another discourse effect on prosody is *contrastive stress*, which can occur on almost any word, phrase or clause which the speaker considers to contradict or contrast with one that was previously stated or implied in the discourse. For instance, one says, "I'll GIVE it to you" when one believes that some other verb (like "sell") was incorrectly assumed by the listener.

Still another aspect of phrasal stress pertains to lexical stress contrasts. English has many noun/verb pairs like *'import* versus *im'port*, in which the stress pattern is the major spoken contrast. Another lexical effect is the pattern on compounds versus phrases. For example, the compound noun *'blackboard* contrasts with the noun phrase *black `board* (board that is black). Stress in English, whether contrastive or lexical, is not merely a matter of intensity but involves all three acoustic parameters— duration, intensity, and fundamental frequency—of which duration may be the most salient and reliable (Adams & Munro, 1978; Fry, 1955; Sluijter & van Heuven, 1996). Although intensity seems to be less important than fundamental frequency or duration in most published studies, vocal effort may be a cue that listeners use to identify stressed syllables. One acoustic cue for vocal effort is spectral balance, or the relative amount of energy at high frequencies (above 0.5 kHz) versus low frequencies (Sluijter & van Heuven, 1996). However, the role of spectral tilt in stress is far from clear. Although Sluijter and van Heuven (1996) concluded that tilt is an important acoustic feature in lexical stress contrasts, van Kuijk and Boves (1999) found that tilt was less effective than either duration or energy in such contrasts. van Kuijk and Boves determined that the best feature was one that integrates energy over the duration of a vowel.

Stress also affects segmental properties such as vowel and consonantal articulation (Kent & Netsell, 1971; de Jong, 1991). Segments in stressed syllables tend to have larger articulatory movements than syllables in unstressed syllables. In a sense, the movements in stressed syllables are more contrastive, and this contrastivity is also realized in the acoustic patterns of speech. Therefore, a vowel in a stressed syllable usually has a distinctive formant pattern, that is, one that resembles the presumed target pattern for the vowel as might be defined in an isolated production. Acoustic distinctiveness usually decreases in unstressed syllables.

Some linguistic accounts distinguish types of stress-like effects such as stress and *accent* (Lehiste, 1970); however, a unifying theory (Beckman, 1986; Beckman & Edwards, 1991) proposes a representation with four levels:

Level 1: syllables with reduced nuclei, such as the second syllable in *vita*.

Level 2: syllables similar to those above except that they have full vowels (e.g., *veto*).

Level 3: syllables may be selectively given more stress by assigning to them a pitch accent.

Level 4: syllables can receive a marking called *nuclear accent* (or *phrase accent*) in which the last accented item in a phonologic grouping assumes the most prominent accent.

This proposal illustrates the complexity of stress, which may involve several differ-

ent, interacting phenomena. Consider a speaker who wants to place pitch accent on the word *tuba*. The accent cannot be placed on the second syllable, which is a reduced nucleus. Rather, the accent must be placed on the stressed syllable. In this way, the various levels of the stress representation can interact without destroying essential phonologic patterns

Prosodic boundary cues

At the level of syntax, too, prosody plays essential roles. At this level, we encounter juncture and pause phenomena marking multiword units. One of the best-known and most important of these in English is phrase-final lengthening, in which the last stressable syllable in a major syntactic phrase or clause is lengthened. For example, if we contrast the two sentences,

1. Grapes, melons, and apples are my favorite fruits.

2. Apples, grapes, and melons are my favorite fruits.

the first syllable of *apples* will be longer in (1) than (2) because in the former this word is at the end of the subject noun phrase. (Although the word *apples* contains two syllables, only the first one can be stressed.) To an even greater degree, *fruits* will be longer in both sentences than it would be if it stood in the middle of a phrase. Klatt (1976) provides a classic survey of this and related phenomena that determine durations of speech elements. Read and Schreiber (1982) showed that listeners use phrase-final lengthening to recognize the structure of (that is, to parse) spoken sentences. They argued that children rely more on this prosodic cue than adults do, and in fact that prosody provides the language-learner with an accessible starting point for learning the complex syntactic structures of language.

Also at the level of syntax, the fundamental frequency contour typically declines across clauses or comparable units. The origin, nature, and measurement of this fundamental-frequency tilt are the subjects of argument (Cohen, Collier, & t'Hart, 1982). One view is that declination is linear—fundamental frequency falls gradually and linearly throughout a sentence (Maeda, 1976; Sorensen & Cooper, 1980; Thorsen, 1985). This pattern often is described as a universal property of spoken language. Other writers have disputed the linear declination hypothesis, especially for spontaneous speech (Lieberman et al., 1985). Lieberman (1967) proposed a *breath-group theory of intonation* in which variation is allowed in the non-terminal part of the fundamental-frequency contour. That is, if a declarative sentence is divided into non-terminal and terminal parts, the former can take various forms whereas the latter typically shows a rapid fall in fundamental frequency. Support for this proposal comes from studies showing that an important acoustic cue for syntactic structure is the fall in fundamental frequency and intensity at the end of the breath group (Landahl, 1980; Lieberman & Tseng, 1981; Lieberman et al, 1985). Additional support for this more flexible view of intonation was reported by Umeda (1982), who described declination as situation-dependent: the pattern of fundamental frequency becomes more complex as the complexity of contextual information increases.

The f_0 declination appears as a downward slope of the fundamental frequency contour. It has been observed that the differences between the onset and offset frequencies are nearly constant regardless of the duration of the utterance. Therefore, the rate (r) of declination becomes greater with decreasing utterance length. Maeda (1976) computed r as follows:

$$r = \wedge f / t,$$

where $\wedge f$ is the average f_0 declination for an individual speaker (about 20–30 Hz for males).

The *top-line rule* assumes a negative slope of f_0 peaks over time and is used primarily to predict one or more f_0 values intermediate to the initial and final values. An effect called f_0 *resetting* occurs at an observed f_0 peak which is higher than the peak preceding it. In order for resetting to occur:

f_0 declination should be present before and after the resetting; and

the resetting is between sentences or at clause boundaries of a multi-clause sentence.

P_1 effect is a property of f_0 which accounts for general length of a sentence when programming the first f_0 peak; that is, longer sentences have higher P_1 values so that the f_0 declination slope remains fairly constant on single-clause sentences. The higher P_1 value for longer sentences allows the speaker an adequate range of f_0 values.

Sentence final f_0 fall or sentence-final lengthening refers to the largest f_0 fall in a given word occurring sentence finally. This marks the end of an utterance—minor falls preceding it signal that the speaker intends to continue an utterance.

Boundary cues also are called *edge effects*, which are asymmetries in phonetic form that occur between internal positions and the edges of prosodic domains, that is, a segment assumes somewhat different characteristics in internal versus edge position. In general, acoustic cues for segments are enhanced at the edges of these domains. The enhancements take the form of lengthening of segments or pauses (Beckman & Edwards, 1991; de Pijper & Sanderman, 1994; Klatt, 1975b, 1976; Oller, 1973; Wightman et al., 1992), strengthening (Fourgeron & Keating, 1997), alteration of the degree of overlap with adjacent segments (Byrd, 1996; Byrd & Saltzman, 1998), and the likelihood of glottalization of word-initial vowels (Dilley, Shattuck-Hufnagel, & Ostendorf, 1996). These effects might be likened to oral punctuation because they help the listener to determine phrase and clause boundaries that are often represented by commas, semicolons, and other punctuation marks in written text. The perceptual salience of these cues was studied by de Pijper and Sanderman (1994), who referred to their collective effects as *perceptual boundary strength*. Their experiments showed that untrained listeners could reliably judge prosodic boundaries even when the lexical contents of the utterances were made unrecognizable. It appears that prosodic boundaries are quite salient and could be very helpful in understanding spoken discourse.

Meter (Rhythm)

It is often asserted that speech has a rhythmic quality. As noted earlier in this chapter, rhythm is one component of the prosody of language. Rhythm is especially notable in the recitation of poetic verse, but even ordinary conversational speech seems to have a rhythm, and, to some degree, different languages have different rhythms. Simply defined, rhythm is the distribution of various levels of stress across a series of syllables (Kent, Adams, & Turner, 1996). This definition of rhythm in speech accords with a more general definition of rhythmic behavior in which the "experience of rhythm involves movement, regularity, grouping, and yet accentuation and differentiation" (Handel, 1989, p. 384). At the heart of the matter for rhythm in speech is a sequence of units (presumably syllables) that cohere together in an overall stress pattern that can be analyzed as levels of stress assigned to the individual units.

The rhythm of speech can be defined in two general ways that carry quite different implications for empirical study (Guaitella, 1999). First, rhythm can be defined metrically, for example, as "an assimilation tendency involving the regulation of intervals" (Guaitella, 1999, p. 509). The concept of isochrony (equalized time intervals) is an example of this metric approach. Second, rhythm can be defined to emphasize a dissimilarity tendency over the events of speech. Guaitella explains the difference in

approach as follows: "Metric analysis is based on the premise that a temporal continuum can be analyzed by quantification, while rhythmic analysis approaches temporal organization through the mechanisms of perception." (p. 509) A certain tension exists between the metric and rhythmic approaches, because they are not easily synthesized in a common analysis of rhythm. In an analysis of eight languages, Ramus, Nespor, and Mehler (1999) concluded that intuitive rhythm types reflect specific phonologic properties, and these, in turn, are associated with acoustic/phonetic features of speech. Perhaps an approach of this kind will be useful in establishing the acoustic correlates of rhythm across different languages. It should be emphasized also that rhythm is relational, in the sense that the same rhythm can apply to different rates of production, much as the same melody can apply to lyrics sung at different rates.

To make things very simple, the meter of American English could be described as an alternating pattern of strong and weak (SW) syllables. This simple approach has enough descriptive adequacy that it is taken as a convenient starting point in the analysis of meter or rhythm. If a rhythmic structure of SW syllables applies to American English, then it might be expected that the interval between two stressed syllables (the metrical foot) would be fairly uniform. This proposal has been evaluated in several studies (Bolinger, 1965; Hoequist, 1983; Nakatani, O'Connor, & Aston, 1981). Although the results were not compelling, they provide at least weak evidence for a tendency for constancy (isochronicity) in some types of metrical feet. But as explained earlier, rhythm could be a perceptual phenomenon that is not closely tied to actual temporal measures of the physical signal of speech. Another approach is based on the theory of metric phonology (Selkirk, 1984). The idea is that, in effort to maintain rhythmic constancy, speakers manipulate the placement of stress to avoid strings of adjoining stressed syllables (e.g., SS) or adjoining unstressed syllables (e.g., WW). Presumably, speakers alternate S and W syllables. One test of this hypothesis is to determine if there is a shift of syllable stress in phrases where "stress clashing" (such as two adjacent strong stress syllables) occurs. If Selkirk's hypothesis holds true, speakers should try to adjust the metrical pattern of the second stressed syllable. This hypothesis was evaluated by Cooper and Eady (1986) and Kelly and Bock (1988). Cooper and Eady measured the duration and pitch change associated with the stress clash but did not observe an acoustic reduction in stress (reduced duration and pitch) for either syllable of the stress clash pair. Kelly and Bock (1988), in a perceptual experiment, concluded that speakers did tend to change the metrical feet so as to impose alternating stress rhythm. It is sufficient to say that the search continues for evidence of the SW pattern in American English.

Putting it all together: The large picture of prosody

For convenience of discussion, the foregoing information about prosody was described in respect to the three general categories of phrasal stress, boundary cues, and meter. To the prosodic effects at these levels of formal linguistic description, we could add sociolinguistic patterns, such as those of geographic and social dialects. For example, a British pronunciation of "Are you going?" may have level pitch on the first two words, with pitch accent on *go* while an American pronunciation may have rising pitch on the first three syllables, followed by a sharper rise on *-ing*. Like many such transatlantic differences, this one may covary with social status, actual or desired. Affect (attitude, commitment, mood, emotion) also can strongly affect prosody. One example is the occurrence of rising intonation on what is intended as a declarative utterance, a pattern of which may suggest a lack of certainty, a desire to elicit a response from the listener, or even a

lower social status than one's listener. More will be said about affect later in this chapter.

The point here is simply that prosody interweaves several different types of information that have been studied in linguistics and experimental phonetics. When we contemplate the possible interactions of all these (and more) sources of prosodic variation, we can readily understand why prosody is generally understood less well than segment structure. We can describe quite well (although not completely) the formant structure of the vowel [a], but we have scarcely begun to describe the prosodic differences between using that vowel as an exclamation of sudden discovery ("Ah!") and as a listener's interjection, warning the speaker that he seems to be about to say something controversial or offensive. Still less have we systematically compared the uses of prosody across languages.

What is clear, however, is that prosody is not merely the melodic and rhythmic decoration of language. It is true that arhythmic, monotone speech can be understood if other cues are intact, but it is equally true that segments can be obliterated without affecting intelligibility (Warren, 1970, 1976) and that "intact" words extracted from conversation can be unintelligible when presented in isolation (Craig & Kim, 1990). These observations merely show that no one aspect of speech is essential, given the redundancy of the whole. More adequately, prosody might be regarded as the fabric of speech, within which segments are the individual stitches or fibers. Prosodic patterns span the linguistic levels, holding together the many influences that make up the rich tapestry of language in context. Prosody serves essential, if sometimes subtle, functions in communication, and its acoustic foundations are no less important in the speech signal than those which distinguish segments. Cutler, Dahan, and VanDonselaar (1997) discussed the role of prosody in the comprehension of spoken language, and their paper is an excellent summary of the ways in which listeners rely on prosodic information to understand a spoken message.

Representations of prosody

There are many different approaches to the problem of representing prosody, but we select one for discussion here because it can be validated by acoustic methods. The approach is called *close-copy stylization*, which is defined as "a synthetic approximation of the natural course of pitch, meeting two criteria: it should be perceptually indistinguishable from the original, and it should contain the smallest possible number of straight-line segments with which this perceptual equality can be achieved" (Nooteboom, 1997, p. 646). Although it is not absolutely necessary to use straight lines, this approach offers a simplifying advantage to description.

How do we know that this method is valid? Supporting evidence comes from the use of analysis-by-synthesis techniques. Analysis-by-synthesis determines how a speech pattern is composed by generating the pattern through synthetic speech. Studies have shown that replacing the original pitch course of an utterance with an artificial one derived though close-copy analysis can give a highly satisfactory result, even when the pitch pattern is simplified as a series of straight-line segments. This can be done with LPC-analysis-resynthesis or a method known as Pitch Synchronous Overlap and Add method (PSOLA) (Nooteboom, 1997).

The next two sections address what many consider to be additional aspects of prosody: speaking rate and vocal effort/loudness. These effects are summarized under a separate heading primarily for ease of writing and not to suggest that speaking rate or vocal effort and loudness are distinct from prosody.

Speech Rate (Tempo)

Obviously, when a person speaks faster, the overall duration of an utterance decreases. However, what is not clear is how the alteration affects the various components of an utterance, including vowels versus consonants, stressed versus unstressed syllables, and movement durations versus steady-state durations. Part of a speaker's competence is the ability to produce an utterance at various rates, ranging from very slow to moderate to very fast. Acoustic studies of rate changes reveal how speakers accomplish variations in rate, how these changes are signaled to listeners, and how these alterations affect various classes of speech sounds.

As speaking rate increases, the durations of the components of speech necessarily get smaller. What is not so obvious is the manner in which reductions of duration are distributed across the components. The reduction is not constant. Generally, pauses and steady state segments for vowels and consonants tend to be sacrificed more than transitional or dynamic aspects of the speech signal. However, at very fast speaking rates, segments and even unstressed syllables may be deleted. Rapid rates also tend to be accompanied by undershoot, as described in Chapter 4. Particularly for vowels, it appears that the actual production can deviate from the spatial configuration that occurs for an isolated production of the sound.

Some examples of speaking rate variations are shown in Figure 7–4, which contains spectrograms for a slow and rapid rate of speech for the sentence, "It starts at six o'clock." The difference in overall duration is immediately evident from the spectrograms. The rapid-rate production takes only about half as long as the slow-rate production. Other differences can be detected by a careful examination of the spectrographic features.

Changes in speaking rate also can affect a number of phonetic characteristics of speech, including the actual deletion of segments or even syllables (Dalby, 1986). Attempts to use acoustic measures to study the effect of speaking rate obviously must be used with recognition of changes in phonetic structure of the speech signal.

Because changes in speaking rate can affect the base duration of segments, it is

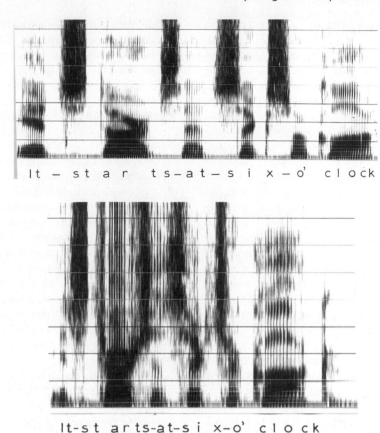

FIGURE 7–4. Spectrograms of the sentence "*It starts at six o'clock*" produced at two rates: moderate and rapid.

important to know how other duration-related phenomena, such as phrase-final lengthening and contrastive emphasis, relate to variations in speaking rate. An experiment by Cummins (1999) showed that over a large range of speaking rates, phrase-final lengthening and contrastive emphasis combined additively to determine segment durations.

Vocal Effort and Loudness

Speakers can readily adjust the *vocal effort* with which speech is produced. These adjustments are commonly used for some emotional expressions (e.g., anger), to be heard over a long distance or against a noisy background, or for certain stylistic purposes. It may seem that vocal effort, loudness, and sound pressure level would refer very much to the same phenomenon, but, in fact, they are not identical. First, it is important to distinguish vocal effort from loudness. Traunmuller and Eriksson (2000) defined vocal effort as "the quantity that ordinary speakers vary when they adapt their speech to the demands of increased or decreased communication distance" (p. 3438). That is, most variations in vocal effort occur when speakers adjust to changes in interlocutor distance, although vocal effort may be used for other purposes noted earlier.

Loudness is defined as the perception of the magnitude or strength of a sound, and is scaled from soft to loud. The unit of loudness is the *sone*, defined as the loudness of a 1 kHz tone 40 dB above threshold. The *loudness level* of a sound is expressed in *phons* and is numerically equal to the sound pressure level of a 1 kHz tone that is judged to be equally loud. Although the perceptual attribute of loudness is related especially to the intensity or sound pressure level of a sound, loudness also varies with the frequency and composition of sounds (Beranek, 1988; Handel, 1989; Neuhoff, McBeath, & Wanzie, 1999). Because loudness relates fairly directly to sound pressure level, it may seem intuitive that speakers make primary adjustments in loudness and sound pressure level when they need to be heard over varying distances from a listener. A very simple hypothesis in this regard is that speakers follow the inverse square law, which implies that speakers increase or decrease their vocal intensity by 6 dB for every doubling or halving of distance from the listener (Warren, 1968). However, subsequent studies have not confirmed this relationship (Johnson et al., 1981; Markel, Prebor, & Brandt, 1972; Michael, Siegel, & Pick, 1995).

Indeed, recent perceptual studies have shown that sound pressure level (or intensity) does not play a major role in judgments of vocal effort (Traunmuller & Eriksson, 2000). Although sound pressure level may change as speakers adjust their vocal effort, the relationship is not invariant and may be much smaller than predicted from the inverse square law. The most consistent changes that occur with increased vocal effort are increased f_0 (Rostolland, 1982; Traunmuller & Eriksson, 2000), increased formant frequencies, especially for F1 (Huber et al., 1999; Junqua, 1993; Lienard & Di Benedetto, 1999; Rostolland, 1982; Schulman, 1989; Traunmuller & Eriksson, 2000), increased vowel duration (Bonnot & Chevrie-Muller, 1991; Fonagy & Fonagy, 1966), and changes in spectral emphasis or tilt (Traunmuller & Eriksson,

2000). Vocal effort, then, is associated with several possible acoustic features, but sound pressure level is not chief among them.

Speech Affect (Emotion)

Speech affect is considered by some writers to be a suprasegmental property of speech, but other writers place it in a separate domain such as paralinguistics. We regard affect as a separate aspect although in its expression it shares many acoustic attributes with the suprasegmentals previously discussed. An individual's personality or emotional state can be determined to some degree from patterns of speech. Particularly for people we know well—but sometimes even for complete strangers—we can assess the emotions that lie behind an utterance. What are the cues by which we make these decisions?

Several studies have shown that vocal fundamental frequency and speech rate are associated with personality variables such as extroversion, assertiveness, competence, or activity (Brown, Giles, & Thakerar, 1985; Brown, Strong, & Rencher, 1974; Ziegler & Hartmann, 1996). Studies of the perceptual evaluation of f_0 excursions have shown that ratings of liveliness vary with power functions of speech rate and the magnitude of f_0 excursions (Traunmuller & Eriksson, 1995). A lively speaker tends to use a faster rate and has substantial variations in f_0.

Because listeners can judge a speaker's emotions at rates far greater than chance (Bachorowski, 1999), it may be supposed that emotions have specific acoustic correlates. Several studies have been performed to identify these correlates, but it is not easy to draw a simple set of conclusions, partly because of differences in procedures. Murray and Arnott (1993) reviewed the literature on the speech correlates of emotional states. Their major findings are summarized in Table 7–1. More recent studies have examined emotional expression in different types of speech material. Even a one-word utterance can carry an emotional quality, and such simple vocal expressions provide an opportunity to identify acoustic correlates of stress (Leinonen et al., 1997). As the speech materials become more complex, different combinations of acoustic cues may be used. Sobin and Alpert (1999) concluded that although a certain degree of acoustic differentiation of emotions is possible, the classic acoustic variables may not be sufficient to identify those factors used by human decoders of emotion in speech.

The combination of Segmental and Suprasegmental Information

As an example of the complexity of the acoustic signal as it relates to the various information sources in speech, consider the duration of a given phonetic segment, such as a vowel or even a pause. What are the factors that govern duration? The following list is a compilation of factors drawn in part from information presented in this and previous chapters.

1. Inherent phonologic differences in vowel duration. Short (lax) and long (tense) vowels differ by as much as 40% in duration. Especially when formant pattern is similar, these durational differences can be influential in phonetic recognition.

2. Duration as a cue to voicing in fricatives. Generally, longer durations of frication noise are associated with voiceless cognates.

3. Duration as a cue to phonetic distinctions based on manner. Duration of noise can be a significant cue for decisions regarding whether a sound is a stop, affricate, or fricative. Noise duration increases across the sound classes listed.

4. Phrase-final lengthening. Words or syllables are lengthened when they occur phrase-finally, both for internal and

TABLE 7-1
Selected speech and voice correlates of human vocal emotion. Based on data from I. R. Murray and J. L. Arnott (1993). Toward the simulation of emotion in synthetic speech, *Journal of the Acoustical Society of America, 93,* 1097–1108.

	ANGER	HAPPINESS	SADNESS	FEAR	DISGUST
SPEECH RATE	slightly faster	faster or slower	slightly slower	much faster	very much slower
PITCH AVERAGE	very much higher	much higher	slightly lower	very much higher	very much lower
PITCH RANGE	much wider	much wider	slightly narrower	much wider	slightly wider
INTENSITY	higher	higher	lower	normal	lower
VOICE QUALITY	breathy, chest tone	breathy, blaring	resonant	irregular voicing	grumbled chest tone
PITCH CHANGES	abrupt, on smooth, stressed syllables	upward inflections	downward inflections	normal	wide, downward terminal inflections
ARTICULATION	tense	normal	slurring	precise	normal

sentence-final phrase boundaries. Lengthening can occur even for the final item in lists of words.

5. Stress-related effects. Duration is one correlate of phrasal, lexical, or emphatic stress.

6. Vowel duration as a cue to the voicing of a postvocalic consonant. Vowels are longer preceding voiced, as opposed to voiceless, consonants.

7. Shortening of elements in consonant clusters. Segments in clusters tend to be shortened relative to their durations as singletons. There is a general tendency for segment durations to decrease as the number of syllables in a word increases.

8. New versus given information. New information in a discourse is typically associated with lengthening of the relevant words.

9. Speaking rate. As speaking rate increases, segment durations generally decrease. The effect is most pronounced for vowels and pauses.

10. Vocal effort. Increased vocal effort may be associated with an increased duration of segments, especially vowels.

11. Emotion. Changes in emotion can affect segment durations along with other acoustic properties of the signal.

So it is that the acoustic signal of speech reflects a number of different levels of information that are integrated in the act of speaking. This is one of the challenges and potentials of acoustic analysis.

Speech Synthesis

Purposes and Applications

With a few billion people on the planet who can produce natural speech more or less fluently, why would anyone want to create synthetic speech? This question seems especially pertinent considering the poor quality of some earlier attempts to produce synthetic speech. However, synthetic speech has several good uses, some of which are actually quite important, and others of which we have only begun to imagine.

Toys that Speak

One of the first widely known uses for synthetic speech was in toys and games, such as the Texas Instruments *Speak & Spell*™, which (in one of its several modes) pronounces words for a child to spell on its keyboard. When it was introduced in 1978,

this toy surprised many speech scientists as well as business competitors; few people were aware that synthetic speech of commercial quality could be produced by an integrated circuit (a "chip") so low in price that it could be at the heart of a toy. Industrial Research/Development selected the *Speak & Spell*™ as one of the 100 most significant products of 1979. Another toy, the *Julie Doll*™, extended the use of speech technology by incorporating speech synthesis, speech recognition, and a control algorithm that managed speech and hardware sensor functions, all of this in a lifelike interactive doll. Another popular toy is an interactive virtual pet called *Furby*™. This toy not only talks (in Furbish) but gradually seems to "learn" English words. It has a vocabulary of more than 800 words and phrases. It is equipped with sensors so that it can respond to light, sound, and touch. It can wiggle its ears, blink its eyes, and move its mouth.

The potential for talking toys and games is now limited only by our imaginations. Synthetic speech is easily incorporated in a variety of items designed for entertainment and recreation. With the miniaturization of speech technology, it is almost certain that a variety of toys will be equipped with the ability to produce and recognize speech.

Reading Instruction

A short step from a talking toy for young spellers is a word processor which reads back what one has written. Most primary school teachers today encourage children to write while, or even before, they learn to read. In the process, children frequently ask, "What did I write?" Upon command, a talking word processor attempts to speak what a child has written. This same feedback can be helpful to older writers, too—even to adults, and especially to the visually impaired. An extension of this idea is the reading machine, of which one notable example is the Kurzweil Personal Reader™, sold by Xerox Imaging Systems. A reading machine, also known as a **text-to-speech system**, links a scanner which can recognize printed characters to a synthesizer which takes those characters as input and produces speech as output.

Communication Aids for the Nonvocal

Not everyone can speak fluently, or speak at all. Those who have not developed or have lost the capability may nonetheless be able to control a speech synthesizer, which enables them to interact with other people via spoken language, face-to-face or over the telephone. This replacement can be vital in a world in which most communication, including most urgent communication, is oral. For a review of speech synthesis as an aid, see Edwards (1991), who gives particular attention to the interface, that is, the ways in which a person can control a synthesizer. Edwards includes several case

studies of devices, as well as appendices listing equipment and manufacturers. Speech synthesis is one technology used in the field of augmentative and assistive communication systems.

Voice-controlled Machines

In many situations, workers' eyes and hands are fully occupied; examples are aircraft pilots during takeoffs and landings, as well as factory workers who are controlling a machine that demands their attention. In such cases, spoken messages from the aircraft or other machine, rather than more lights, gauges, and beeps, can be essential to getting a crucial message across. Such applications do not necessarily require *synthetic* speech; if the messages are relatively few and brief, they can be recorded digitally and played back on command. It is this approach which telephone companies use today to answer "directory assistance" requests or to provide error messages. The same technique is used in systems for telephone inquiries about bank balances, reports to the home office from sales representatives on the road, and course registration at universities. When the potential messages become extremely numerous or unpredictable (as with word processing), recorded speech is no longer feasible and synthetic speech becomes necessary. As systems for information and control become more complex and the quality of synthetic speech improves, we may well find ourselves listening more often to machines that talk.

Multilingual Communication Systems

Machine-based multilingual voice communication is a challenging goal, but substantial progress has been made toward the development of systems that enable a speaker of one language to transmit a translated spoken message to a speaker of another language. This application requires automatic speech recognition (to represent the message from the sender), machine translation (to convert the message from one language to another), and speech synthesis (to produce the translated message in the language of the receiver).

Speech Science

Despite this growing list of commercial applications, the use of synthetic speech that is most important to speech science is the ultimate check on our analysis of speech. In fact, analysis and synthesis are often paired complementary parts of an investigation. If we conclude from spectrographic analysis that a certain formant pattern is crucial to the production and comprehension of [æ], for instance, the real test of that hypothesis is to synthesize that pattern and see whether it sounds like [æ]. After the development of the sound spectrograph, one of the most important steps in modern speech research was the development of the "pattern playback" synthesizer at Haskins Laboratories in the 1950s. This device was simply the inverse of a spectrograph: given a spectrogram as input, it produced the corresponding speech as output. That is, it scanned a spectrogram and produced sound at the indicated frequencies and intensities over time. What made the device so important was that the spectrographic pattern at the input could be hand-drawn instead of printed by a spectrograph. Thus researchers tested the hypothesis that the first two or three formants are crucial to the quality of vowels by drawing just those formants and listening to the corresponding synthetic speech. In this way researchers discovered the importance of formant transitions in conveying the place of articulation of stop consonants, for example. It would be difficult to test such ideas by analyzing natural speech because brief events like formant transitions cannot be manipulated separately from the vowels to which they are attached. When we listen to formant transitions by themselves, they sound like chirps, not stop consonants.

Synthesis is essential not only in studies of the speech signal and its production, but also in studies of how people perceive speech. For example, as we have seen, there are several acoustic differences between "voiced" and "voiceless" stops: in the occurrence of aspiration, the duration of the stop and of a preceding vowel, the fundamental frequency of a following vowel, and the occurrence of voicing during the closure, to name a few. Which of these most affects listeners' ability to hear this distinction? Is any one of them necessary? We could scarcely have studied such questions without synthetic speech, because we could not control these features individually by editing natural speech.

In modern synthesis, we can control almost any feature of speech that is thought to be important, including qualities of the voice source as well as of articulation and resonance. Given the rapidity with which change occurs in the speech signal, such control can be tedious, but it is the ultimate test of our understanding.

Speech Synthesis Methods

The remainder of this chapter describes different types of speech synthesis. Most of these are based on acoustic models of the speech signal and are most commonly used today. Because many of these have been implemented on ordinary microcomputers, anyone with a personal computer and some ancillary equipment can experiment with synthetic speech. This fact has certainly accelerated progress in the field.

There are two major ways of synthesizing a speech waveform: **parametric approaches** and **concatenative approaches**. The former is a rule-based strategy that synthesizes speech using either acoustic information (time-domain and frequency-domain characteristics of speech sounds) or articulatory information (physiologic properties of speech sounds). The acoustic-phonetic information summarized in Chapters 4, 5, 6, and 7 is the kind of acoustic knowledge needed for successful rule-based synthesis. Parametric synthesis that relies on acoustic information is called *signal-based* (bottom-up) *synthesis* because it specifies acoustic properties of speech such as formants, durations of segments, and types of noise for fricatives. This type of synthesis is sometimes called *terminal analog*, because it attempts to produce an analog of the terminal (acoustic) level of speech and pays little or no attention to articulatory aspects of speech. As applied to synthesis of an individual vowel, such as [i] in *he*, signal-based synthesis typically defines the sound in terms of its formant structure, the duration of its periodic energy, and the f_0 pattern.

The other parametric approach is *articulatory* (top-down) *synthesis* which attempts to model the physical properties of the human vocal tract. Articulatory synthesis typically produces speech with a set of parameters that simulate human speech articulation. For the vowel /i/, for example, an articulatory synthesizer might specify jaw position, tongue position, and lip configuration. Articulatory synthesis creates speech from a model of the changing shape of the vocal tract during articulation. This method is considered by many to have the best potential for natural-sounding synthetic speech because it incorporates the properties of human speech production. However, it is correspondingly more intricate and demanding than signal-based synthesis. Only recently has it become possible to create computer models of articulation that run relatively rapidly. The first articulatory synthesizers generally used phonemes as the input units, but recent work emphasizes articulatory gestures, or abstract representations of movements. These gestures can be used in a phonologic representation of an utterance, so that phonemes are not used at all. The gestures specify vocal tract adjustments in an articulatory synthesizer. For example, the word *had* might be represented with gestures for vocal fold abduction (for [h]), vocal adduction (for [æ] and [d]), advanced tongue root (for [æ]), and coronal constriction (for [d]). These gestures can be organized in a table called a gestural score, that shows the timing (and overlap) of the component gestures. Note that the word *hand* would use the same gestures described for *had* but would add a gesture of velopharyngeal opening (for [n]) followed by a gesture of velopharyngeal closing (for [d]). An advantage of this approach is that the overlapping gestures will quite naturally reflect coarticulatory patterns in natural speech. If the gestures are prescribed to have the timing characteristics of natural speech, then they should be suitable to simulate the dynamics of human speech articulation.

Concatenative synthesis creates speech by drawing from a library of prerecorded units that are assembled into a desired speech message. The phoneme is a possible unit. After all, given that American English has about 45 phonemes, it should be possible to produce just about any utterance by using the right combinations of phoneme-sized units. However, it turns out that the phoneme can be problematic as a unit of synthesis, especially because the transitions from one unit to the next are very difficult to specify. Transitions reflect both coarticulatory adjustments between adjacent phones and prosodic phenomena such as speaking rate and stress pattern. Unless these matters are considered in detail, the synthetic speech can be highly unnatural and even difficult to understand.

Concatenative synthesis (also called **copy synthesis**) can be accomplished with other units, such as the syllable, **diphone**, demisyllable, or even pieces of speech waveform. The syllable is discussed in Chapter 7. For present purposes, it is sufficient to note that the syllable is an appealing unit because it includes within its boundaries a number of steady states and transitions for individual phones and because it can be combined with other syllables to form words of varying length. It might seem that the number of syllables needed for synthesis would be forbiddingly large, given that the phonemes of American English can form over 4 billion arbitrary sequences of 1 to 6 members. But the number diminishes quickly when one considers the actual composition of admissible and actual syllables. There are only about 100,000 possible (pronounceable) monosyllabic words, and only one tenth of these are actual monosyllabic words. Furthermore, syllables differ greatly in their frequency of occurrence. Dewey (1923), who analyzed the frequency of occurrence of different units in human speech, reported that the 12 most frequently used syllables account for about a quarter of our verbal behavior, that 70 different syllables make up half of our speech, and that fewer than 1,500 syllables are sufficient for over 90% of what we say.

Diphones are produced by dividing the speech waveform into phone-sized units with the cuts made at the middle (steady state) of the phones. Each diphone contains the transition between two phones. For example, the word *ballgame* [b a l g eI m] would have the diphone constituents [b-a], [a-l] [l-g], [g-eI], and [eI-m]. The [b-a] diphone could be used for any word beginning with that phone combination (e.g., *box*, *bond*, *boss*, *bog*). In general, it is relatively easy to connect steady states, which are the points of junction in diphone concatenation. Because diphones include transitions, they avoid many of the complexities that confront rule-based synthesis with phone-sized units. Approximately 2,000 diphones are required for concatenative synthesis of American English. Although this number is considerably greater than the number of phonemes in the language, it is by no means a burdensome number for modern computers.

The demisyllable is similar to the diphone insofar as it includes transitional information within the unit. **Disyllables** are obtained by dividing the speech wave into syllable segments, with the cuts made in the middle of the syllables. For example, the word *streetlights* would consist of the disyllables [stri], [it], [laI], and [aIts]. The

number of demisyllables is about the same as the number of diphones. One advantage to this unit is that it includes consonant clusters in either syllable-initial or syllable-final positions. It also represents coarticulatory effects occurring within syllables.

There are still other possibilities for units in concatenative synthesis. One is to use units of different sizes in a synthesis system. For example, diphones may be used as a kind of default unit, but frequently occurring and highly coarticulated sequences can be represented by multiphone sequences. For example, a common phrase such as *I don't know* or *Would you repeat that, please?* would be a candidate for a multi-phone unit. A relatively recent method is that of **waveform** synthesis, which uses a time-domain representation of speech segments. The waveform pieces are then connected to form longer utterances.

Statistical properties of speech are important in designing most methods of concatenative synthesis. The object is to identify units that are economic to store and that can be effectively used in the assembly of arbitrary speech sequences. The units so selected need not correspond to those traditionally recognized in phonology and phonetics.

Formant Synthesis

The most basic acoustic synthesis is simply to recreate the changing formants of speech, each one being specified as a frequency and bandwidth, updated every 5 ms or so during an utterance. A few such formants (resonances) together with suitable inputs, namely periodic and noise sources to mimic voicing and frication respectively, have proven sufficient to produce recognizable speech. In essence, this was the approach of the pattern playback synthesizer although it was primitive compared to modern devices; for example, its voice source did not vary in f_0 or other parameters. Formant synthesis received a big boost in 1980 with Dennis Klatt's publication of a more elaborate model, complete with a computer program which synthesized speech on a laboratory computer (Klatt, 1980). Because speech synthesis had commercial value, this publication was a generous contribution on Klatt's part. Variants of this model are now available as working computer programs from several sources at little or no cost. Klatt updated the model, especially as to voice quality, in Klatt and Klatt (1990), and Sensimetrics Corporation offers a microcomputer program based on this second model.

The basis for Klatt's model is the **source–filter theory**, as discussed in chapter 2. This a good example of the way in which theory leads to applications. Figure 8–1 is Klatt's block diagram of his (1980) cascade/parallel formant synthesizer. There are two sound sources, one for voicing (labeled "voicing source") and one for frication (labeled "noise source"). These drive two resonating systems, a cascade (or serial) resonator for vowels and a parallel resonator for fricatives. In the cascade resonator, the output of the first formant res-

onator (R1) becomes the input to the second formant resonator (R2), and so on. Thus the formants influence each other: the relative amplitude of each depends partly on how close it is in frequency to other formants, as in the natural articulation of vowels (discussed in Chapter 2). There is no need for a separate amplitude control for each formant as there is in the parallel resonator, in which each formant is developed independently. The cascade synthesizer models the production of speech sounds in which the excitation source is at the larynx and the entire vocal tract serves as a resonator, while the parallel synthesizer models the production of fricatives, in which the noise source is higher, usually in the oral cavity, and only that part of the vocal tract which is in front of the source serves as the resonator.

Let us trace the cascade system in Figure 8–1 from source to output. The voicing source generates a train of impulses such as that produced by the vocal folds. The boxes labeled RGP, RGZ, and RGS are essentially

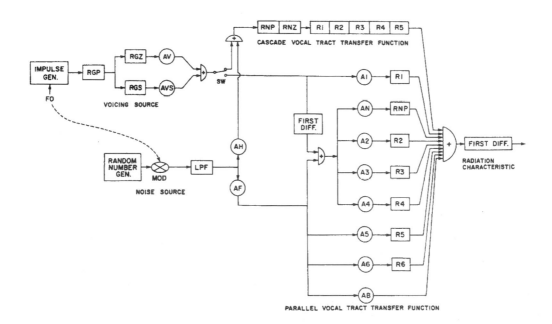

FIGURE 8–1. Block diagram of cascade/parallel formant synthesizer (Klatt, 1980).

filters that smooth this simulated glottal waveform and shape its spectrum. AV controls the amplitude of voicing; it is set to zero during voiceless sounds or pauses. This source then enters the resonating system, in which RNP and RNZ represent nasal pole and nasal zero, respectively, and R1 to R5 represent formants 1 through 5. For each formant, the user specifies a frequency and bandwidth for every few ms of speech.

Tracing the parallel system, we find a noise source which begins with a random number generator, as frication noise begins with turbulence that is quasi-random in frequency and amplitude. MOD provides for mixing the noise and voicing sources for voiced fricatives. LPF is a low-pass filter which shapes the source spectrum, and AH and AF control the amplitude of aspiration and of frication, respectively. Aspiration noise goes to the cascade resonator because aspiration generated at the larynx, like voicing, uses the entire vocal tract as a resonator. Aspiration can be mixed with the voice source to produce (among other things) a breathy voice quality, as is common in female voices. The noise source for fricatives goes through the parallel resonators, each with its own amplitude control. The boxes labeled "First Diff" are high-pass filters; the one at the output simulates the emphasis given to higher frequencies as sound radiates from the lips.

Altogether, the 1980 Klatt model has 39 parameters (control values), of which 19 are fixed. The user must specify the other 20 for every 5 ms of speech to be produced. Thus, for a syllable of, say, 250 ms, the 20 variable parameters must be set 50 times, for a total of 1,000 specifications. Most of these values do not change constantly. For example, during a vowel, AF (amplitude of frication) and the amplitudes of all the parallel formants can be set to zero and remain there. In principle, f_0 and AV (amplitude of voicing) could be set to constant values during a syllable in which fundamental frequency does not change. However, even in such a syllable, more life-like speech will result if these two values vary a little, as they do in natural speech. In some implementations of the Klatt synthesizer, the user can set key parameters at points of major change, and the program will fill in the rest, using linear or other interpolations. For example, one might set the fundamental frequency at the beginning and end of the voiced portion of a syllable, and the program would fill in f_0 at all points in between, creating a linear or nonlinear slope and perhaps introducing slight variation in the fundamental period (jitter).

Table 8–1 lists suggested values for F1, F2, F3, and duration for most phonemes of English, as produced by an adult male speaker. (As discussed in previous chapters, these values must be adjusted if the object is to produce women's or children's speech.) These are "default" values, in the sense that they might be used as starting points in synthesis before one takes context and individual variation into account. Note also that Table 8–1 gives only part of the information needed for intelligible and natural speech. Many sounds need not only specification of formants, but also specification of noise bursts or intervals of frication.

Figure 8–2 shows two spectrograms of utterances of *seep*. The lower one is of natural speech, and the upper one of speech produced with the Klatt and Klatt (1990) synthesizer as implemented by Sensimetrics. Only moderate efforts were made to shape the synthetic speech. Note that it has little sound energy above 5 kHz, while in the natural speech the [s] has intense energy up to the 8 kHz range of the spectrogram. The synthetic speech has less variable amplitude, more abrupt transitions, more intense aspiration of the [p], and less noise in the higher frequencies than the natural speech. Generally, the synthesized pattern has a greater regularity and simplicity.

Figure 8–3 shows an amplitude spectrum taken near the middle of the [i] in each utterance; the lighter trace is for the natural speech. Notice that the synthetic vowel has a wider bandwidth for F2, and a considerably higher F3. In fact, the tilt of the spectrum in the higher frequencies is wrong.

TABLE 8-1

Suggested values for formant synthesis of phonetic segments. Shown for each IPA phoneme are: CPA—computer phonetic alphabet, Keyword—keyword for pronunciation of the sound, F1—frequency of first formant in Hz, F2—frequency of second formant in Hz, F3—frequency of third formant in Hz, and DUR—inherent duration in ms. When two values are listed for a formant, they indicate the onglide (initial) and offglide (terminal) values for a diphthong pattern.

IPA	CPA	Keyword	F1	F2	F3	DUR
Vowels and Diphthongs							
/i/	IY	beet	300	2200	3000	160
/I/	IH	bit	400	1900	1550	130
/e/	EY	bait	550–400	1800–2100	2650–2700	190
/ɛ/	EH	bet	525	1800	2500	150
/ae/	AE	bat	650	1750	2400	230
/ɑ/	AA	Bob	750	1150	2400	240
/ɔ/	AO	bought	575	850	2400	240
/oU/	OW	boat	575–450	900–800	2400–2350	220
/U/	UH	book	450	1050	2250	160
/u/	UW	boot	300	900	2200	180
/ə/	AX	above	600	1300	2450	120
/ʌ/	AH	above	650	1200	2400	140
/ɜ/	RR	bird	500	1350	1700	180
/aI/	AY	bite	750–400	1250–2000	2500–2700	250
/ɔI/	OY	boy	550–400	850–1900	2525–2700	280
/aU/	AW	bout	750–575	1325–900	2700–2250	260
Sonorant Consonants							
/w/	W	wet	300	600	2200	80
/r/	R	red	425	1300	1600	80
/l/	L	let	375	875	2575	80
/j/	Y	yet	300	2200	3050	80
/m/	M	met	275	900	2200	70
/n/	N	net	275	1700	2600	65
/ð/	NG	sing	275	2300	2750	80
Fricative Consonants							
/f/	F	fin	150	1100	2400	120
/v/	V	van	150	1100	2400	60
/θ/	TH	thin	200	1600	2200	110
/ð/	DH	this	200	1600	2200	50
/s/	S	sip	200	1800	2600	125
/z/	Z	zip	200	1800	2600	75
/ʃ/	SH	ship	200	1300	2400	125
/ʒ/	ZH	azure	200	1300	2400	70
/h/	H	hat	— — — — —- set to match adjacent vowel — — — — —-			
Affricate Consonants							

For affricates, use values for a similar fricative, but include stop gap to represent the closure portion and possibly shape the noise segment to have a short rise time.

(continued)

IPA	CPA	Keyword	F1	F2	F3	DUR
			Stop consonants			
/p/	P	pat	150	800	1750	85
/b/	B	bat	150	800	1750	80
/t/	T	tip	150	1800	2600	85
/d/	D	dip	150	1800	2600	65
/k/	K	come	150	2350	2750	65
/g/	G	gum	150	3250	2750	65
/ʕ/	DX	butter	150	1800	2600	20

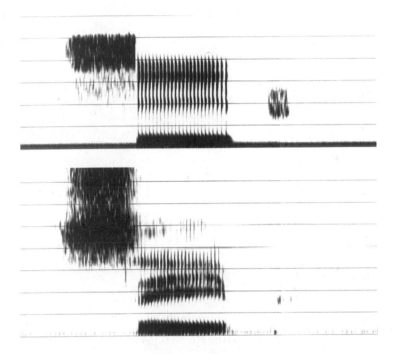

FIGURE 8–2. Spectrograms of two utterances of *"seep."* Lower channel: natural speech; upper channel: synthetic speech by the Klatt and Klatt (1990) synthesizer.

Figure 8–4 shows the waveforms and f_0 contours of each utterance; counting from the top, channels 1 and 3 are the natural speech, which has more gradual change in both amplitude and f_0. In principle, all these differences could have been eliminated if we had tailored the relevant parameters in sufficient detail.

Table 8–2 lists the 60 parameters of this synthesizer, with a brief description of each. The default values are those for a "neutral"

schwa-like vowel. Column 2, headed V/C, indicates whether that parameter is variable or constant; the "constant" ones can be changed, but are set only once for each utterance. For example, DU (duration) is a constant, in this sense. Among the variable parameters, some may be changed almost continually while others may be adjusted only occasionally, depending on the requirements of the synthesis.

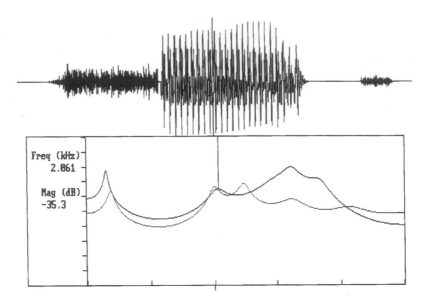

FIGURE 8–3. Spectra of the vowel [i] shown in Figure 8–2. The lighter trace is for the natural speech. The cursor points to F2 in the synthetic speech (darker trace). The waveform above the spectra is of the synthetic speech, with the cursor at the position from which the spectrum was calculated.

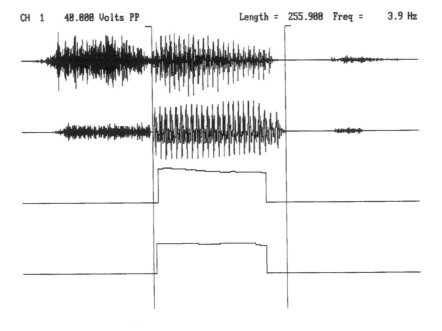

FIGURE 8–4. Waveforms and f_0 contours of the utterances shown in Figure 8–2. Channels 1 and 3 are the waveform and f_0 contour, respectively, of the natural speech.

TABLE 8–2

The 60 parameters of the Klatt and Klatt (1990) synthesizer, as implemented by Sensi-metrics. Each row is one parameter; the columns are the symbol (SYM), whether vari-able or constant (V/C) during synthesis of a particular utterance, the minimum (MIN) value, current (VAL) value, maximum (MAX) value, and a description of the parame-ter. The current value is either a default value or one selected for a particular applica-tion. *Note:* the parameters identified as variable are not necessarily updated in the same way. Some will vary throughout an utterance, whereas others may be set to an initial value that does not change. For example, F2, the second-formant frequency may change while B2, the second-formant bandwidth, is kept at a constant value.

SYM	V/C	MIN	VAL	MAX	DESCRIPTION
DU	C	30	700	5000	Duration of the utterance, in ms
UI	C	1	5	20	Update interval for parameter reset, in ms
SR	C	5000	10000	20000	Output sampling rate, in samples/s
NF	C	1	5	6	Number of formants in cascade branch
SS	C	1	2	3	Source switch (1 = impulse, 2 = natural, 3 = LF model
RS	C	1	8	8191	Random seed (initial value of random number generator)
SB	C	0	1	1	Same noise burst, reset RS if AF = AH = 0, 0 = no, 1 = yes
CP	C	0	0	1	0 = cascade, 1 = parallel tract excitation by AV
OS	C	0	0	20	Output selector (() = normal, 1 = voicing source, ...)
GV	C	0	60	80	Overall gain scale factor for AV, in dB
GH	C	0	60	80	Overall gain scale factor for AG, in dB
GF	C	0	60	80	Overall gain scale factor for AF, in dB
F0	V	0	1000	5000	Fundamental frequency in tenths of a Hz
AV	V	0	60	80	Amplitude of voicing, in dB
OQ	V	10	50	99	Open quotient (voicing open-time/period), in %
SQ	V	100	200	500	Speed quotient (rise/fall time, LF model), in %
TL	V	0	0	42	Extra tilt of voicing spectrum, dB down at 3 kHz
FL	V	0	0	100	Flutter (random fluctuation in F0), in% of maximum
DI	V	0	0	100	Diplophonia (alternate periods closer), in % of maximum
AH	V	0	0	80	Amplitude of aspiration, in dB
AF	V	0	0	80	Amplitude of frication, in dB
F1	V	180	500	1300	Frequency of first formant, in Hz
B1	V	30	60	1000	Bandwidth of first formant, in Hz
DF1	V	0	0	100	Change in F1 during open portion of period, in Hz
DB1	V	0	0	400	Change in B1 during open portion of period, in Hz
F2	V	550	1500	3000	Frequency of second formant, in Hz
B2	V	40	90	1000	Bandwidth of second formant, in Hz
F3	V	1200	2500	4800	Frequency of third formant, in Hz
B3	V	60	150	1000	Bandwidth of third formant, in Hz
F4	V	2400	3250	4990	Frequency of fourth formant, in Hz
B4	V	100	200	1000	Bandwidth of fourth formant, in Hz
F5	V	3000	3700	4990	Frequency of fifth formant, in Hz
B5	V	100	200	1500	Bandwidth of fifth formant, in Hz
F6	V	3000	4990	4990	Frequency of sixth formant, in Hz (applies if NH=6)
B6	V	100	500	4000	Bandwidth of sixth formant, in Hz (applies if NH=6)
FNP	V	180	280	500	Frequency of nasal pole, in Hz
BNP	V	40	90	1000	Bandwidth of nasal pole, in Hz

(continued)

TABLE 8-2 (continued)

SYM	V/C	MIN	VAL	MAX	DESCRIPTION
FNZ	V	180	280	800	Frequency of nasal zero, in Hz
BNZ	V	40	90	1000	Bandwidth of nasal zero, in Hz
FTP	V	300	2150	3000	Frequency of tracheal pole, in Hz
BTP	V	40	180	1000	Bandwidth of tracheal pole, in Hz
FTZ	V	300	2150	3000	Frequency of tracheal zero, in Hz
BTZ	V	40	180	2000	Bandwidth of nasal zero, in Hz
A2F	V	0	0	80	Amplitude of frication-excited parallel second formant, in dB
A3F	V	0	0	80	Amplitude of frication-excited parallel third formant, in dB
A4F	V	0	0	80	Amplitude of frication-excited parallel fourth formant, in dB
A5F	V	0	0	80	Amplitude of frication-excited parallel fifth formant, in dB
A6F	V	0	0	80	Amplitude of frication-excited parallel sixth formant, in dB
AB	V	0	0	80	Amplitude of frication-excited parallel bypass path, in dB
B2F	V	40	250	1000	Bandwidth of frication-excited parallel second formant, in Hz
B3F	V	60	300	1000	Bandwidth of frication-excited parallel third formant, in Hz
B4F	V	100	320	1000	Bandwidth of frication-excited parallel fourth formant, in Hz
B5F	V	100	360	1500	Bandwidth of frication-excited parallel fifth formant, in Hz
B6F	V	100	1500	4000	Bandwidth of frication-excited parallel sixth formant, in Hz
ANV	V	0	0	80	Amplitude of voice-excited parallel nasal formant, in dB
A1V	V	0	60	80	Amplitude of voice excited parallel first formant, in dB
A2V	V	0	60	80	Amplitude of voice excited parallel second formant, in dB
A3V	V	0	60	80	Amplitude of voice excited parallel third formant, in dB
A4V	V	0	60	80	Amplitude of voice excited parallel fourth formant, in dB
ATV	V	0	0	80	Amplitude of voice-excited parallel tracheal formant, in dB

How good can formant synthesis be? Essentially, as good as one has patience to make it. If one starts with a spectrogram to match, for example, and specifies many parameters at each update, listening to the output occasionally and revising accordingly, a painstaking investigator can shape the output closer and closer to the target. Holmes (1973) managed to produce speech which listeners could not reliably distinguish from a natural recording. Two main sources of unnaturalness in synthetic speech are the lack of small variations in fundamental frequency and other parameters and the difficulty of creating a voice source which mimics that produced by the larynx, particularly during rapid changes in f_0.

Given the demands made on one's patience, formant synthesizers have been useful mainly in research, especially perceptual research comparing the effects of changing one or two parameters within a relatively small number of syllables. Clearly, setting 60 rather technical parameters every 5 ms is not a practical way of meeting the more commercial needs for speech synthesis, even with the aid of automatic interpolation. There certainly would have been no *Speak & Spell*™ if users had to know about formant frequencies and bandwidths. Conversely, however, there would have been no *Speak & Spell*™ or other practical synthesis if researchers using formant synthesizers had not painstakingly discovered the parameter settings which are now programmed into the commercial products.

Synthesis by Rule

A key step toward making synthesis of wider practical value is the realization that many parameters are roughly predictable over syllables, words, and utterances if one knows the sequence of phonemes to be produced. Fundamental frequency declines slowly over utterances and rapidly at the end of a declarative sentence; vowels are lengthened before voiced consonants; vowels are nasalized before nasal consonants; low vowels are generally longer than high vowels: these are a few rules of thumb that are well-known bits of the phonology of English and other languages. Phonologists write such rules in precise forms, taking into account the effect of one upon another. The classic book *The Sound Pattern of English* by Noam Chomsky and Morris Halle (1968) inspired an approach to synthesis based on rewrite rules. These were used to construct special rule compilers for text-to-speech synthesis. If we can quantify those rules, we can automate much of the parameter-setting in synthesis. For example, how *much* longer are vowels before voiced conso-

nants, and how does that factor interact with vowel height? Earlier chapters, especially Chapters, 4, 5, and 7 presented information of the kind that can be used to formulate rule-based synthesis. This information is the product of many studies in acoustic phonetics, coupled with principles of phonology.

In such a system, the user might type in the sequence of phonemes in an utterance. The synthesizer would then start with a table of default values for each phoneme, for example, for each vowel, the intrinsic duration, f_0, and formant frequencies and bandwidths. It would then automatically tailor each of those values according to the context of each phoneme. The variety of rules which might be included, at least in principle, ranges from prosodic rules like "increase the duration and pitch change on the last stressed syllable in an utterance" to detailed acoustic specifications which are not found in phonology books, such as, "F2 changes toward a value of about 1800 Hz before alveolar consonants." Interestingly, one might seek to make the speech more natural by expanding this range of rules on both ends. At a higher level, one might try to formulate discourse rules, such as "increase the prominence (amplitude and duration) of a noun if this is the first time it has been mentioned in the discourse." At the other extreme, one might introduce small random fluctuations in fundamental frequency and amplitude during the longer syllables to simulate vocal jitter and shimmer.

Obviously, such a set of rules might be very formidable indeed, and even so might not capture the subtle ways in which natural speech varies in relation to context at all linguistic levels. Nonetheless, speech researchers have created synthesis-by-rule programs which produce reasonably natural-sounding speech and yet operate rapidly on inexpensive hardware. That development has made possible the practical applications of synthesis, from toys to speech prostheses to reading machines.

Clearly, these applications depend on one more step, however. Most users cannot be expected to type in a representation of a string of phonemes. A reading machine must start with ordinary print. In virtually all the practical applications, one prior translation is needed before synthesis by rule can operate: from ordinary spelling to a sequence of phonemes. Anyone acquainted with English spelling knows that for English, at least, such a translation is no trivial matter. However, with the aid of a built-in "dictionary," together with rules for words which are not in the dictionary, synthesizers can make this first translation. The result is reasonably natural-sounding speech, produced almost instantly from typed (or scanned) ordinary spelling.

One of the best commercial examples of such a synthesizer is DECtalk™, produced by Digital Equipment Corporation, and based on rules developed by Dennis Klatt. This device, first marketed in about 1983, takes ordinary spelling (from a keyboard, a computer file, or a scanner) as input and produces highly intelligible and reasonably natural English speech as output. In its earlier version, it had built-in voices (male, female, and child), plus one which could be tailored to the user's needs, selecting 13 specifications ranging from sex and average pitch to head size and breathiness. Figure 8–5 is a flow chart, showing the sequence of operations by which DECtalk™ arrives at a pronunciation, taking account of punctuation as well as spelling.

Note that DECtalk™ searches its dictionary first and then applies its spelling-to-sound rules only to words not found there; thus, the dictionary is a list of words with exceptional spellings. If a string of letters fails to match any word in its dictionary or its spelling-to-sound rules, DECtalk™ simply names the letters. If DECtalk's™ pronunciation is not satisfactory, the user may type in phonemic symbols instead of standard spelling. For example, DECtalk™ mispronounces *shoebench* as [bɛn]. One solution is simply to hyphenate the word, but another is to replace the spelling with ['shuwbehnch]. What one cannot control with DECtalk™ is precisely what one *must*

control with a formant synthesizer, namely the formant frequencies and bandwidths over time.

Figure 8–6 shows two spectrograms of "We show speech," the upper one uttered by DECtalk™ from standard spelling and the lower one by an adult male speaker at approximately the same rate. The most obvious difference is in frequency range. DECtalk™ produces very little sound above 5 kHz (the scale of the spectrogram is 0 to 8 kHz), whereas the natural speech has a great deal of sound energy above 5 kHz in the three fricatives (including the second part of [tʃ] in "speech"). However, this restriction is of no consequence in commercial applications, especially over the standard telephone network, which transmits only up to about 3.3 kHz.

Note the extensive shaping of the second and third formants in DECtalk's™ utterance, not only in the glide [w] of "we," but also in transitions at the beginning of the vowels of "show" and "speech." These contrast with the minimally specified synthetic speech shown in Figure 8–2. Note also that the duration of each segment closely resembles that in the natural speech at a similar overall rate. In both of these respects, DECtalk™ has taken the context of each phoneme into account.

There are also differences other than the frequency range that allow us to make inferences about DECtalk's™ built-in rules. The [p] in "speech" is considerably more aspirated in DECtalk's™ utterance than in the natural sample. DECtalk™ does know, however, that /p/ after initial /s/ is relatively unaspirated; it would produce /p/ in "peach" with much longer aspiration. Note also the falling f_0 during the vowel of "speech," as shown by the distance between the vertical striations. Those striations become farther apart in DECtalk's™ production, but to a lesser degree than in the natural one. As with most synthetic speech, DECtalk™ produces less amplitude variation than this human speaker. Particularly at the ends of the vowels of "show" and "speech," amplitude decreases

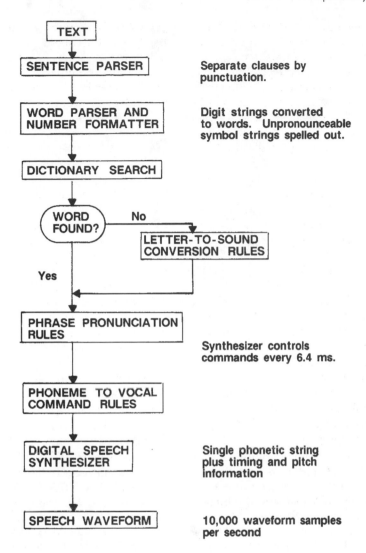

FIGURE 8–5. Flowchart of operations in the DECtalk™ synthesizer, from the DECtalk™ User Manual. The chart begins at the top with the input of standard spelling and ends with the production of synthetic speech.

markedly in the natural speech, especially notable in the higher formants.

However, these differences may have little significance for intelligibility or even naturalness. Logan, Greene, and Pisoni (1989) studied the intelligibility of 10 synthesis-by-rule systems. DECtalk's™ default voice ("Paul") yielded the lowest error rate; on syllable-initial consonants, it was equiv-

alent to natural speech. Under good listening conditions (words in context, low ambient noise), one rarely notices difficulty in comprehending DECtalk™. For further description of DECtalk,™ see Bruckert (1984). For a description of the rules built into its predecessor, see Allen, Hunnicutt, and Klatt (1987). But the superiority of DECtalk's™ male voice "Paul" now has

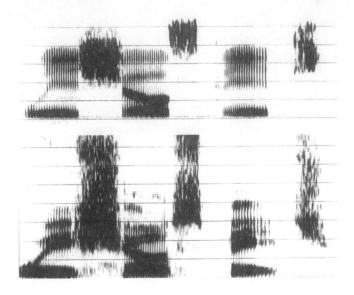

FIGURE 8–6. Spectrograms of two utterances of "*We show speech.*" Lower channel: natural speech by an adult male; upper channel: synthetic speech by the DECtalk™ synthesizer.

some competitors, especially in Mac-inTalk™ (Hustad, Kent, & Beukelman, 1998).

Considering that it produces its utterances almost instantaneously once it encounters a final punctuation mark (a period, question mark, or exclamation point), DECtalk's™ speech is audible testimony to the accomplishments of contemporary speech science. We should bear in mind that the recent achievements, such as Klatt's remarkable synthesizer and his detailed rules, are built upon fundamental understandings that have been developing for most of this century, such as the source-filter theory presented in Chapter 2. Progress in speech science has been additive and has sometimes surprised even those who take part in it.

Linear Predictive Synthesis

A third type of synthesis begins with linear predictive coding (LPC), which was described in Chapter 3. LPC parameterizes the speech signal, that is, it analyses the

complex, constantly changing speech signal into a few values called parameters, which change relatively slowly. The model is the source-filter view described in Chapter 2; the parameters that represent the signal are the frequencies and bandwidths of a set of filters that produce that signal, given a certain excitation. This analysis is reversible; given an LPC analysis, one can produce (or synthesize) the signal which it describes. If the LPC analysis were perfect, the resynthesized signal would exactly match the original. An advantage to LPC synthesis is that its structure is simpler than that of formant synthesis, given that the spectral properties of speech (except periodicity) are represented in the LPC coefficients that are automatically calculated from normal speech.

Of course, the LPC analysis is never perfect. For one thing, most LPC models are *all-pole* models, meaning that they provide for resonances only. As a result, they have difficulty in describing nasal and lateral sounds, which have anti-resonances (zeroes) as well. For another, the model describes the filter but not the source; the glottal waveform in voiced speech and the noise source in fricatives are not well described. However, resynthesizing speech from an LPC analysis is at least a check on how good the analysis was. Another limitation is that interpolation of LPC parameters at segment boundaries can be difficult, because each coefficient affects a range of speech frequencies in a complicated way.

If that were all it could do, linear predictive synthesis probably would not qualify for inclusion in this chapter. However, it has one additional feature which makes it interesting: having represented the speech signal as a small set of parameters, one can edit those parameters before resynthesizing. For instance, we can change the frequency or bandwidth of F1 independently of all other formants and then listen to the effect. We have no way of performing such an operation on the natural speech signal. We cannot edit one formant or ask a live

speaker to vary just F1. In a sense, LPC synthesis is like having a formant synthesizer that starts with an analysis of real speech, so we do not have to build each signal from scratch. A typical experiment, for example, is to start with a recording of the vowel /i/; perform LPC analysis; then edit that analysis, moving F1 up and F2 down in ten steps; synthesize the resulting ten variants; and play them in random order for listeners, to determine at what point the /i/ begins to sound more like /e/ or /æ/.

As an example, we will use ASL™, an LPC analysis/synthesis program sold by Kay Elemetrics Corp. as an addition to their digital spectrograph and as part of a speech analysis program known as CSL™. Figure 8–7 is one of ASL's™ basic displays. The upper channel shows the waveform of the phrase "speech synthesis," spoken by a male speaker. Under the voiced part of each

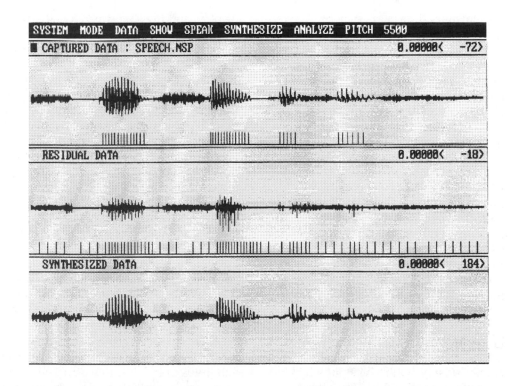

FIGURE 8–7. Three waveforms in display of ASL, a program for LP analysis and synthesis. The phrase is "*speech synthesis*" spoken by an adult male. Upper channel: speech waveform; middle channel: residual signal; lower channel: synthesized speech.

syllable, a series of short vertical ticks marks the glottal periods. These ticks become farther apart during the last two syllables because f_0 was falling at the end of the utterance. ASL™ can perform such an analysis of fundamental periods automatically and then the user can edit it if necessary. Its importance is that LPC analysis (and thus resynthesis) is more accurate if it is *pitch-synchronous*, that is, if (in the voiced portions only) the unit of analysis is a glottal period.

After a linear predictive analysis, there is a part of the signal which remains unaccounted for by the sequence of digital filters which the analysis has developed. This part is known as the *error* or *residual* signal. For our example utterance, the waveform of the residual signal is shown in the middle panel of Figure 8–7. Ideally, the residual should represent just the source: the glottal waveform and the noise excitation. The residual may be a very weak signal; its apparent amplitude has been normalized to fill the panel in Figure 8–7. However, it is evident that the residual in the voiced parts of syllables is not just a glottal waveform; it is too complex. In fact, listening to a residual signal, one may hear traces of the original vowels if all the formant structure was not captured in the analysis.

Having done the LPC analysis, we can then resynthesize the signal. We have a choice of using or not using the residual signal to complete the synthesis. Using it means adding back that part of the signal which the analysis did not account for; the resulting synthesized signal should be identical to the original. We get excellent synthesis but a poor test of the analysis.

In this example, we did not use the residual. The lowest panel of Figure 8–7 shows the resulting synthesized utterance. Comparing the waveform to the original (top panel), one can see that it is different. In a general way, one can even see that the synthesized waveform plus the residual would more closely approximate the original.

Figure 8–8 is a spectrographic view of a similar comparison. The lower channel is a spectrogram of "seven," spoken by a female talker; the upper channel is that same utterance after LPC analysis and resynthesis without the residual. Note that the formant structure of both vowels is rather well reproduced in the synthesis, but that there are difficulties at the transitions between the fricatives and the vowels. Such transitions are major changes, not only in the source, but also in the shape and resonance of the vocal tract. Because LPC analysis operates on frames (in this case, 20 ms long during the voiceless parts of the signal), it has difficulty in representing rapid transitions between voiceless and voiced speech.

ASL™ provides two modes in which the user can edit the analysis before synthesizing. Figure 8–9 shows the full-screen graphic display of an analysis of "spurious," spoken by a male speaker. The top panel is the waveform, with glottal periods marked; the middle panel is the formant display; and the lowest panel is the f_0 contour during the voiced part of the word. In the middle panel, the short horizontal bars represent the formant center frequencies, and the vertical lines intersecting them represent bandwidths. One can readily track the first five formants during most of the voiced portion; during the fricatives, the formant frequencies change rapidly and the bandwidths are often wide, so that the vertical lines predominate. In this display, one can use a mouse to draw new formants or a new f_0 contour for synthesis. An experienced user with a steady hand can create quite dramatic changes in the signal, although the results sometimes include noisy transitions or other unpredictable effects of interaction among these variables.

Figure 8–10 shows the numeric editor's display for the same utterance. Each row represents one analysis frame and each column one parameter. RES is the frame number (of the residual), PK stands for peak amplitude, LEN for the duration of the frame, B1 for the bandwidth of F1, and so on. Frame 26, just below the middle of the table, is marked by a box in the waveform.

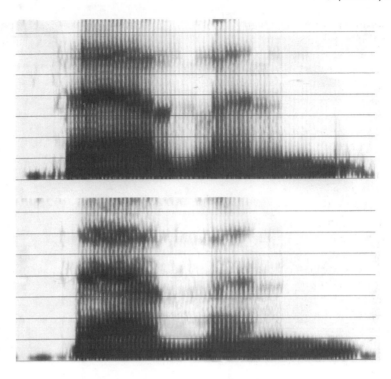

FIGURE 8–8. Spectrograms of two utterances of the word *seven*. Lower channel: natural speech by an adult female; upper channel: that utterance after LP analysis and resynthesis.

It is near the [ɪ], so that F2 (highlighted in the table) is low, at 1442 Hz. The user can edit any of the parameters, taking advantage of interpolation to produce changes at linear and nonlinear rates. In this mode one has precise control over every aspect of a spoken utterance represented by LPC parameters. This degree of control is not practical for the commercial applications of speech synthesis, but it opens important doors for research. For example, if one suspected that the rate of formant transitions after stop consonants is an important part of what makes certain dysarthric speech difficult to comprehend (Kent et al., 1989), one could edit just that characteristic and see what difference it makes. In a formant synthesizer, one has the same kind of control, but not starting with a parametric analysis of natural speech.

Looking Back

One gauge of the progress in speech synthesis is to look at spectrograms of synthetic speech over the last 50 years. Pattern Playback synthesis (about 1951) of the words *four hours* is represented by wideband and narrow-band spectrograms in Figure 8–11. *Speak & Spell*^{TM} output (about 1980) is illustrated for the words *now spell* in Figure 8–12. The standard male voice of DECtalk^{TM} (about 1990) is illustrated, appropriately enough, with the words *standard male voice* in Figure 8–13. By comparing the spectrograms in Figures 8–11, 8–12, and 8–13, you can probably detect improvements in the naturalness of the speech patterns. Notice, in particular, the smoothness of the harmonics and formants in Figure 8–13, which compare favorably with the spectrograms of natural human speech

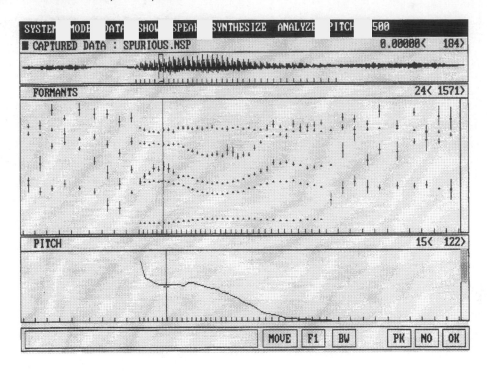

FIGURE 8–9. Formant display in ASL of the word *"spurious"* spoken by an adult male. Upper channel: speech waveform with fundamental periods marked by vertical ticks; middle channel: formants (horizontal lines) and bandwidths (vertical lines); lower channel: f₀ contour.

shown in other chapters of this book. In the last five decades, synthesized speech has improved considerably in both its intelligibility and naturalness.

Table 8–3 lists a number of watershed accomplishments in speech analysis and speech technology. This list is highly selective but it indicates a strong record of progress, beginning with early attempts to visualize speech as waveforms and spectrograms and leading up to sophisticated computer systems that can recognize human speech and produce synthetic speech of high quality and naturalness. See also Campbell (1999), Flanagan (1972) and Venkatagiri (1996).

Looking to the Future

Speech synthesis is a good example of progress in technology. The first efforts produced speech that was decidedly unnatural and not very easy to understand. Contemporary synthetic speech is both natural and intelligible, and we truly have reached the point at which listeners may be hard pressed to say whether the speech they hear over a telephone or other communication system was produced by a human or by a machine. The future is likely to hold progress in miniaturization, personalization, and globalization.

Miniaturization will come about partly because the input/output device for speech can be a small microphone/speaker, as opposed to a keyboard or tablet. Although microphones are fairly small now, the prospect is for even smaller ones. A particularly promising technology is the development of microphones carved into silicon integrated circuits (Ouellette, 1999). These microphones may well replace the electret-condenser microphones that are commonly

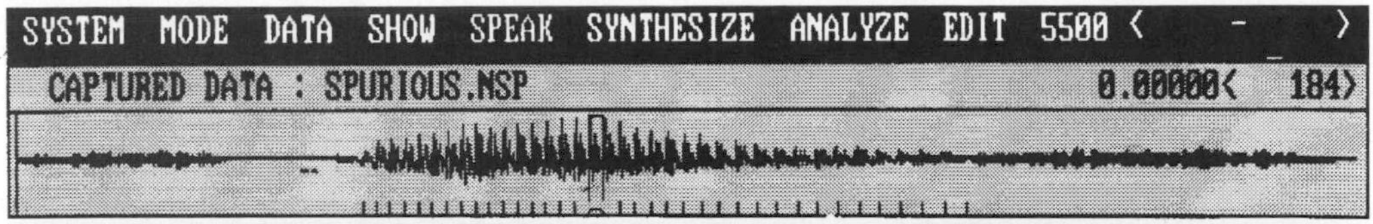

```
SYSTEM  MODE  DATA  SHOW  SPEAK  SYNTHESIZE  ANALYZE  EDIT  5500 <      -      >
  CAPTURED DATA : SPURIOUS.NSP                              0.00000<     184>
```

#	M	RES	PK	F0	LEN	F1	B1	F2	B2	F3	B3	F4	B4
17	0	17	11768	126	79	377	27	1837	31	2264	188	3316	87
18	0	18	11600	126	79	397	26	1815	37	2091	129	3315	71
19	0	19	10776	125	80	419	21	1769	21	2110	44	3192	46
20	0	20	10784	120	78	433	25	1673	15	2110	30	3103	65
21	0	21	11336	128	78	450	33	1601	16	2047	39	3046	76
22	0	22	11328	126	79	469	52	1553	19	1940	70	3003	82
23	0	23	12304	125	80	477	43	1505	17	1901	54	2928	57
24	0	24	13472	123	81	485	43	1467	15	1859	56	2873	75
25	0	25	13656	121	82	490	49	1454	20	1844	62	2934	134
26	0	26	13664	120	83	493	44	1442	18	1849	47	2935	184
27	0	27	13880	117	85	496	51	1448	18	1822	55	2881	143
28	0	28	12088	116	86	497	48	1467	20	1878	48	3104	427
29	0	29	10024	113	88	492	38	1495	32	1918	36	3021	299
30	0	30	9752	111	90	487	23	1513	16	1933	68	2853	202
31	0	31	9360	107	93	487	34	1544	19	1999	39	2905	164
32	0	32	8544	104	96	484	29	1640	29	2120	60	2931	134

FIGURE 8–10. Numeric editor display in ASL™ of the same utterance shown in Figure 8–9. The rows are frames; the columns are results of the LPC analysis, including amplitude (PK), the frame length (LEN), and formant frequencies and bandwidths (F1, B1, etc.).

used today in handheld consumer products such as cellular phones. The new microphones could be placed into large arrays that would permit hands-free usage in automobiles or conference calls. These arrays could detect a speaker's voice but could also be used with signal processing techniques to cancel noise and interference. Significant advantages accrue with the incorporation of microphones into silicon integrated circuits, and we may well see within a short time a revolution in the use of speech as input to miniaturized computer systems.

Personalization is facilitated by miniaturization because we can easily transport the system as we move about. Speech technologies such as synthesized speech also will become personalized because they can be (1)

adjusted to individual characteristics (e.g., vocabulary, speaking rate, and emotion) (2) adapted to various environments (e.g., noisy backgrounds or hazardous conditions), and (3) equipped with types of information specific to a given user (e.g., a database of technical information, customer accounts, or summaries of published articles). Telephony coupled with a Global Positioning System (GPS) can ensure communication virtually anywhere in the world.

Global refers not only to distance but also to universal communication across language barriers. Therefore, globalization depends on the multinational (across both distance and language barriers) development of speech systems that offer automatic translation as well as speech synthesis. The day may not be far away when it will be

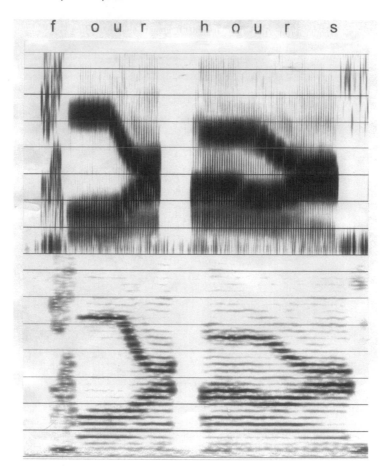

FIGURE 8–11. Wide-band (top) and narrow-band (bottom) spectrograms of the phrase *four hours* produced with the Pattern Playback speech synthesizer in about 1950.

commonplace to speak into a machine that will recognize the linguistic message as one language (say English), translate it into another language (say Hindi), and then use speech synthesis to produce the message in the translated language. With enough effort, the translated and synthesized output may even reflect the emotional state of the speaker.

Conclusion

Current speech synthesis offers a panoply of options. One can start with ordinary English text, a sample of recorded speech to be edited, or a screen full of blank rows and columns to be filled in. The user may have no technical knowledge at all or an understanding of the acoustic structure of speech in immense detail. Instead of absolute limits, we face tradeoffs between time and degree of control.

In whatever form, speech synthesis today illustrates the idea that one truly understands a process only when one can reproduce it. That all of these types of synthesis can produce comprehensible speech must indicate that we understand a considerable part of the nature of speech—that they are all imperfect indicates that there is

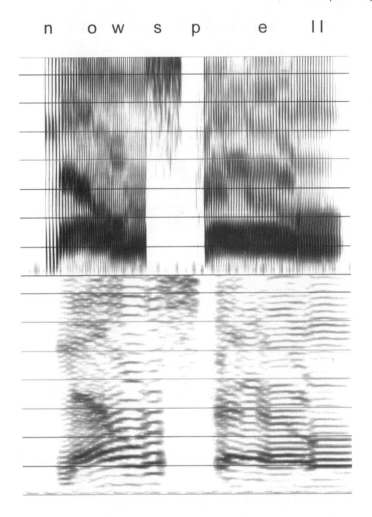

n   o   w   s   p   e   ll

FIGURE 8–12. Wide-band (top) and narrow-band (bottom) spectrograms of the phrase *now spell* produced with *Speak & Spell*™ toy in about 1980.

important work yet to be done. Rapid progress is being made in the area of prosody and emotional expression. Synthetic speech in the near future may not only be highly intelligible but may have humanlike emotional attributes.

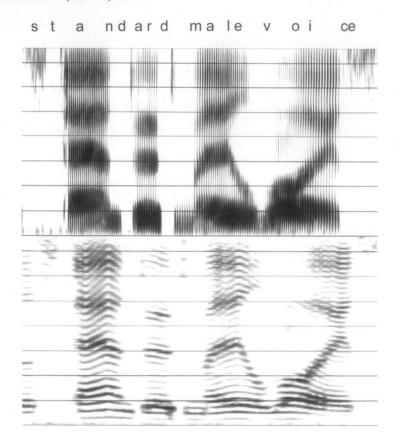

FIGURE 8-13. Wide-band (top) and narrow-band (bottom) spectrograms of the phrase *standard male voice* produced with DECtalk™ in about 1990. Note the unaspirated [t] in *standard*, the smooth variations in the formants, and the intonation contour.

TABLE 8–3
Some watershed advances in speech analysis and technology.

Year	Accomplishment
1920	Development of the oscillograph, permitting waveform analyses of speech.
1930	Electronics technology emerges for application to telecommunications and related fields; this technology overcame many of the limitations of mechanical systems; the VODER demonstrated at the 1939 World's Fair was one of the earliest examples of synthesized speech.
1940	Fourier analysis performed with the Henrici Analyzer; Dudley, Riesz and Watkins described a "synthetic speaker" in 1939. World War II stimulates research into telecommunications and speech analysis.
1950	Development of the sound spectrograph and filter-bank analysis techniques; development of the Pattern Playback speech synthesizer at Haskins Laboratories. In 1952, publication of Peterson and Barney's classic paper, "Control methods used in a study of the vowels" (*Journal of the Acoustical Society of America, 27*, 338–352).
1960	Publication of Gunnar Fant's *Acoustic Theory of Speech Production* (The Hague: Mouton). In 1967, publication of A. M. Liberman, F. S. Cooper, D. P. Shankweiler, and M. Studdert-Kennedy's "Perception of the speech code" (*Psychological Review, 74*, 431–461).
1970	Digital signal processing begins to be widely applied to speech. Linear predictive coding (LPC) introduced as a tool to derive vocal tract parameters from the speech signal. Linear predictive coding first used for speaker recognition. Dynamic time warping used in automatic speech recognition to cope with variations in speaking rates. Demonstration that synthetic speech generated by a vocal tract model can be indistinguishable from natural speech. Active development of full text-to-speech systems. Development and demonstration of articulatory synthesizers. Reading machines for the blind become practical. In 1978, introduction of Texas Instruments *Speak 'n Spell*™ talking toy.
1980	Introduction of Hidden Markov Models in automatic speech recognition. Publication of D. H. Klatt's "Software for a cascade/parallel formant synthesizer" (*Journal of the Acoustical Society of America, 67*, 971–995). Vector quantization used as a solution for narrow-band speech coding systems. Development of speaker-independent recognition systems for isolated words. Development of a cochlear implant that uses speech feature processing (Nuclear 22-channel cochlea implant system).
1990	Connectionist networks used for automatic speech recognition. Construction of speech databases; for example, Defense Advanced Research Projects Agency (DARPA). Introduction of speech recognition processing into hearing aids. Publication in 1998 of K. N. Stevens' *Acoustic Phonetics* (Cambridge, MA: MIT Press). Advances in digital signal processing, including wavelet analysis, chaos models, and connectionist networks. Development and marketing of several low-cost speech analysis systems based on digital signal processing. Introduction of *Furby*™, a toy that not only talks (in Furbish) but gradually seems to "learn" English words. Development of the video game *Seaman*™ (for Sega's Dreamcast game console), which is the first of its kind to use voice recognition. It also talks, by selecting from its library of 12,000 lines of dialogue.

Appendix A: Phonetic Symbols for Vowels and Consonants; Abbreviations Used in the Text

TABLE A–1
Symbols used for vowels of American English, by traditional articulatory categories.

	Front	Central	Back
High	i ɪ	ʊ	u
Mid	e ɛ	ə	o ɔ
Low	æ	a	ɑ

Monophthongs

Example words containing these vowels in Northern Midwestern American English:

[i]: beat		[u]: boot
[ɪ]: bit		[ʊ]: book
[e]: bait	[ə]: about	[o]: boat
[ɛ]: bet	[a]: (see below)	[ɔ]: bought
[æ]: bat	[ɑ]: pot	

Major diphthongs based on these nuclei are:

Note: In this dialect, [a] does not occur as a monophthong, but occurs as the nucleus of two diphthongs.

aɪ: bite

aʊ: bout

ɔɪ boy

Rhotacized ("r-colored") vowels include [ə^], a rhotacized shwa, as in father.

TABLE A–2
**Symbols used for consonants of American English,
by traditional articulatory categories.**

	Bilabial	Labio-dental	Inter-dental	Alveo-lar	Retro-flex	Alveo-palatal	Velar	Glottal
Stop	p b			t d			k g	ʔ
Fricative		f v	θ ð	s z		ʃ ʒ		h
Affricate						tʃ dʒ		
Nasal	m			n			ŋ	
Liquid				l	r			
Glide	w					j	w	

Notes:

(1) Among the obstruents (the stops, fricatives, and affricates), the symbol on the left is for the voiceless sound while that on the right is for the voiced one.

(2) In other books, [h] is sometimes classified as a glide, apporoximant, or semivowel.

(3) [w] is labiovelar; that is, it is articulated at both places.

(4) [j] is actually palatal; in other American books, it is often written [y].

Example words containing these consonants in Northern Midwestern American English:

[p]: *pet*, ti*p*
[b]: *bet*, ri*b*
[t]: *t*ip, pe*t*
[d]: *d*ip, be*d*
[k]: *c*ap, ba*ck*
[g]: *g*ap, ba*g*
[ʔ]: "unh-unh" (negative

[f]: *f*at, lau*gh*
[v]: *v*at, ha*v*e
[θ]: *th*in, ba*th*
[ð]: *th*en, ba*the*
[s]: *s*ip, le*ss*
[z]: *z*ip, red*s*

[ʃ]: *sh*ip, me*sh*
[ʒ]: mea*s*ure, rou*g*e
[h]: *h*eat

[tʃ]: *ch*urch
[dʒ]: *j*udge

[m]: *m*ean, la*mb*
[n]: *n*ear, wi*n*
[ŋ]: si*ng*

[l]: *l*ive, a*ll*
[r]: *r*ed, ca*r*

[w]: *w*et
[j]: *y*et

TABLE A–3
Abbreviations used in this book.

Frequency:

Hz	hertz, or cycles per second
kHz	kilohertz (1000 hertz)
cps	cycles per second
f_0	fundamental frequency
F1	first formant; F2 = second formant, and so forth

Time:

s	second
cs	centisecond (0.01 second)
ms	millisecond (0.001 second)
μs	microsecond (0.000001 second)

Amplitude:

dB	decibel
v	volt
mv	millivolt (0.001 volt)

Length:

m	meters
cm	centimeters (0.01 meter)
mm	millimeters (0.001 meter)
l	length

Speech sounds:

[p]	A phonetic symbol in brackets represents a phone, that is, a speech sound.
/p/	A phonetic symbol in slashes represents a phoneme, that is, a linguistically significant class of speech sounds.
IPA	The International Phonetic Alphabet

Acoustic analyses:

LPC	Linear predictive coding
FFT	Fast Fourier Transform
DFT	Discrete Fourier Transform

Digital Sampling:

A/D	analog to digital conversion or converter
D/A	digital to analog conversion or converter

Speed:

c	the speed of sound in air at sea level

Appendix B: Elementary Physics of Sound

Acoustics is the branch of physics that deals with sound. *Psychoacoustics* is the study of the psychological response to sound; it is a division of psychophysics, or the general study of psychological responses to physical stimuli. The study of speech acoustics has both a physical and psychophysical side. The physical side pertains to the physical structure of the sounds of speech. The psychophysical side is concerned with the perception of these sounds. A proper understanding of speech requires knowledge of both of these aspects of speech acoustics. A well-known riddle asks, "If a tree falls in the forest, but there is no one to hear it, does it make a sound?" Of course, the answer depends on the definition of terms. If *sound* is defined with respect to human perception, then no sound could be verified. But if *sound* is defined as a physical disturbance in the air, then sound must have occurred. A riddle more apropos to speech might be: "If speech is made visible as patterns on paper (or a video monitor), but no one hears it, is it really speech?"

Sound is vibration. Vibration is a repetitive to-and-fro motion of a body. Usually, we do not directly hear the actual vibrations in a sound source such as an engine, but rather we hear the vibrations that are propagated, or transmitted, in a medium like air. When we stand next to a humming machine, we hear the vibrations produced by the machine at a distance and air is the medium of propagation. Figure B–1 shows a simple physical arrangement to demonstrate the nature of sound. The sound source is a stretched rubber band that can be plucked to set it into vibration. The band undergoes a series of to-and-fro vibrations after it is plucked. The initial vibrations are of large

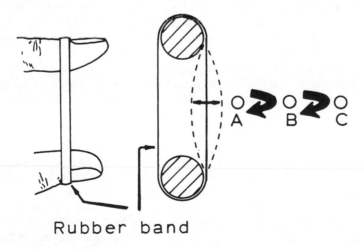

Rubber band

FIGURE B–1. Sound generation with a rubber band. When the band is plucked, it vibrates. As it does so, it causes a chain reaction of collisions for the adjacent air particles, A, B, and C. Because air is elastic, each particle returns to its original position following the collision. Therefore, each particle moves in a to-and-fro manner.

amplitude, meaning that the to-and-fro swings have a relatively great motion. The amplitude diminishes until motion eventually stops altogether. The reduction in amplitude reflects *damping*, or the loss of energy. In the natural world, vibrations do not continue indefinitely after the energy source responsible for the vibration has ceased. Rather, vibrations die out. The rate at which they die out is a measure of damping, which is the rate at which energy is absorbed. When a coin is dropped on a hard tile floor, the sound seems to "ring" for a short time. When the coin is dropped on a sofa cushion, the sound is more like a dull thud that quickly dies out. The coin and tile combination produces a low rate damping, so that sound energy continues for a time beyond the initial impact of the coin on the floor. Therefore, the coin rings. In contrast, the coin and cushion produce a sound that is quickly damped and we hear a thud.

How do we hear the vibrations of the rubber band in the example described earlier? To answer this question, we consider first the way in which the vibrating rubber band interacts with air molecules immediately adjacent to it. Air is made up of particles that move in response to applied energy. When the rubber band vibrates, its outward motion pushes against the adjacent air molecules, compressing them. If air were a rigid body, then the entire air mass would move back and forth with the rubber band, like a giant piston. But air is elastic, so that its molecules can move relative to one another, as though they were interconnected by tiny springs. Molecules that have been displaced tend to return to their original position. By virtue of this elasticity, the vibratory energy imparted by the rubber band is transmitted from air molecule to air molecule in a kind of chain reaction. Let us suppose that we have three air molecules, A, B, and C, as shown schematically in Figure B–1. Molecule A is closest to a sound source, B is intermediate, and C is farthest. The following sequence would occur in response to vibratory energy: A is pushed so that it collides with B. B in turn collides with C but at the same time A returns to its original position (because of elasticity). In this sequence, a pattern of *compressions* and *rarefactions* is developed. Molecule collision produces compression as particles are pressed together. However, the return motion of a particle in the elastic medium produces a rarefaction in which particle density is momentarily reduced at a particular point in space.

Sound is thus a series of condensations and rarefactions. A given particle in the path of the propagating sound wave will be subjected to an impulse of condensation and rarefaction. For the particles A, B, and C introduced above, short time lags would occur between their motion: Molecule A moves first, then B, and then C. When we watch lightning and hear thunder, we have a common example of this time lag. We see the flash of lightning immediately because light travels very fast, at about 186,000 miles per second. But the accompanying sound of thunder reaches our ears after a delay, sometimes of several seconds, because sound moves more slowly through the air medium at about one-fifth of a mile per second. Sound travels slowly enough that we often hear evidence that the "sound barrier" has been broken. When a jet aircraft exceeds the speed of sound, we hear a sonic boom. The same things happens when we crack a whip—the rapid movement of the end of the whip catches up with the sound wave and, in so doing, makes a small sonic boom.

What we hear as sound is the response of the human ear to vibrations in the surrounding medium, usually air, but, for example, which could be water if we are swimming. The ear detects particle excursions as small as 0.0001 inch. In fact, the sensitivity of the ear falls just short of responding to the random movements of air particles. Small pressure fluctuations in the air give rise to sound. These fluctuations move in a wave-like fashion, and sound is therefore described in terms of wave motion.

There are two major types of wave motion. Sound moves as a *longitudinal wave*, meaning that the particles move back and forth along the direction of the wave. Recall the particles A, B, and C described above: They moved in succession, to and fro, along the path of the sound wave. In contrast, the waves that are produced when a stone is dropped into the middle of the pond are *transverse waves*, in which the particles move up and own, or perpendicular to the advancing wave. The longitudinal wave of sound is not as easily seen as the transverse waves in a pool of water. However, the nature of the longitudinal wave of sound can be imagined with the demonstration illustrated in Figure B–2. This is a *Gedanken* (thought) experiment that would actually be very difficult to perform. Suppose that a pencil is attached to the tine of a tuning fork. When the tuning fork is struck to set it into vibration, the pencil at the end of the fork's tine will vibrate to and fro with the fork. The to-and-fro motion would be drawn by the pencil as a repeating motion, so that the pencil's line would be drawn on itself over and over again. Now if we smoothly pull the vibrating fork across the sheet of writing paper, the result would be a pattern in which the to-and-fro motions appear as a line that smoothly varies up and down. Because the tuning fork vibrates at a single frequency, that is, it has a simple periodic to-and-fro motion, the pattern produced on paper takes the shape of a *sinusoid* (named for the sine function in geometry).

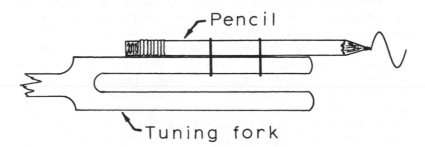

FIGURE B–2. A *Gedanken* (thought) experiment to illustrate sinusoidal vibration. A pencil is attached to the tine of a tuning fork. When the tuning fork is struck, it vibrates a particular frequency. The idea of this illustration is that as that vibrating tuning fork with attached pencil is drawn across a piece of paper, a sinusoidal waveform would be traced out.

The graph shown in Figure B–3 is called a *waveform*, which is a graph of amplitude versus time. All sounds can be represented in a two-dimensional graph of amplitude and time. The waveform in Figure B–3 is especially important, because the sinusoid is a basic waveform that can be used as a kind of analysis unit. The idea is that all sounds can be decomposed into a number of sinusoidal components. To see how this is possible, we need to examine some features of the waveform and introduces some additional concepts.

One complete *cycle* of vibration of the tuning fork (a to-and-fro motion) is represented on the sinusoidal waveform as a sequence of up and down motion. The time required for this cycle is called the *period*. The frequency of vibration is measured as the number of cycles in a second (called hertz, abbreviated Hz). If a tuning fork vibrates at 256 Hz, it completes 256 cycles of vibration in one second. The period, or duration of one cycle, can be computed simply by dividing the number of cycles into one second. That is, the period is the reciprocal of frequency. The period of a 256 Hz tone is about 0.004 seconds, or 4 milliseconds (ms). The physical measure of frequency correlates highly with the perceptual phenomenon of pitch. A high-pitched sound has a high frequency, and a low-pitched sound has a low frequency. The range of frequencies that the human ear can detect is about 20–20,000 Hz, corresponding to a range of periods of 50 msec to 0.5 ms. Dogs and many other animals can hear an extended range of frequencies, which is why dogs can hear whistles that humans cannot. Sounds also vary in loudness. The primary physical correlate of loudness is amplitude. As amplitude of vibration increases, we tend to hear a louder sound.

The sound wave also can be represented spatially. Because sound propagates longitudinally, a cycle of vibration covers a certain distance in space. The distance is called a *wavelength* and is determined by dividing the speed of sound (about 1100 ft/s) by the frequency of the sound. A sound of low frequency has a long wavelength and a sound of high frequency has a short wavelength.

The sinusoid is an elemental waveform that is basic to acoustic analysis because various types of sounds can be analyzed into component sinusoids of specified frequency, amplitude, and phase. Frequency and amplitude already have been described as a measure of rate of vibration and a measure of the magnitude of excursion, respectively. Sounds of different frequency but same amplitude are illustrated as waveforms in Figure B–3A. Tones of different amplitudes but same frequency are illustrated in Figure B–3B. Phase specifies the time relationship among the components of a sound wave and is most effectively demonstrated with a *complex tone*, or a tone that is composed of two or more harmonics. Each harmonic is a sinusoid and the different harmonics are related as integer multiples. For example, the third harmonic of a 100 Hz tone is a tone of 300 Hz (the harmonic number, 3, is multiplied by the fundamental, or lowest, tone).

We have seen that the waveform is a graph of amplitude versus time. It may be interpreted to reflect the displacement of an air molecule during sound propagation. An alternative way of viewing sound is the *spectrum*, which is a graph of amplitude versus frequency. The spectrum indicates the amplitude of each sinusoidal component in a

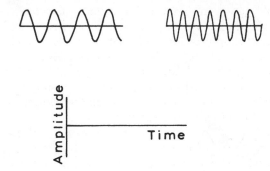

FIGURE B–3A. Wave forms of sinusoids with same amplitude but different frequency (number of complete vibrations per unit of time), conventionally expressed as hertz (or number of cycles per second). The wave form at the left has a lower frequency than the one at the right.

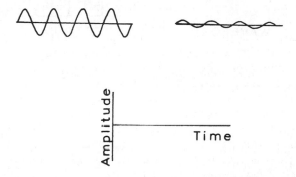

FIGURE B–3B. Waveforms of sinusoids with same frequency but different amplitudes. The waveform at the left has a greater amplitude than the one at the right.

sound. Figure B–4 shows several waveform and spectrum pairs. Note that a single sinusoid has one line in its spectrum because all the sound energy is concentrated at one frequency. As more sinusoidal components are added, more lines appear in the spectrum. The most complex pattern in Figure B–4 resembles the sound of the human voice, that is, the sound generated by the vocal folds. This sound is harmonically rich, and the harmonics are spaced at intervals corresponding to the fundamental frequency of vocal fold vibration. The spectra in Figure B–4 are all *line spectra*, so called because the spectra are composed of lines.

So far the discussion has been restricted to complex tones, or sounds having a harmonic composition. Harmonics are integer multiples. If the first harmonic is 100 Hz, then the second harmonic is 200 Hz, the third is 300 Hz, and so on. Sounds with harmonic structure are periodic, meaning that some basic vibratory pattern recurs repeatedly

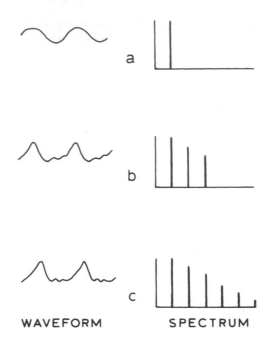

WAVEFORM   SPECTRUM

FIGURE B–4. Waveform and spectrum pairs: (A) sinusoid, (B) complex tone with three harmonics, and (C) complex tone with six harmonics.

at a fixed interval. The fixed interval is the fundamental period, or the period of the lowest harmonic. In the example just cited, the fundamental period of a harmonic sequence of 100, 200, and 300 Hz would be 10 msec, the period of the lowest harmonic. But not all sounds in the world, or even in speech, are harmonic complexes. Many sounds are noiselike and do not have a regularly recurring pattern of vibration. Noise is much more random in its nature. This randomness is shown in Figure B–5 in both a waveform and spectrum. The waveform looks "noisy"—the amplitude varies with no detectable pattern. The spectrum shows that the noise is composed of energy at many different frequencies. This kind of spectrum is called a *continuous spectrum.*

The waveform and spectrum are alternative ways of representing a sound. The two representations are mathematically related by an operation called the *Fourier transform.* A spectrum is sometimes called a Fourier spectrum, and Fourier analysis is a very common type of spectral analysis. The basic objective of this spectral analysis is to convert the amplitude-by-time pattern of the waveform into an alternative pattern which reveals the amount of energy in the various sinusoidal components of the sound. Note that phase has been neglected in this simplified discussion. To make a waveform and spectrum completely interchangeable, phase information would have to be included with the spectral analysis. This information would describe the time relationships among the spectral components. Although phase cannot be neglected in the study of sound, phase generally is ignored in studies of speech acoustics because phase does not contribute critically to the perception of speech.

The unit of frequency measurement was defined as the hertz, which is a linear measure of frequency as the number of vibrations occurring in one second. However, the human ear does not perceive pitch in a way that is linear in frequency. For example, on a piano keyboard, an equivalent increase in pitch is judged to occur in proceeding from middle C, to the next higher C, and so on. These intervals are called *octaves* and they correspond to multiplying the linear frequency values by two. If we go up one octave from 220, the corresponding linear frequency is 440 Hz.

To this point, the unit of amplitude measurement has been neglected. That neglect must now be remedied. Amplitude conceivably could be measured in terms of the actual excursions of molecules, but the measurement would be implausibly difficult for most applications. In addition, the human response to sound is such that loudness judgments change roughly with the logarithm of the actual physical changes in the signal. For example, with a base 10 logarithm, powers of ten would be represented with the log values of 0 for 1 or unity, 1 for a

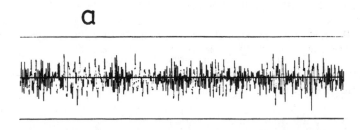

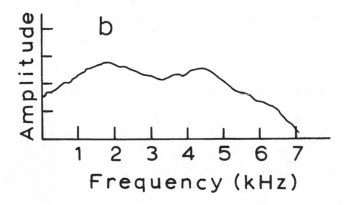

FIGURE B–5. Waveform (a) and spectrum (b) of noise. Note diffuse energy distribution in spectrum.

value of 10, 2 for a value of 100, 3 for a value of 1,000, and so on. Because the range of amplitudes to be considered in human hearing is vast, the logarithmic scale is convenient to represent this dimension of sound.

The unit typically used to measure sound energy is *decibel*. The decibel has a rather complicated derivation, but the following sequence should help to clarify it.

The *decibel* is one tenth of a *bel*. Because the bel is too large to be a practical unit of measurement, the decibel (*deci* = one-tenth) is used instead.

The bel is a logarithm of a ratio. Recall that a logarithmic scale is advantageous because of the large range of sound amplitudes that need to be considered. Going from a linear to logarithmic scale helps to keep the numbers of convenient size, for example, logarithm of 4 corresponds to a linear value of 10,000 (10 to the fourth power). The ratio enters the picture because sound energy is measured relative to a reference value. That is, the variable sound energy V is described relative to a standard energy S:

Sound energy in bels = log(base 10) V/S

Because 1 bel (B) equals 10 decibels (dB),

Sound energy in decibels = 10 log(base 10) V/S

Both intensity and sound pressure are commonly used as the actual physical measurement of sound energy. For intensity measurement, or intensity level (IL),

Sound intensity in dB IL = 10 log(base 10) Iv/Is

where Iv is the variable intensity and Is is the standard intensity.

Because sound pressure is equal to the square of intensity, sound pressure level in dB introduces a factor of 2:

Sound pressure in dB SPL = 20 log(base 10) Pv/Ps,

where Pv is the variable sound pressure and Ps is the standard sound pressure.

In this book, sound magnitude usually will be expressed in either dB intensity level or dB sound pressure level. Therefore, a spectrum of a sound will have the horizontal axis of frequency (in Hz or kHz, where k is a multiplier of 1,000) and a vertical axis of intensity or sound pressure level in dB. An interesting property of the logarithmic dB scale is that addition of dB values corresponds to multiplication of the original (antilog) values. This is a useful feature, as it simplifies some calculations in acoustics.

We have seen that sound is a wave phenomenon in which the vibratory energy is propagated in a medium. This wave property can be represented graphically as a waveform (amplitude of displacement versus time) or a wavelength (amplitude of a displacement versus distance). One of the most useful ways to analyze sound is by means of the spectrum (energy versus frequency). A fundamental appeal of the spectrum is that even very complex sounds can be analyzed as a combination of elemental sounds, such as sinusoids. The Fourier spectrum accomplishes this kind of analysis, enabling us to describe various types of sounds in terms of their energy distributions across frequency. A general rule for relating waveform and spectral representations is as follows (assuming that the waveforms are plotted on the same time scale): The more peaked (sharp-cornered) the waveform, the greater the energy in the higher frequencies of the spectrum. This relation holds because sharp features in the waveform require high frequencies for their definition.

Speech sounds usually have energy distributed widely over frequency, but some energy regions are more important than others. Part of the goal of acoustic analysis of speech, then, is to determine how sounds differ in their spectra and to describe the most important spectral regions for each sound or sound class. The chapters in this book describe modern approaches to making speech visible, an enterprise that has occupied the labors of speech scientists for several decades. Almost a half-century ago, Potter, Kopp, and Green (1947) published a book, *Visible Speech*. The present book could be similarly subtitled and reports on about fifty years of progress in this quest.

Appendix C: Nonlinear Frequency Scales for Speech Analysis

The scales described in this section have been proposed as alternatives to linear frequency for the representation of speech sounds. A major argument for the use of these nonlinear frequency scales is that they come closer than a linear scale to the analysis performed by the ear. Although these nonlinear scales have been particularly important for vowels, they also can be used for consonents.

In each of the equations that follow, f designates a value of frequency. Equations are defined for mels, Barks, and Koenig values.

Technical mels (TM), were defined by Fant (1973),

$$TM = (1000 / \log 2) \log(f/1000 + 1)$$

The Bark transform (B for Bark), is calculated according to Zwicker and Terhardt's (1980) equation,

$$B = 13 \arctan (0.76f / 1000) + 3.5 \arctan (f / 7500)^2$$

Koenig values (K), from Koenig (1949) are calculated with the equations,

$$K = 0.002f \quad \text{for } 0 \leq f < 1000.$$
$$K = (4.5 \log f) - 11.5 \quad \text{for } 1000 < f \leq 10,000.$$

For a graphical comparison of these scales, see Miller (1989).

References

Abberton, E. R. M., Howard, D. M., & Fourcin, A. J. (1989). Laryngographic assessment of normal voice: A tutorial. *Clinical Linguistics and Phonetics, 3,* 281–296.

Abramson, A. S. (1977). Laryngeal timing in consonant distinctions. *Phonetica, 34,* 295–303.

Adams, C., & Munro, R. R. (1978). In search of the acoustic correlates of stress: Fundamental frequency, amplitude, and duration in the connected utterance of some native and non-native speakers of English. *Phonetica, 35,* 125–156.

Adams, S. G. (1990). *Rate and clarity of speech: An X-ray microbeam study.* Ph.D. dissertation, University of Wisconsin-Madison, Madison, WI.

Ahmadi, S., & Spanias, A. S. (1999). Cepstrum-based pitch detection using a new statistical V/UV classification algorithm. *IEEE Transactions on Speech & Audio Processing, 7,* 333–338.

Al-Bamerni, A. (1975). *An instrumental study of the allophonic variation of /l/ in RP.* Master of Arts dissertation, University College of North Wales, Bangor, UK.

Allen, G. D. (1978). Vowel duration measurement: A reliability study. *Journal of the Acoustical Society of America, 63,* 1176–1181.

Allen, G. D., & Hawkins, S. (1980). Phonological rhythm: Definition and development. In G. H. Yeni-Komshian, J. F. Kavanagh, & C. A. Ferguson (Eds.), *Child phonology* (Vol. 1, pp. 227–256). New York: Academic Press.

Allen, J., Hunnicutt, M. S., & Klatt, D. H. (1987). *From text to speech: The MITalk system.* Cambridge, UK: Cambridge University Press.

Ali, L., & Daniloff, R. (1972). A contrastive cine-fluorographic investigation of the articulation of emphatic-nonemphatic cognate consonants. *Studia Linguistica, 18,* 81–105.

Alwan, A. (1989). Perceptual cues for place of articulation for the voiced pharyngeal and uvular consonants. *Journal of the Acoustical Society of America, 86,* 549–556.

Alwan, A., Narayanan, S., & Haker, K. (1997). Toward articulatory-acoustic models for liquid approximants based on MRI and EPG data. II. The rhotics. *Journal of the Acoustical Society of America, 101,* 1078–1089.

Andrianopoulos, M. V., Darrow, K., & Chen, J. (in press). Multimodal standardization of voice among four multicultural populations: Formant structures. *Journal of Voice.*

Aronson, L., Rosenhouse, J., Rosenhouse, G., & Podoshin, L. (1996). An acoustic analysis of modern Hebrew vowels and voiced consonants. *Journal of Phonetics, 24,* 283–293.

Arsland, L. M., & Hansen, J. H. L. (1997). Study of temporal features and frequency characteristics in American English foreign accent. *Journal of the Acoustical Society of America, 102,* 28–40.

Assman & Katz, W. F. (2000). Time-varying spectral change in the vowels of children and adults. *Journal of the Acoustical Society of America, 108,* 1856–1866.

Assman, P., Nearey, T., & Hogan, J. (1982). Vowel identification: orthographic, perceptual, and acoustic aspects. *Journal of the Acoustical Society of America, 71,* 975–989.

Atal, B. S., & Hanauer, S . L. (1971). Speech analysis and synthesis by linear prediction of the speech wave. *Journal of the Acoustical Society of America, 50,* 637–655.

Atal, B. S., & Schroeder, M. R. (1970). Adaptive predictive coding of speech signals. *Bell System Technical Journal, 49,* 1973–1986.

Azou, P., Ozsancak, C., Morris, R. J., Jan, M., Eustache, F., & Hannequin, D. (2000). Voice onset time in aphasia, apraxia of speech and dysarthria: A review. *Clinical Linguistics & Phonetics, 14,* 131–150.

Bachety, M. (1998, September). Bouncing reverb out of the lab. *Sound Communications, 44,* 96–97 and 126.

Bachorowski, J.-A. (1999). Vocal expression and perception of emotion. *Current Directions in Psychological Science, 8,* 53–57.

Bachorowski, J.-A., & Owren, M. J. (1999). Acoustic correlates of talker sex and individual talker identity are present in a short vowel segment produced in running speech. *Journal of the Acoustical Society of America, 106,* 1054–1063.

Badin, P., Perrier, P., Boe, L.-J., & Abry, C. (1990). Vocalic nomograms: Acoustic and articulatory considerations upon formant convergences. *Journal of the Acoustical Society of America, 87,* 1290–1300.

Baken, R. (1987). *Clinical measurement of speech and voice.* Boston: Little, Brown & Co.

Baken, R. (1990). Irregularity of vocal period and amplitude: A first approach to the fractal analysis of voice. *Journal of Voice, 4,* 185–197.

Baken, R., & Daniloff, R. (Eds.) (1990). *Readings in clinical spectrography of speech.* San Diego: Singular Publishing Group.

Banbrook, M., McLaughlin, S., & Mann, I. (1999). Speech characterization and synthesis by nonlinear methods. *IEEE Transactions on Speech & Audio Processing, 7,* 1–17.

Baranek, L. (1988). *Acoustical measurements.* Woodbury, NY: Acoustical Society of America.

Barry, W. (1979). Complex encoding in word-final voiced and voiceless stops. *Phonetica, 36,* 361–372.

Bauer, H. R., & Kent, R. D. (1987). Acoustic analysis of infant fricative and trill vocalizations. *Journal of the Acoustical Society of America, 81,* 505–511.

Baum, S. R., & Blumstein, S. E. (1987). Preliminary observations on the use of duration as a cue to syllable-initial fricative voicing in English. *Journal of the Acoustical Society of America, 82,* 1073–1077.

Beckman, M. E. (1986). *Stress and non-stress accent. Netherlands Phonetic Archives, 7.* Dordrecht: Foris.

Beckman, M. E., & Edwards, J. (1990). Lengthenings and shortenings and the nature of prosodic constituency. In J. Kingston & M. E. Beckman (Eds.), *Between the grammar and physics of speech* (pp. 152–214). Cambridge: Cambridge University Press.

Beckman, M. E., & Edwards, J. (1991). Prosodic categories and duration control. *Journal of the Acoustical Society of America, 87,* (Suppl. 1), S65.

Behne, D. (1989). *Acoustic effects of focus and sentence position on stress in English and French.* Ph.D. dissertation, University of Wisconsin-Madison.

Behrens, S., & Blumstein, S. E. (1988a). On the role of the amplitude of the fricative noise in the perception of place of articulation in voiceless fricative consonants. *Journal of the Acoustical Society of America, 84,* 861–867.

Behrens, S., & Blumstein, S. E. (1988b). Acoustic characteristics of English voiceless fricatives: A descriptive analysis. *Journal of Phonetics, 16,* 295–298.

Bennett, S. (1981). Vowel formant frequency characteristics of preadolescent males and females. *Journal of the Acoustical Society of America, 69,* 231–238.

Beranek, L. (1988). *Acoustical measurements.* New York: American Institute of Physics.

Berg, J. W. van den (1955). Transmission of the vocal cavities. *Journal of the Acoustical Society of America, 27,* 161–168.

Bergem, D. R. van, Pols, L. C. W., & Koopmans-van Beinum, F. J. (1988). Perceptual normalization of the vowels of a man and a child in various contexts. *Speech Communication, 7,* 1–20.

Bettagere, R., & Fucci, D. (1999). Magnitude-estimation scaling of computerized (digitized) speech under different listening conditions. *Perceptual and Motor Skills, 88,* 1363–1378.

Bladon, A. (1983). Two-formant models of vowel perception: shortcomings and enhancements. *Speech Communication, 2,* 305–313.

Bladon, R. A. W., & Fant, G. (1978). A two-formant model and the cardinal vowels. Royal Institute of Technology Speech Transmission Laboratory (Stockholm), *Quarterly Progress and Status Reports, 1,* 1–8.

Bless, D. M., Biever, D., & Shaikh, A. (1986). Comparisons of vibratory characteristics of young adult males and females. *Proceedings of International Conference on Voice,* Kurume, Japan, Vol. 2, 46–54.

Blomgren, M., & Robb, M. (1998). How steady are vowel steady-states? *Clinical Linguistics & Phonetics, 12,* 405–415.

Blumstein, S. E. (1986). On acoustic invariance in speech. In J. Perkell & D. H. Klatt (Eds.), *Invariance and variability in speech processes.* Hillsdale, NJ: Lawrence Erlbaum & Associates.

Blumstein, S. E., & Stevens, K. N. (1979). Acoustic invariance in speech production: Evidence from measurements of the spectral characteristics of stop consonants. *Journal of the Acoustical Society of America, 66*, 1001–1017.

Blumstein, S. E., & Stevens, K. N. (1980). Perceptual invariance onset spectra for stop consonants in different vowel environments. *Journal of the Acoustical Society of America, 67*, 648–662.

Bogert, B. P. (1953). On the bandwidth of the vowel formants. *Journal of the Acoustical Society of America, 25*, 791–792.

Bolinger, D. L. (1965). Pitch accent and sentence rhythm. In I. Abe. & T. Kanekiyo (Eds.), *Forms of English* (pp. 123–141). Cambridge, MA: Harvard Press.

Bolt, R. H., Cooper, F. S., David, E. E., Denes, P. B., Pickett, J. M., & Stevens, K. N. (1970). Speaker identification of speech spectrograms: A scientists' view of its reliability for legal purposes. *Journal of the Acoustical Society of America, 47*, 597–612.

Bolt, R. H., Cooper, F. S., David, E. E., Denes, P. B., Pickett, J. M., & Stevens, K. N. (1973). Speaker identification by speech spectrograms: Some further observations. *Journal of the Acoustical Society of America, 54*, 531–534.

Bond, Z. S., & Moore, T. J. (1994). A note on the acoustic-phonetic characteristics of inadvertently clear speech. *Speech Communication, 14*, 325–337.

Bonneau, A., Djezzar, L., & Laprie, Y. (1996). Perception of the place of articulation of French stop bursts. *Journal of the Acoustical Society of America, 100*, 555–564.

Bonnot, J. -F. P., & Chevrie-Muller, C. (1991). Some effects of shouted and whispered conditions on temporal organization. *Journal of Phonetics, 19*, 473–483.

Bosch, L., Costa, A., & Sebastian-Galles, N. (2000). First and second language vowel perception in early bilinguals. *European Journal of Cognitive Psychology, 12*, 189–221.

Bradlow, A. R. (1995). A comparative acoustic study of English and Spanish vowels. *Journal of the Acoustical Society of America, 97*, 1916–1924.

Bradlow, A. R., Torretta, G. M., & Pisoni, D. B. (1996). Intelligibility of normal speech. 1. Global and fine-grained acoustic-phonetic talker characteristics. *Speech Communication, 20*, 255–272.

Brancazio, L., & Fowler, C. A. (1998). On the relevance of locus equations for production and perception of stop consonants. *Perception and Psychophysics, 60*, 24–50.

Brown, B. L., Giles, H., & Thakerar, J. N. (1985). Speaker evaluations as a function of speech rate, accent and context. *Language and Communication, 5*, 207–220.

Brown, B. L., Strong, W. J., & Rencher, A. C. (1974) Fifty-four voices from two: The effects of simultaneous manipulations of rate, mean fundamental frequency and variance of fundamental frequency on ratings of personality from speech. *Journal of the Acoustical Society of America, 55*, 313–318.

Bruckert, E. (1984/January/February). A new text-to-speech product produces human-quality voice. *Speech Technology*, 114–119.

Buder, E. H. (2000). Acoustic analysis of voice quality: A tabulation of algorithms 1902-1990. In R. D. Kent & M. J. Ball (Eds.), *Voice quality measurement* (pp. 119–244). San Diego: Singular/Thomson Learning.

Busby, P. A., & Plant, G. L. (1995). Formant frequency values of vowels produced by preadolescent boys and girls. *Journal of the Acoustical Society of America, 97*, 2603–2606.

Byrd, D. (1996). Influences on articulatory timing in consonant sequences. *Journal of Phonetics, 24*, 209–244.

Byrd, D., & Saltzman, E. (1998). Intragestural dynamics of multiple prosodic boundaries. *Journal of Phonetics, 26*, 173–199.

Byrne, D., Dillon, H., Tran, K., Arlinger, S., Wilbraham, K., Cox, R., Hagerman, B., Hetu, R., Kei, J., Lui, C., Kiessling, J., Kotby, M. N., Nasser, N. H. A., El Kholy, W. A. H., Nakanishi, Y., Oyer, H., Powell, R., Stephens, D., Meredith, R., Sirimanna, T., Tavartkiladze, G., Frolenkov, G. I., Westerman, S., & Ludvigsen., C. (1994). An international comparison of long-term average speech spectra. *Journal of the Acoustical Society of America, 96*, 2108–2120.

Cairns, D. A., Hansen, J. H. L., & Riski, J. E. (1996). Noninvasive technique for detecting hypernasal speech using an nonlinear operator. *IEEE Transactions on Biomedical Engineering, 43*, 35–45.

Campbell, N. (1999). Speech synthesis. In Webster, J. G. (Ed.), *Wiley encyclopedia of electrical and electronics engineering* (Vol. 20), (pp. 243–260)). New York: Wiley.

Carlson, R., Fant, G., & Granstrom, B. (1975). Two-formant models, pitch and vowel perception. In G. Fant & M. A. A. Tatham

(Eds.), *Auditory analysis and perception of speech* (pp. 55–82). London: Academic Press.

Castleman, W. A., & Diehl, R. L. (1996). Effects of fundamental frequency on medial and final [voice] judgments. *Journal of Phonetics, 24,* 383–398.

Chen, M. (1970). Vowel length variation as a function of the voicing of the consonant environment. *Phonetica, 22,* 129–159.

Chen, M. Y. (1997). Acoustic correlates of English and French nasalized vowels. *Journal of the Acoustical Society of America, 102,* 2360–2370.

Cheveigne, A. de, & Kawahara, H. (1999). Missing-data model of vowel identification. *Journal of the Acoustical Society of America, 105,* 3497–3508.

Chiba, T., & Kajiyama, M. (1958). *The vowel: Its nature and structure.* Tokyo: Phonetic Society of Japan.

Childers, D. G., Hicks, D. M., Moore, G. P., Eskenazi, L., & Lalwani, A. L. (1990). Electroglottography and vocal fold physiology. *Journal of Speech and Hearing Research, 33,* 245–354.

Childers, D. G., & Wu, K. (1991). Gender recognition from speech. Part II: fine analysis. *Journal of the Acoustical Society of America, 90,* 1841–1856.

Chistovich, L. A., & Lublinskaja, V. V. (1979). The "centre of gravity" effect in vowel spectra and critical distance between the formants: Psychoacoustical study of the perception of vowel-like stimuli. *Hearing Research, 1,* 185–195.

Chistovich, L. A., Sheikin, R. L., & Lublinskaja, V. V. (1979). Centres of gravity and spectral peaks as the determinants of vowel quality. In Lindblom, B. & Ohman, S. (Eds.), *Frontiers of speech communication research* (pp. 143–158). London: Academic Press.

Cho, T. & Ladefoged, P. (1999). Variation and universals in VOT: Evidence from 18 languages. *Journal of Phonetics, 27,* 207–229.

Chomsky, N., & Halle, M. (1968). *The sound pattern of English.* New York: Harper & Row.

Claes, T., Dologlou, I., Tenbosch, L., & Vancompernolle, D. (1998). A novel feature transformation for vocal tract length normalization in automatic speech recognition. *IEEE Transactions on Speech & Audio Processing, 6,* 549–557.

Cohen, A., Collier, R., & t'Hart, J. (1982). Declination: Construct or intrinsic feature of speech pitch? *Phonetica, 39,* 254–273.

Coker, C. (1976). A model of articulatory dynamics and control. *Proceedings of the Institute of Electrical and Electronic Engineering, 64,* 452–460.

Cole, R. A., & Scott, B. L. (1974). Toward a theory of speech perception. *Psychological Review, 81,* 348–374.

Collier, R., Bell-Berti, F., & Raphael, L. (1982). Some acoustic and physiological observations on diphthongs. *Language & Speech, 25,* 305–323.

Colton, R. H., & Steinschneider, A. (1980). Acoustic relationships of infant cries to the Sudden Infant Death syndrome. In Murry, T. & Murry, J. (Eds.), *Infant communication: Cry and early speech* (pp. 183–208). Houston, TX: College-Hill.

Cooper, F. S., Delattre, P. C., Liberman, A. M., Borst, J. N., & Gerstman, L. J. (1952). Some experiments on the perception of synthetic speech sounds. *Journal of the Acoustical Society of America, 24,* 597–606.

Cooper, W. E., & Eady, S. J. (1986). Metrical phonology in speech production. *Journal of Memory and Language, 25,* 369–384.

Craig, C. H., & Kim, B. W. (1990). Effects of time gating and word length on isolated word recognition performance. *Journal of Speech and Hearing Research, 33,* 808–815.

Crowther, C. S., & Mann, V. (1992). Native language factors affecting use of vocalic cues to final consonant voicing in English. *Journal of the Acoustical Society of America, 92,* 711–722.

Crowther, C. S., & Mann, V. (1994). Use of vocalic cues to consonant voicing and native language background: the influence of experimental design. *Perception & Psychophysics, 55,* 513–525.

Crystal, T. H., & House, A. S. (1988). A note on the durations of fricatives in American English. *Journal of the Acoustical Society of America, 84,* 1932–1935.

Cummins, F. (1999). Some lengthening factors in English combine additively at most rates. *Journal of the Acoustical Society of America, 105,* 476–480.

Cutler, A., Dahan, D., & Van Donselaar, W. (1997). Prosody in the comprehension of spoken language: A literature review. *Language & Speech, 40,* 141–201.

Dalby, J. M. (1986). *Phonetic structure of fast speech in American English.* Bloomington, IN: Indiana University Linguistics Club.

Damper, R. I., Gunn, S. R., Gore, M. O. (2000). Extracting phonetic knowledge from learning systems: Perceptrons, support vector machines and linear discriminants. *Applied Intelligence, 12,* 43–62.

Dang, J., & Honda, K. (1997). Acoustic characteristics of the piriform fossa in models and humans. *Journal of the Acoustical Society of America, 101,* 456–465.

Delattre, P., Liberman, A. M., & Cooper, F. S. (1955). Acoustic loci and transitional cues for consonants. *Journal of the Acoustical Society of America, 27,* 769–774.

Dembowski, J. S. (1998). *Articulator point variability in the production of oral stop consonants.* Unpublished Ph.D. Dissertation, University of Wisconsin-Madison.

Dewey, G. (1923). *Relative frequency of speech sounds.* Cambridge, MA: Harvard University Press.

DiBenedetto, M. G. (1989a). Vowel representation: Some observations on temporal and spectral properties of the first formant frequency. *Journal of the Acoustical Society of America, 86,* 55–66.

DiBenedetto, M. G. (1989b). Frequency and time variations of the first formant: Properties relevant to the perception of vowel height. *Journal of the Acoustical Society of America, 86,* 67–78.

Diehl, R. L., & Kluender, K. R. (1989). On the objects of speech perception. *Ecological Psychology, 1,* 121–144.

Diehl, R., Lindblom, L., Hoemeke, K. A., & Fahey, R. P. (1996). On explaining certain male-female differences in the phonetic realization of vowel categories. *Journal of Phonetics, 24,* 187–208

Diehl, R. L., & Walsh, M. A. (1986). An auditory basis for rate normalization in stops and glides. *Journal of the Acoustical Society of America, 80* (Suppl. 1), S125.

Dilley, L., Shattuck-Hufnagel, S., & Ostendorf, M. (1996). Glottalization of word-initial vowels as a function of prosodic structure. *Journal of Phonetics, 24,* 423–444.

Disner, S. F. (1980). Evaluation of vowel normalization procedures. *Journal of the Acoustical Society of America, 67,* 2453–261.

Dorman, M. F., Raphael, L. C., & Eisenberg, D. (1980). Acoustic cues for a fricative-affricate contrast in word-final position. *Journal of Phonetics, 8,* 397–405.

Dorman, M. F., Studdert-Kennedy, M., & Raphael, L. F. (1977). Stop consonant recognition: Release bursts and formant transitions as functionally equivalent, context-dependent cues. *Perception & Psychophysics, 22,* 109–122.

Edwards, A. D. N. (1991). *Speech synthesis: Technology for disabled people.* London: Paul Chapman Publishing Ltd.

Eek, A., & Meister, E. (1994). Acoustics and perception of Estonian vowel types. *Phonetic Experimental Research, Institute of Linguistics, University of Stockholm (PERILUS),* No. XVIII, pp. 55–90.

Eguchi, S., & Hirsch, I. J. (1969). Development of speech sounds in children. *Acta Otolaryngologica* (Suppl. 257).

El-Halees, Y. (1985). The role of F1 in the place of articulation distinction in Arabic. *Journal of Phonetics, 13,* 287–298.

Endres, W., Bambach, W., & Flosser, G. (1971). Voice spectrograms as a function of age, voice disguise, and voice imitation. *Journal of the Acoustical Society of America, 49,* 1842–1848.

Erickson, M. L. (2000). Simultaneous effects on vowel duration in American English: A covariance structure modeling approach. *Journal of the Acoustical Society of America, 108,* 2980–2995.

Espy-Wilson, C. Y. (1992). Acoustic measures for linguistic features distinguishing the semivowels / w j r l/ in American English. *Journal of the Acoustical Society of America, 92,* 736–757.

Espy-Wilson, C. Y., Boyce, S. E., Jackson, M., Narayanan, S., & Alwan, A. (2000). Acoustic modeling of American English /r/. *Journal of the Acoustical Society of America, 108,* 343–356.

Evers, V., Reetz, H., & Lahiri, A. (1998). Crosslinguistic acoustic categorization of sibilants independent of phonological status. *Journal of Phonetics, 26,* 345–370.

Fant, G. (1960). *Acoustic theory of speech production.* The Hague: Mouton.

Fant, G. (1961). The acoustics of speech. In *Proceedings of the Third International Congress on Acoustics* (Stuttgart). Vol. 1 (Amsterdam), pp. 188–201. (Cited by Hawkes & Miller [1995]).

Fant, G. (1962). Formant bandwidth data. *Speech Transmission Laboratory, Quarterly Progress and Status Reports,* STL/QPSR-1, 1–2.

Fant, G. (1973). *Speech sounds and features.* Cambridge, MA: MIT Press.

Fant, (1975). Non-uniform vowel normalization. *Speech Transmission Laboratory Quarterly Progress and Status Report* (Royal Institute of Technology, Stockholm), 2–3, 1–9.

Farnetani, E. (1997). Coarticulation and connected speech processes. In W. J. Hardcastle & J. Laver (Eds.), *The handbook of phonetic sciences* (pp. 371–404). Cambridge MA: Blackwell.

Feijoo, S., Fernandez, S., & Balsa, R. (1999). Acoustic and perceptual study of phonetic integration in Spanish voiceless stops. *Speech Communication, 27*, 1–18.

Fell, H. J., Macauslan, J., Ferrier, L. J., & Chenausky, K. (1999). Automatic babble recognition for early detection of speech related disorders. *Behavior & Information Technology, 18*, 56–63.

Fischer-Jorgensen, E. (1954). Acoustic analysis of stop consonants. *Miscellanea Phonetica, 2*, 42–49.

Flanagan, J. L. (1955). Difference limen for vowel formant frequency. *Journal of the Acoustical Society of America, 27*, 613–617.

Flanagan, J. L. (1972). *Speech analysis, synthesis and perception*. New York: Springer-Verlag.

Flege, J. E., MacKay, I. R. A., & Meador, D. (1999). Native Italian speakers' perception and production of English vowels. *Journal of the Acoustical Society of America, 106*, 2973–2987.

Flege, J. E., Yeni-Komshian, G. H., & Liu, S. (1999). Age constraints on second-language acquisition. *Journal of Memory & Language, 41*, 78–104.

Fonagy, I., & Fonagy, J. (1966). Sound pressure level and duration. *Phonetica, 15*, 14–21.

Forrest, K., Weismer, G., Milenkovic, P., & Dougall, R. N. (1988). Statistical analysis of word-initial voiceless obstruents: preliminary data. *Journal of the Acoustical Society of America, 84*, 115–123.

Fort, A., Ismaelli, A., Manfredi, C., & Bruscaglioni, P. (1996). Parametric and non-parametric estimation of speech formants—application to infant cry. *Medical Engineering & Physics, 18*, 677–691.

Fourakis, M., Botinis, A., & Katsaiti, M. (1999). Acoustic characteristics of Greek vowels. *Phonetica, 56*, 28–43.

Fourgeron, C., & Keating, P. A. (1997). Articulatory strengthening at edges of prosodic domains. *Journal of the Acoustical Society of America, 101*, 3728–3740.

France, D. J., Shiavi, R. G., Silverman, S., Silverman, M., & Wilkes, D. M. (2000). Acoustical properties of speech as indicators of depression and suicidal risk. *IEEE Transactions on Biomedical Engineering, 47*, 829–837.

Frisch, U., & Orszag, S. A. (1990/January). Turbulence: Challenges for theory and experiment. *Physics Today*, 24–32.

Fruchter, D., & Sussman, H. M. (1997). The perceptual relevance of locus equations. *Journal of the Acoustical Society of America, 102*, 2997–3008.

Fry, D. (1955). Duration and intensity as physical correlates of linguistic stress. *Journal of the Acoustical Society of America, 27*, 765–768.

Fry, D. B., Abramson, A. S., Eimas, P. D., & Liberman, A. M. (1962). The identification and discrimination of synthetic vowels. *Language & Speech, 5*, 171–189.

Fujimura, O. (1962). Analysis of nasal consonants. *Journal of the Acoustical Society of America, 34*, 1865–1875.

Fujimura, O., & Lindqvist, J. (1971). Sweep-tone measurements of vocal-tract characteristics. *Journal of the Acoustical Society of America, 49*, 541–558.

Garofolo, J. S., Lamel, L. F., Fisher, W. M., Fiscus, J. G., Pallett, D. S., & Dahgren, D. L. (1993). *The DARPA TIMIT acoustic-phonetic continuous speech corpus CDROM*, NTIS order number PB91-100354.

Gates, S. (1989/February). Analog to digital converters in the laboratory. *Scientific Computing and Automation*, 49–56.

Gauvin, J. L., Lamel, L. F., & Eskenazi, M. (1990). Design considerations and text selection for BREF, a large French read-speech corpus. *Proceedings of 1990 International Conference on Speech Processing*.

Gay, T. (1968). Effect of speaking rate on diphthong formant movements. *Journal of the Acoustical Society of America, 44*, 1570–1573.

Gerken, L., & McGregor, K. (1998). An overview of prosody and its role in normal and disordered child language. *American Journal of Speech-Language Pathology, 7*, 38–48.

Gilbert, H. R., Robb, M. P., & Chen, Y. (1997). Formant frequency development—15 to 36 months. *Journal of Voice, 11*, 260–266.

Giles, S. B. (1971). *A study of articulatory characteristics of /l/ allophones in English*. Ph.D. Dissertation, University of Iowa, Iowa City, Iowa.

Glasberg, B. R., & Moore, B. C. J. (1990). Derivation of auditory filter shapes from notched-noise data. *Hearing Research, 47*, 103–138.

Gopal, H. S. (1995). Technical issues underlying the development and use of a speech research laboratory. In A. Syrdal, R. Bennett & S. Greenspan (Eds.), *Applied speech technology* (pp. 315–342). Boca Raton, FL: CRC Press.

Greenwood, D. D. (1990). A cochlear frequency-position function for several species—29 years later. *Journal of the Acoustical Society of America, 87*, 2592–2605.

Guaitella, I., (1999). Rhythm in speech: What rhythmic organizations reveal about cognitive processes in spontaneous speech production versus reading aloud. *Journal of Pragmatics, 3*, 509–523.

Haggard, M. (1973). Abbreviation of consonants in English pre- and post-vocalic clusters. *Journal of Phonetics, 1*, 9–24.

Hagiwara, R. (1995). Acoustic realization of American /R/ as produced by women and men. *University of California-Los Angeles Working Papers in Phonetics* (Phonetics Laboratory, University of California- Los Angeles), No. 90.

Hagiwara, R. (1997). Dialect variation and formant frequency: The American English vowels revisited. *Journal of the Acoustical Society of America, 102*, 655–658.

Halle, M., Hughes, G. W., & Radley, J. P. (1957). Acoustic properties of stop consonants. *Journal of the Acoustical Society of America, 29*, 107–116.

Handel, S. (1989). *Listening: An introduction to the perception of auditory events*. Cambridge, MA: MIT Press.

Hanson, H. M. (1997). Glottal characteristics of female speakers—acoustic correlates. *Journal of the Acoustical Society of America, 101*, 466–481.

Hanson, H. M., & Chuang, E. S. (1999). Glottal characteristics of male speakers: acoustic correlates and comparison with female data. *Journal of the Acoustical Society of America, 106*, 1064–1077.

Harper, P., Kraman, S. S., Pasterkamp, H., & Wodicka, G. R. (2001). An acoustic model of the vocal tract. *IEEE Transactions on Biomedical Engineering, 48*, 543–550.

Harris, K. (1958). Cues for discrimination of American English fricatives in spoken syllables. *Language & Speech, 1*, 1–17.

Harshman, R., Ladefoged, P., & Goldstein, L. (1977). Factor analysis of tongue shapes. *Journal of the Acoustical Society of America, 62*, 693–707.

Hawkes, J. W. (1994). Difference limens for formant patterns of vowel sounds. *Journal of the Acoustical Society of America, 95*, 1074–1084)

Hawkes, J. W., & Miller, J. D. (1995). A formant bandwidth estimation procedure for vowel synthesis. *Journal of the Acoustical Society of America, 97*, 1343–1344.

Hayes, B. (1984). The phonology of rhythm in English. *Linguistic Inquiry, 15*, 33–74.

Hedrick, M. (1997). Effect of acoustic cues on labeling fricatives and affricates. *Journal of Speech, Language, and Hearing Research, 40*, 925–938.

Heinz, J. M., & Stevens, K. N. (1961). On the properties of voiceless fricative consonants. *Journal of the Acoustical Society of America, 33*, 589–596.

Henton, C. G., & Bladon, R. A. W. (1985). Breathiness in normal female speech: Inefficiency versus desirability. *Language & Communication, 5*, 221–227.

Hermes, D. J., & van Gestel, J. C. (1991). The frequency scale of speech intonation. *Journal of the Acoustical Society of America, 90*, 97–102.

Hertegard, S., & Gauffin, J. (1995). Glottal area and vibratory patterns studied with simultaneous stroboscopy, glow glottography, and electroglottography. *Journal of Speech and Hearing Research, 38*, 85–100.

Hess, W. J. (1982). Algorithms and devices for pitch determination of speech signals. *Phonetica, 39*, 219–240.

Hess, W. J. (1992). Pitch and voicing determination. In S. Furui & M. M. Sondhi (Eds.), *Advances in speech signal processing* (pp. 3–48). New York: Marcel Dekker, Inc.

Hillenbrand, J., Clark, M. J., & Houde, R. A. (2000). Some effects of duration on vowel recognition. *Journal of the Acoustical Society of America, 108*, 3013–3022.

Hillenbrand, J., & Gayvert, R. T. (1993). Identification of steady-state vowels synthesized from the Peterson and Barney measurements. *Journal of the Acoustical Society of America, 94*, 668–674.

Hillenbrand, J., Getty, L. A., Clark, M. J., & Wheeler, K. (1995). Acoustic characteristics of American English vowels. *Journal of the Acoustical Society of America, 97*, 3099–3111.

Hillenbrand, J. M., & Houde, R. A. (1996). Role of f_0 and amplitude in the perception of intervocalic glottal stops. *Journal of Speech and Hearing Research, 39*, 1182–1190.

Hirahara, T., & Kato, H. (1992). The effect of F_0 on vowel identification. In Y. Tohkura, E. Vatikiotis-Bateson & Y. Sagisaka (Eds.), *Speech perception, production and linguistic structure* (pp. 89–112). Amsterdam: IOS Press.

Hodge, M. M. (1989). *A comparison of spectral-temporal measures across speaker age: Implications for an acoustic characterization of speech maturation.* Unpublished doctoral dissertation, University of Wisconsin-Madison.

Hoequist, C. (1983). Syllable duration in stress-syllable- and mora-timed languages. *Phonetica, 40,* 203–237.

Hogan, J. T., & Rozsypal, A. J. (1980). Evaluation of vowel duration as a cue for the voicing distinction in the following word-final consonant. *Journal of the Acoustical Society of America, 67,* 1764–1771.

Holbrook, A., & Fairbanks, G. (1962). Diphthong formants and their movements. *Journal of Speech and Hearing Research, 5,* 38–58.

Hollien, H., Green, R., & Massey, K. (1994). Longitudinal research on adolescent voice change in males. *Journal of the Acoustical Society of America, 96,* 2646–2654.

Holmberg, E. B., Hillman, R. E., & Perkell, J. S. (1988). Glottal air flow and pressure measurements for soft, normal and loud voice by male and female speakers. *Journal of the Acoustical Society of America, 84,* 511–529.

Holmes, J. N. (1973). Influence of glottal waveform on the naturalness of speech from a parallel formant synthesizer. *IEEE Transactions on Audio & Electroacoustics, AU-21,* 298–305.

Honda, K. (1983). Relationship between pitch control and vowel articulation. In D. M. Bless & J. H. Abbs (Eds.), *Vocal fold physiology: Contemporary research and clinical issues* (pp. 286–297). San Diego: College-Hill.

Honikman, B. (1964). Articulatory settings. In D. Abercrombie (Ed.), *In honour of Daniel Jones* (pp. 73–84). London: Longmans.

House, A. S. (1960). Formant bandwidths and vowel preference. *Journal of Speech and Hearing Research, 3,* 3–8.

House, A. S. (1961). On vowel duration in English. *Journal of the Acoustical Society of America, 33,* 1174–1178.

House, A. S., & Fairbanks, G. (1953). The influence of consonant environment upon the secondary acoustical characteristics of vowels. *Journal of the Acoustical Society of America, 25,* 105–113.

House, A. S., & Stevens, K. N. (1958). Estimation of formant bandwidths from measurements of the transient response of the vocal tract. *Journal of Speech and Hearing Research, 1,* 309–315.

Howell, P., & Rosen, S. (1983). Production and perception of rise time in the voiceless affricate/fricative distinction. *Journal of the Acoustical Society of America, 73,* 976–984.

Hsu, H. C., Fogel, A., & Cooper, R. B. (2000). Infant vocal development during the first 6 months: Speech quality and melodic complexity. *Infant & Child Development, 9,* 1–16.

Huber, J. E., Stathopoulos, E. T., Curione, G. M., Ash, T. A., & Johnson, K. (1999). Formants of children, women, and men: the effects of vocal intensity variation. *Journal of the Acoustical Society of America, 106,* 1532–1542.

Hughes, G. W., & Halle, M. (1956). Spectral properties of fricative consonants. *Journal of the Acoustical Society of America, 28,* 303–310.

Hustad, K., Kent, R. D., & Beukelman, D. (1998). DECtalk and MacinTalk speech synthesizers: Intelligibility differences for three listener groups. *Journal of Speech, Language, and Hearing Research, 41,* 744–752.

Iivonen, A. (1994). A psychoacoustical explanation for the number of major IPA vowels. *Journal of the International Phonetic Association, 24,* 73–90.

Iivonen, A. (1995). Explaining the dispersion of the single-vowel occurrences in an F_1/F_2 space. *Phonetica, 52,* 221–227.

Ingrisano, D. R.-S., Perry, C. K., & Jepson, K. R. (1998). Environmental noise: A threat to automatic voice analysis. *American Journal of Speech-Language Pathology, 7,* 91–96.

Jassem, W. (1995). The acoustic parameters of Polish voiceless fricatives: An analysis of varaince. *Phonetica, 52,* 251–158.

Jenkins, J. (1987). A selective history of issues in vowel perception. *Journal of Memory & Language, 26,* 542–549.

Jenkins, J. J., Strange, W., & Edman, T. R. (1983). Identification of vowels in "vowelless" syllables. *Perception & Psychophysics, 34,* 441–450.

Johns-Lewis, C. (Ed.) (1986). *Intonation in discourse.* Beckenham, Kent, UK: Croon Helm.

Johnson, C. J., Pick, H. L., Siegel, G. M., Cicciarelli, A. W., & Garber, S. R. (1981). Effects of interpersonal distance on children's vocal intensity. *Child Development, 52,* 721–723.

Johnson, K. (1997). *Acoustic and auditory phonetics.* Cambridge, England: Blackwell.

Jong, K. J. de (1991). *The oral articulation of English stress accent.* Ph.D. dissertation, Ohio State University, Columbus, OH.

Jongman, A., & Blumstein, S. E. (1985). Acoustic properties for dental and alveolar stop consonants: A cross-language study. *Journal of Phonetics, 13*, 235–251.

Jongman, A., Wayland, R., & Wong, S. (2000). Acoustic characteristics of English fricatives. *Journal of the Acoustical Society of America, 108*, 1252–1263.

Joos, M. (1948). Acoustic phonetics. *Language Monographs No. 23, 24* (Suppl.).

Junqua, J. -C. (1993). The Lombard reflex and its role on human listeners and automatic speech recognizers. *Journal of the Acoustical Society of America, 93*, 510–524.

Kataoka, R., Michi, K., Okabe, K., Miura, T., & Yoshida, H. (1996). Spectral properties and quantitative evaluation of hypernasality in vowels. *Cleft Palate-Craniofacial Journal, 33*, 43–50.

Keating, P. A. (1990). The window model of coarticulation: Articulatory evidence. In J. Kingston & M. E. Beckman (Eds.), *Papers in laboratory phonology I. Between the grammar and physics of speech* (pp. 451–470). Cambridge, England: Cambridge University Press.

Kelly, M. H., & Bock, J. K. (1988). Stress in time. *Journal of Experimental Psychology: Human Perception and Performance, 14*, 389 403.

Kent (1995). *The speech sciences*. San Diego: Singular Publishing Group, Inc.

Kent, R. D. (1976). Anatomical and neuromuscular maturation of the speech mechanism: Evidence from acoustic studies. *Journal of Speech and Hearing Research, 19*, 421–447.

Kent, R. D., Adams, S. G., & Turner, G. (1996). Models of speech production. In N. J. Lass (Ed.) *Principles of experimental phonetics* (pp. 3–45) St. Louis: Mosby.

Kent, R. D., Atal, B. S., & Miller, J. L. (Eds.) (in press). *Papers in Speech Communication: Speech Production.* Woodbury, NY: Acoustical Society of America.

Kent, R. D., & Ball, M. J. (Eds.) (2000). *Voice quality measurement*. San Diego: Singular/ Thomson Learning.

Kent, R. D., & Bauer, H. R. (1985). Vocalizations of one-year-olds. *Journal of Child Language, 12*, 491–526.

Kent, R. D., & Burkhard, R. (1981). Changes in the acoustic correlates of speech production. In D. S. Beasley. & G. A. Davis (Eds.), *Aging: Communication processes and disorders* (pp. 47–62). New York: Grune & Stratton.

Kent, R. D., & Chial, M. R. (1997). Talker identification. In D. L. Faigman, D. Kaye, M. J. Saks & J. Sanders (Eds.), *Modern scientific evidence: The law and science of expert testi-*mony (pp. 195–224). St. Paul, MN: West Publishing Co.

Kent, R. D., & Forner, L. L. (1980). Speech segment durations in sentence recitations by children and adults. *Journal of Phonetics, 8*, 157–168.

Kent, R. D., Liss, J., & Philips, B. J. (1989). Acoustic analysis of velopharngeal dysfunction in speech. In K. Bzoch (Ed.), *Communicative disorders related to cleft lip and palate,* (Rev. ed.) (pp. 258–270). Boston: Little-Brown.

Kent, R. D., & Murray, A. D. (1982). Acoustic features of infant vocalic utterances. *Journal of the Acoustical Society of America, 72*, 353–365.

Kent, R. D., & Netsell, R. (1971). Effects of stress contrasts on certain articulatory parameters. *Phonetica, 24*, 23–44.

Kent, R. D., & Rosenbek, J. C. (1983). Acoustic patterns of apraxia of speech. *Journal of Speech and Hearing Research, 26*, 231–249.

Kent, R. D., Weismer, G., Kent, J. F., Vorperian, H. K., & Duffy, J. R. (1999). Acoustic studies of dysarthria. *Journal of Communication Disorders, 32*, 141–186.

Kewley-Port, D. (1983a). Time-varying features as correlates of place of articulation in stop consonants. *Journal of the Acoustical Society of America, 73*, 322–335.

Kewley-Port, D. (1983b). Measurement of formant transitions in naturally produced stop consonant-vowel syllables. *Journal of the Acoustical Society of America, 72*, 379–389.

Kewley-Port, D. (1990). Thresholds for formant-frequency discrimination in isolated vowels. *Journal of the Acoustical Society of America, 87* (Suppl. 1), S159.

Kewley-Port, D., & Watson, C. S. (1994). Formant-frequency discrimination for isolated English vowels. *Journal of the Acoustical Society of America, 95*, 485–496.

Kewley-Port, D., & Zheng, Y. J. (1999). Vowel formant discrimination: Towards more ordinary listening conditions. *Journal of the Acoustical Society of America, 106*, 2945–2958.

Khan, I., Gupta, S. K., & Rizvi, H. S. (1994). Formant frequencies of Hindi vowels in /hVd/ and C_1VC_2 contexts. *Journal of the Acoustical Society of America, 96*, 2580–2582.

Klatt, D. H. (1974). Duration of [s] in English words. *Journal of Speech and Hearing Research, 17*, 41–50.

Klatt, D. H. (1975a). Voice onset time, frication and aspiration in word-initial consonant clusters. *Journal of Speech and Hearing Research, 18,* 686–706.

Klatt, D. H. (1975b). Vowel lengthening is syntactically determined in a connected discourse. *Journal of Phonetics, 3,* 129–140.

Klatt, D. H. (1976). Linguistic uses of segmental duration in English: Acoustic and perceptual evidence. *Journal of the Acoustical Society of America, 59,* 1208–1221.

Klatt, D. H. (1979). *Synthesis by rule of consonant-vowel syllables* (Speech Communucation Group Working Papers No. 3, pp. 93–105). Cambridge, MA: MIT Press.

Klatt, D. H. (1980). Software for a cascade/parallel formant synthesizer. *Journal of the Acoustical Society of America, 67,* 971–995.

Klatt, D. H. (1987). Review of text-to-speech conversion for English. *Journal of the Acoustical Society of America, 82,* 737–793.

Klatt, D. H., & Klatt, L. C. (1990). Analysis, synthesis, and perception of voice quality variations among female and male talkers. *Journal of the Acoustical Society of America, 87,* 820–857.

Kluender, K. R., & Walsh, M. A. (1992). Amplitude rise time and the perception of the voiceless affricate/fricative distinction. *Perception and Psychophysics, 51,* 328–333.

Koenig, W. (1949). A new frequency scale for acoustic measurements. *Bell Laboratories Record, 27,* 299–301.

Koenig, W., Dunn, H. K., & Lacy, L. Y. (1946). The sound spectrograph. *The Journal of the Acoustical Society of America, 17,* 19–49. (Reprinted in R. J. Baken & R. G. Daniloff (Eds.), *Readings in clinical spectrography of speech.* San Diego: Singular Publishing Group.)

Krull, D., & Lindblom, B. (1992). Comparing vowel formant data cross-linguistically. PERILUS (Phonetic Experimental Research, Institute of Linguistics, University of Stockholm, Stockholm, Sweden), No. XV, pp. 7–15.

Kuhl, P. K., & Meltzoff, A. N. (1996). Infant vocalizations in response to speech: Vocal imitation and developmental change. *Journal of the Acoustical Society of America, 100,* 2425–2438.

Kuijk, D. van, & Boves, L. (1999). Acoustic characteristics of lexical stress in continuous telephone speech. *Speech Communication, 27,* 95–111.

Kurowski, K., & Blumstein, S. E. (1984). Perceptual integration of the murmur and formant transitions for place of articulation in nasal consonants. *Journal of the Acoustical Society of America, 76,* 383–390.

Ladefoged, P. (1975). *A course in phonetics.* New York: Harcourt, Brace & Jovanovich.

Ladefoged, P. (1993). *A course in phonetics.* New York: Harcourt, Brace & Jovanovich.

Ladefoged, P., & Maddieson, I. (1986). Some of the sounds of the world's languages. University of California Working Papers in Phonetics, 64 (Linguistics Department, University of California at Los Angeles).

Lahiri, A., Gewirth, L., & Blumstein, S. E. (1984). A reconsideration of acoustic invariance for place of articulation in diffuse stop consonants: Evidence from a cross-language study. *Journal of the Acoustical Society of America, 76,* 391–404.

Landahl, K. H. (1980). Language-universal aspects of intonation to children's first sentences. *Journal of the Acoustical Society of America, 67,* (Suppl. 1), S63.

Lang, G. F. (1987). Bits, bytes, baud, Bell and bull. *Sound & Vibration, 21,* 10–14.

LaRiviere, C., Winitz, H., & Herriman, E. (1975). The distribution of perceptual cues in English prevocalic fricatives. *Journal of Speech and Hearing Research, 18,* 613–622.

Laufer, A. (1975). A programme for synthesizing Hebrew speech. *Phonetica, 32,* 292–299.

Laufer, A., & Baer, T. (1988). The emphatic and pharyngeal sounds in Hebrew and Arabic. *Language & Speech, 31,* 181–208.

Lee, S., Potamianos, A., & Narayanan, S. (1999). Acoustics of children's speech: Developmental changes of temporal and spectral parameters. *Journal of the Acoustical Society of America, 105,* 1455–1468.

Leek, M. R. (1995, November). Will a good disc last? *CD-ROM Professional, 8,* 102–110.

Lehiste, I. (1964). Acoustical characteristics of selected English consonants. International *Journal of American Linguistics, 30,* No. 3, 181–223.

Lehiste, I. (1970). *Suprasegmentals.* Cambridge, MA: MIT Press.

Lehiste, I. (1972). The timing of utterances and linguistic boundaries. *Journal of the Acoustical Society of America, 51,* 2018–2024

Lehiste, I., & Peterson, G. E. (1961). Transitions, glides, and diphthongs. *Journal of the Acoustical Society of America, 33,* 268–277.

Lehman, M. E., & Swartz, B. (2000). Electropalatographic and spectrographic descriptions of allophonic variants of /l/. *Perceptual & Motor Skills, 90*, 47–61.

Leinonen, L., Hiltunen, T., Linnankoski, I., & Laakso, M. L. (1997). Expression of emotional-motivational connotations with a one-word utterance. *Journal of the Acoustical Society of America, 102*, 1853–1863.

Lewis, D. (1936). Vocal resonance. *Journal of the Acoustical Society of America, 8*, 91–99.

Liberman, A. M., Cooper, F. S., Shankweiler, D. S., & Studdert-Kennedy, M. (1967). Perception of the speech code. *Psychological Review, 74*, 431–461.

Liberman, A. M., Delattre, P. C., & Cooper, F. S. (1952). The role of selected stimulus variables in the perception of unvoiced stop consonants. *American Journal of Psychology, 65*, 497–516.

Liberman, A. M., Delattre, P. C., Cooper, F. S., & Gerstman, L. J. (1954). The role of consonant-vowel transitions in the perception of the stop and nasal consonants. *Psychological Monographs, 68*, 1–13.

Liberman, A. M., Delattre, P. C., Cooper, F. S., & Gerstman, L. J. (1956). Tempo of frequency change as a cue for distinguishing classes of speech sounds. *Journal of Experimental Psychology, 52*, 127–137.

Lieberman, P. (1967). *Intonation, perception and language.* Cambridge, MA: MIT Press.

Lieberman, P., Katz, W., Jongman, A., Zimmerman, R., & Miller, M. (1985). Measures of the sentence intonation of read and spontaneous speech in American English. *Journal of the Acoustical Society of America, 77*, 649–657.

Lieberman, P., & Tseng, C. Y. (1981). On the fall of the declination theory: Breath-group versus "declination" as the base form for intonation. *Journal of the Acoustical Society of America, 67*, (Suppl.), S63.

Lienard, J. S., & DiBenedetto, M. G. (1999). Effect of vocal effort on spectral properties of vowels. *Journal of the Acoustical Society of America, 106*, 411–422.

Liljencrants, J. (1971). A Fourier series description of the tongue profile. *Speech Transmission Laboratory (Stockholm) Quarterly Progress and Status Reports, 4*, 9-18.

Lindblom, B. E. F. (1963). Spectrographic study of vowel reduction. *Journal of the Acoustical Society of America, 35*, 1773–1781.

Lindblom, B. (1990). Explaining phonetic variation: A sketch of the H&H theory. In W. J. Hardcastle & A. Marchal (Eds.), *Speech production and speech modelling* (pp. 403–439). Amsterdam: Kluwer.

Lindblom, B. E. F., Lubker, J., & Pauli, S. (1977). An acoustic-perceptual method for the quantitative evaluation of hypernasality. *Journal of Speech and Hearing Research, 20*, 485–496.

Lindblom, B. E. F., & Sundberg, J. (1971). Acoustical consequences of lip, tongue, jaw and larynx movement. *Journal of the Acoustical Society of America, 50*, 1166–1179.

Lindqvist, J., & Sundberg, J. (1972). Acoustic properties of the nasal tract. *Phonetica, 33*, 161–168.

Linville, S. E. (1996). The sound of senescence. *Journal of Voice, 10*, 190–200.

Linville, S. E. (2000). The aging voice. In R. D. Kent & M. J. Ball (Eds.), *Voice quality measurement* (pp. 359–376). San Diego: Singular Publishing Group.

Linville, S. E., & Fisher, H. B. (1985). Acoustic characteristics of women's voices with advancing age. *Journal of Gerontology, 40*, 324–330.

Lisker, L. (1957). Minimal cues for separating /w,r,l,j/ in intervocalic position. *Word, 13*, 257–267.

Lisker, L. (1978). Rapid vs. rabid: A catalogue of acoustic features that may cue the distinction. *Status Report on Speech Research*, SR-54, pp. 127–132. Haskins Laboratories, New Haven, CT.

Lisker, L., & Abramson, A. S. (1964). A cross-language study of voicing in initial stops: Acoustical measurements. *Word, 20*, 384–422.

Lisker, L., & Abramson, A. (1971). Distinctive features and laryngeal control. *Language, 47*, 767–785.

Lofqvist, A. (1999). Interarticulator phasing, locus equations, and degree of coarticulation. *Journal of the Acoustical Society of America, 106*, 2022–2030.

Logan, J. S., Greene, B. G., & Pisoni, D. B. (1989). Segmental intelligibility of synthetic speech produced by rule. *Journal of the Acoustical Society of America, 86*, 566–581.

Louth, S. M., Williamson, S., Alpert, M., Pouget, E. R. & Hare, R. D. (1998). Acoustic distinctions in the speech of male psychopaths. *Journal of Psycholinguistics Research, 27*, 375–384.

Lubker, J. F. (1979). Acoustic-perceptual methods for evaluation of defective speech. In Lass, N.J. (Ed.), *Speech and language: Advances in basic research and practice*, Vol. 1, (pp. 49–87). New York: Academic.

Maddieson, I. (1984). *Patterns of sounds. Cambridge studies in speech and communication*. Cambridge, England: Cambridge University Press.

Maeda, S. (1976). *A characterization of American English intonation*. Cambridge, MA: MIT Press.

Maeda, S. (1990). Compensatory articulation during speech: Evidence from the analysis and synthesis of vocal-tract shapes using an articulatory model. In W. J. Hardcastle & A. Marchal (Eds.), *Speech production and speech modelling* (pp. 131–149). Dordrecht, The Netherlands: Kluwer.

Magan, H. S. (1997). The extent of vowel-to-vowel coarticulation in English. *Journal of Phonetics, 25*, 187–205.

Makhoul, J. (1975). Linear prediction: A tutorial review. *Proceedings of the IEEE, 63*, 561–580.

Malecot, A. (1956). Acoustic cues for nasal consonants: An experimental study involving a tape-splicing technique. *Language, 32*, 274–284.

Mandelbrot, B. B. (1982). *The fractal geometry of nature*. San Francisco: W. H. Freeman.

Manrique, A. M. B. de (1979). Acoustic study of /i, u/ in the Spanish diphthongs. *Phonetica, 36*, 194–206.

Manrique, A. M. B., & Massone, M. I. (1981). Acoustic analysis and perception of Spanish fricative consonants. *Journal of the Acoustical Society of America, 69*, 1145–1153.

Markel, N. N., Prebor, L. D., & Brandt, J. F. (1972). Biosocial factors in dyadic communication: Sex and speaking intensity. *Journal of Personality and Social Psychology, 23*, 11–13.

Matthei, E., & Roeper, T. (1983). *Understanding and producing speech*. Bungay, Suffolk, England: Chaucer Press.

McCasland, G. (1979). Noise intensity and spectrum cues of spoken fricatives. *Journal of the Acoustical Society of America, 65* (Suppl. 1), S78-S79.

Mendoza, E., Valencia, N., Munoz, J., & Trujillo, H. (1996). Differences in voice quality between men and women[rm]use of the long-term average spectrum (LTAS). *Journal of Voice, 10*, 59–66.

Mermelstein, P. (1973). Articulatory model for the study of speech production. *Journal of the Acoustical Society of America, 53*, 1070–1082.

Mermelstein, P. (1978). Difference limens for formant frequencieas of steady-state and consonant-bound vowels. *Journal of the Acoustical Society of America, 63*, 572–580.

Michael, D. D., Siegel, G. M., & Pick, H. L., Jr. (1995). Effects of distance on vocal intensity. *Journal of Speech and Hearing Research, 38*, 1176–1183.

Michelsson, K., & Michelsson, O. (1999). Phonation in the newborn, infant cry. *International Journal of Pediatric Otorhinolaryngology, 49*, S297–S301.

Miller, J. D. (1989). Auditory-perceptual interpretation of the vowel. *Journal of the Acoustical Society of America, 85*, 2114–2134.

Miller, J. L., & Baer, T. (1983). Some effects of speaking rate on the production of /b/ and /w/. *Journal of the Acoustical Society, 73*, 1751–1755.

Miller, J. L., & Liberman, A. M. (1979). Some effects of later-occurring information on the perception of stop consonant and semivowel. *Perception & Psychophysics, 25*, 457–465.

Miner, R., & Danhauer, J. L. (1977). Relation between formant frequencies and optimal octaves in vowel perception. *Journal of the American Audiology Society, 2*, 162–168.

Mines, M., Hansen, B., & Shoup, J. (1978). Frequency of occurrence of phonemes in conversational English. *Language & Speech, 21*, 221–241.

Miyazaki, S., Itasaka, Y., Ishikawa, K., & Togawa, K. (1998). Acoustic analysis of snoring and the site of airway obstruction in sleep related respiratory disorders. *Acta Oto-Laryngologica, 537*, (Suppl.) 47–51.

Monsen, R. B., & Engebretson, A. M. (1983). The accuracy of formant frequency measurements: A comparison of spectrographic analysis and linear prediction. *Journal of Speech and Hearing Research, 26*, 89–97.

Moon, S. J., & Lindblom, B. (1989). Formant undershoot in clear and citation-form speech: A second progress report. *Speech Transmission Laboratory, Quarterly Progress and Status Reports, 1/1989*, 121–123.

Moore, H. C. J., & Glasberg, H. R. (1983). Suggested formulae for calculating auditory-filter bandwidths and excitation patterns. *Journal of the Acoustical Society of America, 74*, 750–753.

Munro, M. J., Flege, J. E., & MacKay, I. A. (1996). The effects of age of second language learning on the production of English vowels. *Applied Psycholinguistics, 17,* 313–334.

Murray, I. R., & Arnott, J. L. (1993). Toward the simulation of emotion in synthetic speech: A review of the literature on human vocal emotion. *Journal of the Acoustical Society of America, 93,* 1097–1108.

Nakagawa, T., Saito, S., & Yoshino, T. (1982). Tonal difference limens for second formant frequencies of synthesized Japanese vowels. *Annual Bulletin Royal Institute of Logopedics and Phoniatrics (Tokyo),* No. 16, pp. 81–88.

Nakatani, L. H., O'Connor, K. D., & Aston, C. H. (1981). Prosodic aspects of American English speech rhythm. *Phonetica, 38,* 84–106.

Narayanan, S. S., & Alwan, A. A. (1995). A nonlinear dynamical systems analysis of fricative consonants. *Journal of the Acoustical Society of America, 97,* 2511–2524.

Narayanan, S., & Alwan, A. (2000). Noise source models for fricative consonants. *IEEE Transactions on Speech & Audio Processing, 8,* 328–344.

Narayanan, S., Alwan, A. A., & Haker, K. (1997). Toward articulatory-acoustic models for liquid approximants based on MRI and EPG data. Part I. The laterals. *Journal of the Acoustical Society of America, 101,* 1064–1077.

Nartey, J. N. A. (1982). On fricative phones and phonemes: Measuring the phonetic differences within and between languages. *UCLA Working Papers in Phonetics,* No. 55, Department of Linguistics, University of California at Los Angeles.

Nawka, T., Anders, L. C., Cebulla, M., & Zurakowski, D. (1997). The speaker's formant in male voices. *Journal of Voice, 11,* 422–428.

Nearey, T. M. (1989). Static, dynamic, and relational properties in vowel perception. *Journal of the Acoustical Society of America, 85,* 2088–2113.

Nearey, T. M. (1992). Context effects in a double-weak theory of speech perception. *Language and Speech, 35,* 153–171.

Neuhoff, J. G., McBeath, M. K., & Wanzie, W. C. (1999). Dynamic frequency change influences loudness perception: A central, analytic process. *Journal of Experimental Psychology: Human Perception & Performance, 25,* 1050–1059.

Nittrouer, S. (1993). The emergence of mature gestural patterns is not uniform: Evidence from an acoustic study. *Journal of Speech and Hearing Research, 36,* 959–972.

Nittrouer, S. (1995). Children learn separate aspects of speech production at different rates: Evidence from spectral moments. *Journal of the Acoustical Society of America, 97,* 520–530.

Nittrouer, S., & Studdert-Kennedy, M. (1986). The stop-glide distinction: Acoustic analysis and perceptual effect of variation in syllable amplitude envelope for initial /b/ and /w/. *Journal of the Acoustical Society of America, 80,* 1026–1029.

Nittrouer, S. K., Studdert-Kennedy, M., & McGowen, R. S. (1989). The emergence of phonetic segments: Evidence from the spectral structure of fricative-vowel syllables spoken by children and adults. *Journal of Speech and Hearing Research, 32,* 120–132.

Noll, A. M. (1967). Cepstrum pitch determination. *Journal of the Acoustical Society of America, 41,* 293–309.

Nolan, F. (1983). *The phonetic bases of speaker recognition.* Cambridge, U.K.: Cambridge University Press.

Nooteboom, S. (1997). The prosody of speech: Melody and rhythm. In W. J. Hardcastle & J. Laver (Eds.), *The handbook of phonetic sciences* (pp. 641–673). Oxford, England: Blackwell.

Nord, L., & Sventelious, E. (1979). Analysis and prediction of difference limen data for formant frequencies. *Quarterly Progress Status Report,* No.3–4, Stockholm, Sweden: Speech Transmission Laboratory, Royal Institute of Technology, pp. 60–72.

Nyquist, H. (1928). Certain topics in telegraph transmission theory. *Transactions in Audio, Industrial & Electrical Engineering,* April.

O'Connor, J. D., Gerstman, L. J., Liberman, A. M., Delattre, P. C., & Cooper, F. S. (1957). Acoustic cues for the perception of initial /w, j, r, l/ in English. *Word, 13,* 24–43.

O'Connor, J. D., & Trim, J. L. M. (1953). Vowel, consonant, and syllable: A phonological definition. *Word, 9,* 103–122.

Ohde, R. N., & Sharf, D. J. (1977). Order effect of acoustic segments of VC and CV syllables on stop and vowel identification. *Journal of Speech and Hearing Research, 20,* 543–554.

Ohde, R. N., & Stevens, K. N. (1983). Effect of burst amplitude on the perception of the stop consonant place of articulation. *Journal of the Acoustical Society of America, 74,* 706–714.

Oller, D. K. (1973). The effect of position in utterance on speech segment duration in English. *Journal of the Acoustical Society of America, 54,* 1235–1247.

Oller, D. K. (1986). Metaphonology and infant vocalizations. In B. Lindblom & R. Zetterstrom (Eds.), *Early precursors of speech* (pp. 21–35). Basingstoke: Macmillan.

Oller, D. K. (2000). *The emergence of the speech capacity.* Mahwah, NJ: Lawrence Erlbaum Associates.

Olsson, N., Juslin, P., & Winman, A. (1998). realism of confidence in earwitneess versus eyewitness identification. *Journal of Experimental Psychology: Applied, 4,* 101–118.

Ouellette, J. (1999). The incredible shrinking microphone. *The Industrial Physicist, 5,* 7–9.

Paliwal, K. K., Lindsay, D, & Ainsworth, W. A. (1983). A study of two-formant models for vowel identification. *Speech Communication, 2,* 295–303.

Parsa, V., & Jamieson, D. G. (1999). A comparison of high precision F0 extraction algorithms for sustained vowels. *Journal of Speech, Language, and Hearing Research, 42,* 112–126.

Patterson, R. D. (1976). Auditory filter shapes derived with noise stimuli. *Journal of the Acoustical Society of America, 59,* 640–654.

Paul, D., & Baker, J. (1992). The design for the Wall Street Journal-based CSR corpus. *DARPA Speech and Natural Language Workshop.* New York: Arden House.

Penz, A., & Gilbert, H. (1983). *Comparisons of formants in preadolescent children's vowel productions.* Paper presented in a poster session at the 1983 Annual Convention of the American Speech-Language-Hearing Association.

Peters, H. F. M., Boves, L., & I. C. H. van Dielen (1986). Perceptual judgment of abruptness of voice onset in vowels as a function of the amplitude envelope. *Journal of Speech and Hearing Research, 51,* 299–308.

Peterson, G. E., & Barney, H. E. (1952). Control methods used in a study of vowels. *Journal of the Acoustical Society of America, 24,* 175–184.

Peterson, G. E., & Lehiste, I. (1960). Duration of syllable nuclei in English. *Journal of the Acoustical Society of America, 32,* 693–703.

Peturrson, M. (1972). Peut-on interpreter les donnees de la radiocinematographie en function du tube acoustique a section uniforme? *Travaux de l'Institut de Phonetique de Strasbourg,* No. 4.

Picheny, M. A., Durlach, N. I., & Braida, L. D. (1985). Speaking clearly for the hard of hearing I: Intelligibility differences between clear and conversational speech. *Journal of Speech and Hearing Research, 28,* 96–103.

Picheny, M. A., Durlach, N. I., & Braida, L. D. (1986). Speaking clearly for the hard of hearing II: Acoustic characteristics of clear and conversational speech. *Journal of Speech and Hearing Research, 29,* 434–446.

Picheny, M. A., Durlach, N. I., & Braida, L. D. (1989). Speaking clearly for the hard of hearing III: An attempt to determine the contribution of speaking rate to difference in intelligibility between clear and conversational speech. *Journal of Speech and Hearing Research, 32,* 600–603.

Pickett, J. (1999). Acoustics of speech communication. Boston: Allyn & Bacon.

Piir, H. (1983). Acoustics of the Estonian diphthongs. *Estonian Papers in Phonetics, 82–83,* Tallinn, 5–96.

Pijper, J. R. de, & Sanderman, A. A. (1994). On the perceptual strength of prosodic boundaries and its relation to suprasegmental cues. *Journal of the Acoustical Society of America, 96,* 2037–2047.

Pirello, K., Blumstein, S. E., & Kurowski, K. (1997). The characteristics of voicing in syllable-initial fricatives in American English. *Journal of the Acoustical Society of America, 101,* 3754–3765.

Plante, F., Berger-Vachon, C., & Kauffman, I. (1993). Acoustic discrimination of velar impairment in children. *Folia Phoniatrica, 45,* 112–119.

Polka, L., & Strange, W. (1985). Perceptual equivalence of acoustic cues that differentiate /r/ and /l/. *Journal of the Acoustical Society of America, 78,* 1187–1206.

Pols, L. C. W., Tromp, H. R. C., & Plomp, R. (1973). Frequency analysis of Dutch vowels from 50 male speakers. *Journal of the Acoustical Society of America, 53,* 1093–1101.

Port, R. F., & Dalby, J. (1982). Consonant/vowel ratio as a cue for voicing in English. *Perception & Psychophysics, 32,* 141–152.

Potter, R., Kopp, G., & Green, H. (1947). *Visible speech.* New York: Van Nostrand Reinhold Co. (Reprinted in 1966 by Dover Press, New York).

Price, P.J. (1989). Male and female voice source characteristics: Inverse filtering results. *Speech Communication, 8,* 261–278.

Qi, Y., & Fox, R. A. (1992). Analysis of nasal consonants using perceptual linear prediction. *Journal of the Acoustical Society of America, 91,* 1718–1726.

Rakerd, B., & Verbrugge, R. R. (1985). Linguistic and acoustic correlates of the perceptual structure found in an individual differences scaling study of vowels. *Journal of the Acoustical Society of America, 77,* 296–301.

Ramus, F., Nespor, M., & Mehler, J. (1999). Correlates of linguistic rhythm in the speech signal. *Cognition, 73,* 265–292.

Raphael, L. (1972). Preceding vowel duration as a cue to the perception of the voicing characteristic of word-final consonants in English. *Journal of the Acoustical Society of America, 51,* 1296–1303.

Rastatter, M., & Jacques, R. (1990). Formant frequency structure of the aging male and female vocal tract. *Folia Phoniatrica, 42,* 312–319.

Read, C., Buder, E. H., & Kent, R. D. (1990). Speech analysis systems: A survey. *Journal of Speech and Hearing Research, 33,* 363–374.

Read, C., Buder, E. H., & Kent, R. D. (1992). Speech analysis systems: An evaluation. *Journal of Speech and Hearing Research, 35,* 314–332.

Read, C., & Schreiber, P. A. (1982). Why short subjects are harder to find than long ones. In E. Wanner & L. Gleitman (Eds.), *Language acquisition: The state of the art.* Cambridge, UK: Cambridge University Press.

Remez, R. E., Rubin, P. E., & Pisoni, D. B. (1983). Coding of the speech spectrum in three time-varying sinusoids. *Annals of the New York Academy of Sciences, 405,* 485–489.

Remez, R. E., Rubin, P. E., Pisoni, D. B., & Carrell, T. D. (1981).Speech perception without traditional speech cues. *Science, 212,* 947–950.

Ren, H. (1986). *On the acoustic structure of diphthongal syllables.* Unpublished Ph.D. dissertation, University of California at Los Angeles.

Repp, B. H., & Svastikula, K. (1988). Perception of the [m]-[n] distinction in VC syllables. *Journal of the Acoustical Society of America, 83,* 237–247

Revoile, S., Pickett, J. M., Holden, L. D., & Talkin, D. (1982). Acoustic cues to final stop voicing for impaired- and normal hearing listeners. *Journal of the Acoustical Society of America, 72,* 1145–1154.

Robb, M. P., & Cacace, A. T. (1995). Estimation of formant frequencies in infant cry. *International Journal of Pediatric Otorhinolaryngology, 32,* 57–67.

Robb, M. P., Chen, Y., & Gilbert, H. R. (1997). Developmental aspects of formant frequency and bandwidth in infants and toddlers. *Folia Phoniatrica et Logopaedica, 49,* 88–95.

Robb, M. P., Saxman, J. H., & Grant, A .A. (1989). Vocal fundamental frequency characteristics during the first two years of life. *Journal of the Acoustical Society of America, 85,* 1708–1717.

Robb, M. P., & Saxman, J. H. (1988). Acoustic observations in young children's non-cry vocalizations. *Journal of the Acoustical Society of America, 83,* 1876–1882.

Rostolland, D. (1982). Acoustic features of shouted voice. *Acustica, 51,* 80–89.

Rubin, P., Baer, T., & Mermelstein, P. (1981). An articulatory synthesizer for perceptual research. *Journal of the Acoustical Society of America, 70,* 321–328.

Sabanal, S., & Nakagawa, M. (1996). The fractal properties of vocal sounds and their application in the speech recognition model. *Chaos Solutions & Fractals, 7,* 1825–1843.

Schulman, R. (1989). Articulatory dynamics of loud and normal speech. *Journal of the Acoustical Society of America, 85,* 295–312.

Schwartz, J.-L., Hoe, L.-J., Vallee, N., & Abry, C. (1997). Major trends in vowel system inventories. *Journal of Phonetics, 25,* 233–253.

Schwartz, M. F. (1970). Duration of /s/ in /s/-plosive blends. *Journal of the Acoustical Society of America, 47,* 1143–1144.

Selkirk, E. (1984). *Phonology and syntax: The relation between sound and structure.* Cambridge, MA: MIT Press.

Shadle, C. H. (1990). Articulatory-acoustic relationships in fricative consonants. In W. J. Hardcastle & A. Marchal (Eds.), *Speech production and speech modelling* (pp. 187–209). Dordrecht, Netherlands: Kluwer.

Sharf, D. J., & Ohde, R. N. (1981). Physiologic, acoustic and perceptual aspects of coarticulation: Implications for the remediation of articulatory disorders. In N. J. Lass (Ed,), *Speech and language: Advances in basic research and practice* (Vol. 5, pp. 153–247). New York: Academic Press.

Shinn, P. (1984). *A cross-language investigation of the stop, affricate and fricative manner of articulation.* Ph.D. dissertation, Brown University, Providence, RI.

Shinn, P. C., & Blumstein, S. E. (1984). On the role of the amplitude envelope for the perception of [b] and [w]: Further support for a theory of acoustic invariance. *Journal of the Acoustical Society of America, 75,* 1243–1252.

Shriberg, L. D., & Kent, R. D. (1982). *Clinical phonetics*. New York: Wiley.

Slis, I. H. & Cohen, A. (1969). On the complex regulating the voiced-vocieless distinction. I. *Language & Speech, 1*, 80–102.

Sluijter, A. M. C., & van Heuven, V. J. (1996). Spectral balance as an acoustic correlate of linguistic stress. *Journal of the Acoustical Society of America, 100*, 2471–2485.

Sluijter, A. M. C., van Heuven, V. J., & Pacilly, J. J. A. (1997). Spectral balance as a cue in the perception of linguistic stress. *Journal of the Acoustical Society of America, 101*, 503–513.

Smith, B. L., Hillenbrand, J., & Ingrisano, D. (1986). A comparison of temporal measures of speech using spectrograms and digital oscillograms. *Journal of Speech and Hearing Research, 29*, 270–274.

Smits, R., ten Bosch, L., & Collier, R. (1996). Evaluation of various sets of acoustic cues for the perception of prevocalic stop consonants. I. Perception experiment. *Journal of the Acoustical Society of America, 100*, 3852–3864.

Sobin, C., & Alpert, M. (1999). Emotion in speech: The acoustic attributes of fear, anger, sadness, and joy. *Journal of Psycholinguistic Research, 28*, 347–365.

Son, R. J. J. H. van, & Pols, L. C. W. (1999). Perisegmental speech improves consonant and vowel identification. *Speech Communication, 29*, 1–22.

Sondhi, M. M. (1986). Resonances of a bent vocal tract. *Journal of the Acoustical Society of America, 79*, 1113–1116.

Sorensen, J. M., & Cooper, W. E. (1980). Syntactic coding of fundamental frequency in speech production. In R. A. Cole (Ed.), *Perception and production of fluent speech* (pp. 399–440). Hillsdale, NJ: Lawrence Erlbaum.

Speliotis, D. E., & Peter, K. J. (1991). Corrosion study of metal particle, metal film, and BΛ-ferrite tape. *IEEE Transactions on Magnetics, 27*, 4724–4726.

Stetson, R. H. (1928). *Motor Phonetics. Archives Neerlandaises de Phonetique Experimental, 3.* (2nd Ed.). Amsterdam: North-Holland Publishing (1951). (Reprinted in J. A. S. Kelso & K. G. Munhall [Eds.], *R.H. Stetson's motor phonetics: A retrospective edition*. Boston: Little-Brown [1988].)

Stevens, K. N. (1989). On the quantal nature of speech. *Journal of Phonetics, 17*, 3–45.

Stevens, K. N. (1998). *Acoustic phonetics*. Cambridge, MA: MIT Press.

Stevens, K. N., & Blumstein, S. E. (1975). Quantal aspects of consonant production and perception: A study of retroflex stop consonants. *Journal of Phonetics, 3*, 215–233.

Stevens, K. N., & Blumstein, S. E. (1978). Invariant cues for the place of articulation in stop consonants. *Journal of the Acoustical Society of America, 64*, 1358–1368.

Stevens, K. N., & Blumstein, S. E. (1981). The search for invariant acoustic correlates of phonetic features. In P. Eimas & J. Miller (Eds.), *Perspectives in the Study of Speech* (pp. 1–38). Hillsdale, NJ: Erlbaum.

Stevens, K. N., & House, A. S. (1955). Development of a quantitative description of vowel articulation. *Journal of the Acoustical Society of America, 27*, 484–493.

Stevens, K. N., & House, A. S. (1956). Studies of formant transitions using a vocal tract analog. *Journal of the Acoustical Society of America, 28*, 578–585.

Stevens, K. N., & House, A. S. (1961). An acoustical theory of vowel production and some of its implications. *Journal of Speech and Hearing Research, 4*, 303–320.

Strang, G. (1994)/May–June). Wavelets. *American Scientist, 82*, 250–255.

Strange, W. (1987). Evolving theories of vowel perception. *Journal of the Acoustical Society of America, 85*, 2081–2087.

Strevens, P. (1960). Spectra of fricative noise in human speech. *Language & Speech, 3*, 32–49.

Summers, W. V. (1988). F1 structure provides information for final-consonant voicing. *Journal of the Acoustical Society of America, 84*, 485–492.

Sundberg, J. (1974). Articulatory interpretation of the singing formants. *Journal of the Acoustical Society of America, 55*, 838–844.

Sundberg, J. (1977). The acoustics of the singing voice. *Scientific American, 236*, 81–91.

Sundberg, J. (1987). *The science of the singing voice*. DeKalb, IL: Northern Illinois University Press.

Sundberg, J. (1991). *The science of musical sounds*. New York: Academic Press.

Sussman, H. M., Fruchter, D., & Cable, A. (1995). Locus equations derived from compensatory articulation. *Journal of the Acoustical Society of America, 97*, 3112–3124.

Sussman, H. M., Fruchter, D., Hilbert, J., & Sirosh J. (1998). Human speech—a tinkerer's delight- response. *Behavioral and Brain Sciences, 21*, 287–299.

Sussman, H. M., Hoemeke, K. A., & Ahmed, F. S. (1993). A cross-linguistic investigation of locus equations as a phonetic descriptor for place of articulation. *Journal of the Acoustical Society of America, 94*, 1256–1268.

Sussman, H. M., Hoemeke, K. A., & McCaffrey, H. A. (1992). Locus equations as an index of coarticulation for place of articulation distinctions in children. *Journal of Speech and Hearing Research, 35*, 769–781.

Sussman, H. J., McCaffrey, H. A., & Matthews, S. A. (1991). An investigation of locus equations as a source of relational invariance for stop place categorization. *Journal of the Acoustical Society of America, 90*, 1309–1325.

Sussman, J. E., & Sapienza, C. (1994). Articulatory, developmental, and gender effects on measures of fundamental frequency and jitter. *Journal of Voice, 8*, 145–156.

Syrdal, A. K., & Gopal, H. S. (1986). A perceptual model of vowel recognition based on the auditory representation of American English vowels. *Journal of the Acoustical Society of America, 79*, 1086–1100.

Tabain, M. (1997). Non-sibilant fricatives in English: Spectral information above 10kHz. *Phonetica, 55*, 107–130.

Takagi, N., & Mann, V. (1995). The limits of extended naturalistic exposure on the perceptual mastery of English r and l by adult Japanese learners of English. *Applied Psycholinguistics, 16*, 379–405.

Takagi, T., Seiyama, N., & Miyasaka, E. (2000). A method for pitch extraction of speech signals using autocorrelation functions through multiple window lengths. *Electronics & Communications in Japan, Part Iii: Fundamental Electronic Science, 83*, 67–79.

Tarnoczy, T. (1948). Resonance data concerning nasals, laterals and trills. *Word, 4*, 71–77.

Teager, H. M., & Teager, S. M. (1992). Evidence for nonlinear sound production mechanisms in the vocal tract. In W. J. Hardcastle & A. Marchal (Eds.), *Speech production and speech modelling* (pp. 241–261). Dordrecht, The Netherlands: Kluwer.

Thorsen, N. G. (1985). Intonation and text in standard Danish. *Journal of the Acoustical Society of America, 77*, 1205–1216.

Titze, I. (1989). Physiologic and acoustic differences between male and female voices. *Journal of the Acoustical Society of America, 85*, 1699–1707.

Titze, I. R., & Story, B. H. (1997). Acoustic interactions of the voice source with the lower vocal tract. *Journal of the Acoustical Society of America, 101*, 2234–2243

Titze, I. R., Story, B. H., Burnett, G. C., Holzrichter, J. F., Ng, L. C., Lea, W. A. (2000). Comparison between electroglottography and electromagnetic glottography. *Journal of the Acoustical Society of America, 107*, 581–588.

Tosi, O., Pyer, H., Lashbrook, C., Pedrey, L., Nicol, L., & Nash, E. (1972). Experiment on voice identification. *Journal of the Acoustical Society of America, 51*, 2030.

Traunmuller, H., & Eriksson, A. (1995). The perceptual evaluation of F_0 excursions in speech as evidenced in liveliness estimations. *Journal of the Acoustical Society of America, 97*, 1905–1915.

Traunmuller, H., & Eriksson, A. (2000). Acoustic effects of variation in vocal effort by men, women, and children. *Journal of the Acoustical Society of America, 107*, 3438–3451.

Tyler, A. A., & McOmber, L. S. (1999). Examining phonological-morphological interactions with converging sources of evidence. *Clinical Linguistics & Phonetics, 13*, 131–156.

Umeda, N. (1977). Consonant duration in American English. *Journal of the Acoustical Society of America, 61*, 846–858.

Umeda, N. (1982). Fundamental frequency decline is situation dependent. *Journal of Phonetics, 10*, 279–290.

van Son, R. J. J. H., & Pols, L. C. W. (1999). An acoustic description of consonant reduction. *Speech Communication, 28*, 125–140.

Vandommelen, W. A., & Moxness, B. H. (1995). Acoustic parameters in speaker height and weight identification—sex-specific behavior. *Language & Speech, 38*, 267–287.

Venkatagiri, H. S. (1996). The quality of digitized and synthesized speech: what clinicians should know. *American Journal of Speech-Language Pathology, 5*, 31–42.

Voss, R. J., & Clark, J. (1975). "1/f noise" in music and speech. *Nature, 258*, 317–318.

Walsh, M. A., & Diehl, R. L. (1991). Formant transition and amplitude rise time as cues to the stop/glide distinction. *Quarterly Journal of Experimental Psychology, 43A*, 603–620.

Wardrip-Fruin, C. (1982). On the status of phonetic cues to phonetic categories: Preceding vowel duration as a cue to voicing in final stop consonants. *Journal of the Acoustical Society of America, 71*, 187–195.

Warren R. M. (1968, August). *Vocal compensation for change of distance.* Paper presented at the

Sixth International Congress on Acoustics, Tokyo.

Warren R. M. (1970). Perceptual restoration of missing speech sounds. *Science, 167,* 392–393.

Warren, R. M. (1976). Auditory illusions and perceptual processes. In N. J. Lass (Ed.), *Contemporary issues in experimental phonetics* (pp. 389–417). New York: Academic.

Wayland, R. (1997). Non-native production of Thai—acoustic measurements and accentedness ratings. *Applied Linguistics, 18,* 345–373.

Weismer, G. (1979). Sensitivity of voice-onset time (VOT) to certain segmental features in speech production. *Journal of Phonetics, 7,* 197–204.

Weismer, G. (1984). Acoustic descriptions of dysarthric speech: Perceptual correlates and physiological inferences. In J. D. Rosenbek (Ed.), *Current views of dysarthria. Seminars in speech and language, 5,* 293–314.

Weismer, G., & Liss, J. M. (1991). Speech motor control and aging. In D. Ripich (Ed.), *Geriatric communication disorders* (pp. 205–226). Austin, TX: Pro-ed.

Westbury, J. R., Hashi, M., & Lindstrom, M. J. (1999). Differences among speakers in lingual articulation of American English /r/. *Speech Communication, 26,* 203–226.

Whalen, D. H., & Levitt, A. G. (1995). The universality of intrinsic F_0 of vowels. *Journal of Phonetics, 23,* 349–366.

Whalen, D. H., Levitt, A. G., Hsiao, P. L., & Smorodinsky, I. (1995). Intrinsic F0 of vowel in the babbling of 6-, 9-, and 12-month-old French and English-learning infants. *Journal of the Acoustical Society of America, 97,* 2533–2539.

Whalen, D. H., Wiley, E. R., Rubin, P. E., & Cooper, F. S. (1990). The Haskins Laboratories' pulse code modulation (PCM) system. *Behavior Research Methods, Instruments, and Computers, 22,* 550–559.

White, P. (1999). Formant frequency analysis of children's spoken and sung vowels using sweeping fundamental frequency production. *Journal of Voice, 13,* 570–582.

Whiteside, S. P. (1998). Identification of a speaker's sex—a fricative study. *Perceptual & Motor Skills, 86,* 587–591.

Whiteside, S. P., & Hodgson, C. (2000). Speech patterns of children and adults elicited via a picture-naming task: An acoustic study. *Speech Communication, 32,* 267–285.

Wightman, C. W., Shuttuck-Hufnagel, S., Ostendorf, M., & Price, P. J. (1992). Segmental durations in the vicinity of prosodic phrase boundaries. *Journal of the Acoustical Society of America, 91,* 1707–1717.

Winholtz, W. S, & Titze, I. R. (1997). Miniature head-mounted microphone for voice perturbation analysis. *Journal of Speech, Language, and Hearing Research, 40,* 894–899.

Winitz, H., Scheib, M. E. & Reeds, J. A. (1972). Identification of stops and vowels for the burst portion of the /p,t,k/ isolated from conversational speech. *Journal of the Acoustical Society of America, 51,* 1309–1317.

Wolf, C. G. (1978). Voicing cues in English final stops. *Journal of Phonetics, 6,* 299–309.

Wu, K., & Childers, D. G. (1991). Gender recognition from speech. Part I: Coarse analysis. *Journal of the Acoustical Society of America, 90,* 1828–1840.

Yang, B. (1996). A comparative study of American English and Korean vowels produced by male and female speakers. *Journal of Phonetics, 24,* 245–261.

Zahorian, S. A., & Jagharghi, A. J. (1993). Spectral-shape features versus formants as acoustic correlates for vowels. *Journal of the Acoustical Society of America, 94,* 1966–1982.

Ziegler, W., & Hartmann, E. (1996). Perceptual and acoustic methods in the evaluation of dysarthric speech. In M. J. Ball & M. Duckworth (Eds.), *Advances in clinical phonetics* (pp. 91–114). Amsterdam: John Benjamins.

Zwicker, E., & Terhardt, E. (1980). Analytical expressions for critical-band rate and critical bandwidth as a function of frequency. *Journal of the Acoustical Society of America, 29,* 1523–1525.

Glossary

A/D converter: analog to digital converter; a hardware device that converts an analog (A) signal to a digital (D) form. The conversion involves both **sampling** and **quantization** operations.

Affricate: a speech sound that involves the two phases of a stop (vocal tract obstruction) and a prolonged frication (narrow constriction to produce turbulence noise). These two phases relate to the acoustic events of a stop gap and a noise segment. The English affricates are the initial consonants in the words *joke* and *choke*.

Aliasing: the process in which false or spurious information is created in an analysis, especially because of failure to exclude energy at frequencies higher than one-half of the sampling rate of a digital system. An anti-aliasing filter is used to prevent this problem.

Amplitude: the magnitude of displacement for a sound wave. The waveform of a sound is represented on a two-dimensional graph in which amplitude is plotted as a function of time. To a certain degree, amplitude of sound determines the perceived loudness of the sound.

Analog: a signal that has continuous variations in amplitude as a function of time.

Analog-to-digital conversion: see **A/D converter**.

Antiformant: a property of the vocal tract transfer function in which energy is not passed effectively through the system but is absorbed within it; opposite in effect to a formant. Antiformants, or zeros, arise because of divided passages or constrictions in the vocal tract.

Autocorrelation: an analytic procedure in which a signal is correlated with a time-shifted version of itself (auto = self). If the signal is periodic, the autocorrelation will have a peak (a high correlation) at the time-shift value that corresponds to a fundamental period.

Automatic speech recognition: the process by which natural speech is recognized by a machine.

Bandwidth: a measure of the frequency band of a sound, especially a resonance. Conventionally, bandwidth is determined at the half-power ("3 db down") points of the frequency response curve. That is, both the lower and higher frequencies that define the bandwidth are 3 db less intense than the peak energy in the band.

Bark scale: a nonlinear transformation of frequency that is thought to correspond to the analysis accomplished by the ear. The Bark scale is closely related to the concept of critical band in auditory perception.

Base-of-articulation: the concept that different languages have somewhat different articulatory (and acoustic) characteristics, perhaps even for sounds that are given the same IPA symbol.

Burst: the brief noise created during the release of a stop consonant.

Cepstrum: A Fourier transform of the power spectrum of a signal. The transform is described in terms of **quefrency** (note the transliteration from frequency, which has time-like properties. The cepstrum is used especially to determine the fundamental frequency of a speech signal. Voiced speech tends to have a strong cepstral peak, at the first **rahmonic** (note transliteration from harmonic).

Clear speech: speech that is produced with an attempt to enhance its clarity or intelligibility, as when speaking against a noise background.

Coarticulation: the phenomenon in speech in which the attributes of successive speech units overlap in articulatory or acoustic patterns. That is, one feature of a speech unit may be anticipated during production of an earlier unit in the string (anticipatory or forward coarticulation) or retained during production of a unit that comes later (retentive or backward coarticulation).

Concatenative synthesis: see copy synthesis.

Copy synthesis: a method of speech synthesis in which stored units of speech are retrieved and assembled to form a desired speech pattern. Units typically used are diphones and disyllables.

Coupling: interaction between two or more systems; for example, oral-nasal coupling refers to the degree of interaction between the two resonating cavities. No coupling means no interaction.

Damping: the rate of absorption of sound energy; related to bandwidth.

Digital: a signal or message that is represented as discrete values (a sequence of numbers).

Diphone: a unit of concatenative synthesis defined as the interval from the middle of one phone to the middle of a following phone; as such, it contains the transitional information from one phone to another.

Diphthong: a vowel-like sound involving a gradual change in articulatory configuration from an onglide to offglide position. The usual phonetic symbol is a digraph, or combination of two symbols to represent the onglide and offglide portions.

Discrete Fourier transform (DFT): a Fourier transform that operates on digital (discrete) data.

Disyllable: a unit of concatenative synthesis defined as the interval from the middle of one syllable to the middle of a following syllable; as such, it contains the transitional information from one syllable to another.

Fast Fourier transform (FFT): an algorithm commonly used in microcomputer programs to calculate a Fourier spectrum. The FFT is a special type of DFT (discrete Fourier transform) in which the number of points transformed is a power of 2. The number of points expresses the bandwidth of analysis; the higher the value, the narrower the bandwidth.

Filter: a hardware device or software program that provides a frequency-dependent transmission of energy. Commonly, a filter is used to exclude energy at certain frequencies while passing the energy at other frequencies, A low-pass filter passes the frequencies below a certain cut off frequency; a high-pass filter passes the frequencies above a certain cut-off frequency; and a band-pass filter passes the energy between a lower and upper cut-off frequencies.

Formant: a resonance of the vocal tract. A formant is specified by its center frequency (commonly called formant frequency) and bandwidth. Formants are denoted by integers that increase with the relative frequency location of the formants. F1 is the lowest-frequency formant, F2 is the next highest, and so on.

Formant bandwidth: see **formant**.

Formant frequency: see **formant**.

Formant pattern: a particular combination of formants, as is often used to describe the acoustic characteristics of a vowel.

Formant synthesis: a type of speech synthesis based on the control of formants or modeled resonances.

Formant transition: a change in formant pattern, typically associated with a phonetic boundary; for example, the CV formant transition refers to formant pattern changes associated with the consonant-vowel transition. Formant transitions are often associated with consonant-vowel or vowel-consonant boundaries.

Fourier transform: a mathematical procedure that converts a series of values in the time domain (waveform) to a set of values in the frequency domain (spectrum). The spectrum is the Fourier transform of a waveform; the waveform is the inverse Fourier transform of the spectrum.

Frame: a set of points taken as a single unit of analysis, used, for example, to define the domain of a **short-term analysis**.

Frequency: the rate of vibration of a periodic event; for example a periodic sound has a frequency measured as the number of cycles of vibration per second (expressed in hertz, Hz).

Frequency-domain operation: an operation that is performed in the frequency domain, for example, with a FFT or LPC spectrum.

Fricative: a speech sound characterized by a long interval of turbulence noise. Fricatives are often classified as **stridents** or **nonstridents**, depending on the degree of noise energy.

Fundamental frequency (f_0): The lowest frequency (first harmonic) of a periodic signal. In speech, the fundamental frequency refers to the first harmonic of the voice. Fundamental frequency is the reciprocal of the fundamental period, t_0. Ideally, fundamental frequency is used to refer to a *physical* measure of the lowest periodic

component of vocal fold vibration. *Pitch* should be used to indicate the perceptual phenomenon in which stimuli can be rated along a continuum of low to high. See **Pitch Determination Algorithm.**

Glide: A consonant sound that has a gradual (gliding) change in articulation reflected by a relatively long interval of formant-frequency shift. The glides in English are the initial sounds in the words *we* and *you*, represented by the IPA symbols /w/ and /j/.

Glottis: in the narrow sense, the space between the vocal folds; in the broader sense, pertaining to the vocal folds and their vibration.

Harmonic: an integer multiple of the fundamental frequency in voiced sounds. Ideally, the voice source can be conceptualized as a line spectrum in which energy appears as a series of harmonics.

Laminar flow: a type of airflow in which the air moves in smooth layers. Contrasts with **turbulence**.

Laryngeal (source) spectrum: the spectrum produced by vocal fold vibration.

Linear predictive coding (LPC): a class of methods used to obtain a spectrum. Linear predictive coding uses a weighted linear sum of samples to predict an upcoming value.

Liquid: a cover term for the phonemes /l/ as in *law* and /r/ as in *raw*.

Locus: a characteristic or typical value, especially for the presumed onset value of a formant frequency; an acoustic cue for place of articulation.

Mel: An auditory unit for the measurement of frequency. It follows certain nonlinear properties of the human perception of frequency.

Narrow-band analysis: an analysis in which the analyzing bandwidth is relatively narrow (such as 45 or 29 Hz in speech analysis). A narrow-band analysis is preferred when the interest is to increase frequency resolution, as in the analysis of harmonics for a man's voice.

Nasal: a speech sound that involves a nasal radiation of sound energy, either with or without an accompanying oral radiation.

Nasal formant: the low-frequency resonance associated with the nasal tract. For men's speech, the nasal formant has a frequency of less than 500 Hz.

Nasal murmur: the interval of a nasal consonant in which all sound energy passes through the nasal passage (the oral passage being closed). The murmur is associated with low-frequency spectral energy.

Normalization: a correction for variance. **Speaker normalization** refers to the correction or scaling that reduces variability in acoustic measures such as formant frequencies. **Time normalization** refers to the correction or scaling that reduces variability in the durations of sound sequences.

Nyquist Sampling Theorem: this theorem states that a digital representation requires at least two sampling points for every periodic cycle in the signal of interest. Therefore, the sampling rate of digitization should be at least twice the highest frequency of interest in the signal to be analyzed. Unfortunately, the term *Nyquist Frequency* is inconsistently used. Some use it to indicate the highest frequency of interest in an analysis; others use it to refer to twice the highest frequency of interest, that is to the sampling rate needed to prevent aliasing. See also **sampling theory**.

Parameter synthesis: a method of speech synthesis in which acoustic or articulatory parameters are manipulated to produce speech sounds; compare **concatenative** or **copy synthesis**.

Pitch Determination Algorithm (PDA) (also Pitch Extraction): a procedure used to extract the fundamental frequency of a speech signal. Although the term *pitch* strictly should be used to refer to a percep-

tual phenomenon, it is often used in speech analysis to refer to fundamental frequency.

Pole: a resonance of a system. The term *pole* is used especially in engineering. In speech analysis the term *pole* is synonymous with *formant*.

Pre-emphasis: in speech analysis, a filtering that boosts high-frequency energy relative to low-frequency energy. Because speech normally contains its strongest energy in the low frequencies, these frequencies would dominate analysis results if pre-emphasis were not performed.

Prevoicing: the onset of voicing before the appearance of a supraglottal articulatory event; for example, for stops, prevoicing means that voicing precedes the stop release. Also called voicing lead.

Quantization: the process in analog to digital conversion in which the continuously variable amplitude of an analog signal is converted to a series of discrete amplitude values; typically expressed in bits.

Quefrency: see **cepstrum**.

Radiation characteristic: the term in source–filter theory associated with the radiation of sound from the lips to the atmosphere. It is typically expressed as a 6 dB per octave increase in sound energy (hence, a high-pass filter). It can be modeled as an inductor in an analogous electrical circuit and is sometimes referred to as radiation inductance.

Rahmonic: see **cepstrum**.

Reynold's number: a dimensionless number that serves as an index of the development of turbulence.

Rounding: an articulatory description referring to the rounding (or protrusion) of the lips. As applied to vowels, rounding is associated with a lowering of the frequencies of all formants.

Sampling theorem: this theorem, developed by Nyquist, states that S samples per second are needed to represent a waveform with a bandwidth of $S/2$ Hz.

Segmentation: the delineation of successive sound segments in a speech signal. Typically, segmentation yields units such as phonemes, allophones, or some other phonetic segment.

Short-term transform: a mathematical operation performed on a short time interval of an acoustic sample, usually long enough to include two or three glottal periods. Examples include the fast Fourier transform, linear predictive coding, and autocorrelation.

Source–filter theory: a theory of the acoustic production of speech that states that the energy from a sound source is modified by a filter or set of filters. For vowels, the vibrating vocal folds usually are the source of sound energy and the vocal tract resonances (formants) are the filters.

Source tract interaction: any interaction between the vocal tract and the laryngeal source; for example, the effect of a particular vocal tract configuration on the pattern of vocal fold vibration

Spectral moment: any of the four statistical moments (mean, variance, skewness, kurtosis) that can be calculated from a power spectrum.

Spectrogram: a pattern for sound analysis containing information on intensity, frequency and time. The typical spectrogram provides a three-dimensional display of time on the horizontal axis), frequency on the vertical axis, and intensity on the gray scale. A spectrogram can be printed as hard copy or displayed on a video monitor.

Spectrum: a graph showing the distribution of signal energy as a function of frequency; a plot of intensity by frequency. A Fourier analysis is typically represented as a spectrum.

Speech synthesis: the generation of speech by machine, typically a digital computer.

Stop: a speech sound characterized by a complete obstruction of the vocal tract; usually followed by an abrupt release of air that produces a burst noise.

Stop gap: the acoustic interval corresponding to articulatory closure for a stop or affricate consonant; it is identified on a spectrogram as an interval of relatively low energy, conspicuously lacking in formant pattern or noise.

Strident: a fricative with an intense noise energy; also called a sibilant; /s/ and /ʃ/ are examples. The nonstrident fricatives have less energy; /θ/ is an example.

Synthesis by rule: a synthesis strategy in which rules based on phonologic and phonetic regularities are used to control the synthesizer.

Text-to-speech synthesis: conversion of printed text to synthetic speech.

Time-domain operation: an operation that is performed in the time domain, for example, calculations performed with respect to the waveform of a sound.

Tongue advancement: an articulatory description referring to the relative position of the tongue in the anterior-posterior (front-back) dimension of the vocal tract. As applied to vowels, tongue advancement relates primarily to the relative frequency of F2, or to the frequency difference between F1 and F2. Front vowels tend to have relatively high F2 values and a relatively large value of the F2-F1 difference.

Tongue height: an articulatory description referring to the relative position of the tongue in the inferior–superior (low–high) dimension of the vocal tract. As applied to vowels, tongue height relates primarily to the relative frequency of F1; the higher the vowel, the lower F1 tends to be. Tongue height also varies with jaw position, such that high vowels tend to have a close jaw position.

Transient: the brief noise produced on release of an articulatory closure, as in the case of a stop consonant.

Turbulence: a condition of air flow in which eddies (rotating volume elements of air) are generated. This condition is associated with noise energy (hence we speak of *turbulence noise*). Turbulence contrasts with **laminar flow**.

Vocal tract: usually, the pharyngeal, oral, and nasal cavities of speech production. The vocal tract is an acoustic concept and relates to the sound formation capabilities of the system that extends from the vocal folds to the lips or nose.

Voice bar: a band of energy, typically reflecting the first harmonic of the voice source, that appears on a spectrogram; it is indicative of voicing.

Voice onset time (VOT): a measure of the time between a supraglottal event and the onset of voicing; for stops, VOT is the interval between release of the stop (usually determined acoustically as the stop burst) and the appearance of periodic modulation (voicing) for a following sound.

Waveform: a graph showing the amplitude versus time function for a continuous signal such as the acoustic signal of speech.

Wavelength: the distance that a periodic sound travels in one complete cycle. Wavelength = speed of sound/frequency.

Wavelet: a waveform that can be compressed or expanded to serve as a unit of analysis. A wavelet is an example of a fractal.

Wide-band analysis: an analysis in which a relatively large analyzing bandwidth is used (such as 300 Hz in speech analysis). A wide-band analysis is preferred when the primary concern is to reveal formant pattern or to increase time resolution.

Window: a weighting function applied to a waveform so that its amplitude is shaped in a particular fashion, often to minimize the amplitude at the edges of the window so that the analysis focuses on a representative part of the signal.

Zero: an anti-resonance. The term *zero* is used especially in engineering. In speech analysis, a zero is an antiformant.

Subject Index